Environmental Exposure to Toxic Chemicals and Human Health

Environmental Exposure to Toxic Chemicals and Human Health

Editors

Virgínia Cruz Fernandes
Diogo Pestana

MDPI • Basel • Beijing • Wuhan • Barcelona • Belgrade • Manchester • Tokyo • Cluj • Tianjin

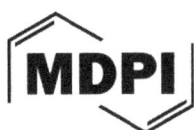

Editors
Virgínia Cruz Fernandes
REQUIMTE/LAQV
Instituto Superior de
Engenharia do Porto,
Instituto Politécnico do Porto
Porto
Portugal

Diogo Pestana
Nutrition & Metabolism
Nova Medical School
Universidade Nova de Lisboa
Lisboa
Portugal

Editorial Office
MDPI
St. Alban-Anlage 66
4052 Basel, Switzerland

This is a reprint of articles from the Special Issue published online in the open access journal *Toxics* (ISSN 2305-6304) (available at: www.mdpi.com/journal/toxics/special_issues/Toxic_Chemicals_Human_Health).

For citation purposes, cite each article independently as indicated on the article page online and as indicated below:

LastName, A.A.; LastName, B.B.; LastName, C.C. Article Title. *Journal Name* **Year**, *Volume Number*, Page Range.

© 2023 by the authors. Articles in this book are Open Access and distributed under the Creative Commons Attribution (CC BY) license, which allows users to download, copy and build upon published articles, as long as the author and publisher are properly credited, which ensures maximum dissemination and a wider impact of our publications.

The book as a whole is distributed by MDPI under the terms and conditions of the Creative Commons license CC BY-NC-ND.

Contents

Preface to "Environmental Exposure to Toxic Chemicals and Human Health" vii

Virgínia Cruz Fernandes and Diogo Pestana
Environmental Chemicals: Integrative Approach to Human Biomonitoring and Health Effects
Reprinted from: *Toxics* 2022, 10, 314, doi:10.3390/toxics10060314 1

Céline Degrendele, Roman Prokeš, Petr Šenk, Simona Rozárka Jílková, Jiří Kohoutek and Lisa Melymuk et al.
Human Exposure to Pesticides in Dust from Two Agricultural Sites in South Africa
Reprinted from: *Toxics* 2022, 10, 629, doi:10.3390/toxics10100629 5

Prakash Thangavel, Kyoung Youb Kim, Duckshin Park and Young-Chul Lee
Evaluation of Health Economic Loss Due to Particulate Matter Pollution in the Seoul Subway, South Korea
Reprinted from: *Toxics* 2023, 11, 113, doi:10.3390/toxics11020113 25

Lilian Calderón-Garcidueñas, Elijah W. Stommel, Ingolf Lachmann, Katharina Waniek, Chih-Kai Chao and Angélica González-Maciel et al.
TDP-43 CSF Concentrations Increase Exponentially with Age in Metropolitan Mexico City Young Urbanites Highly Exposed to $PM_{2.5}$ and Ultrafine Particles and Historically Showing Alzheimer and Parkinson's Hallmarks. Brain TDP-43 Pathology in MMC Residents Is Associated with High Cisternal CSF TDP-43 Concentrations
Reprinted from: *Toxics* 2022, 10, 559, doi:10.3390/toxics10100559 39

Safiye Ghobakhloo, Amir Hossein Khoshakhlagh, Simone Morais and Ashraf Mazaheri Tehrani
Exposure to Volatile Organic Compounds in Paint Production Plants: Levels and Potential Human Health Risks
Reprinted from: *Toxics* 2023, 11, 111, doi:10.3390/toxics11020111 61

José Antonio Varela-Silva, Miguel Ernesto Martínez-Leija, Sandra Teresa Orta-García, Ivan Nelinho Pérez-Maldonado, Jesús Adrián López and Hiram Hernández-López et al.
Differential Expression of *AhR* in Peripheral Mononuclear Cells in Response to Exposure to Polycyclic Aromatic Hydrocarbons in Mexican Women
Reprinted from: *Toxics* 2022, 11, 28, doi:10.3390/toxics11010028 73

Gabriel A. Rojas, Nicolás Saavedra, Kathleen Saavedra, Montserrat Hevia, Cristian Morales and Fernando Lanas et al.
Polycyclic Aromatic Hydrocarbons (PAHs) Exposure Triggers Inflammation and Endothelial Dysfunction in BALB/c Mice: A Pilot Study
Reprinted from: *Toxics* 2022, 10, 497, doi:10.3390/toxics10090497 83

Juliana Guimarães, Isabella Bracchi, Cátia Pinheiro, Nara Xavier Moreira, Cláudia Matta Coelho and Diogo Pestana et al.
Association of 3-Phenoxybenzoic Acid Exposure during Pregnancy with Maternal Outcomes and Newborn Anthropometric Measures: Results from the IoMum Cohort Study
Reprinted from: *Toxics* 2023, 11, 125, doi:10.3390/toxics11020125 97

Jiraporn Chittrakul, Ratana Sapbamrer and Wachiranun Sirikul
Pesticide Exposure and Risk of Rheumatoid Arthritis: A Systematic Review and Meta-Analysis
Reprinted from: *Toxics* 2022, 10, 207, doi:10.3390/toxics10050207 113

Soisungwan Satarug, Aleksandra Buha orević, Supabhorn Yimthiang, David A. Vesey and Glenda C. Gobe
The NOAEL Equivalent of Environmental Cadmium Exposure Associated with GFR Reduction and Chronic Kidney Disease
Reprinted from: *Toxics* **2022**, *10*, 614, doi:10.3390/toxics10100614 . . . . **125**

Ronan Lordan and Ioannis Zabetakis
Cadmium: A Focus on the Brown Crab (*Cancer pagurus*) Industry and Potential Human Health Risks
Reprinted from: *Toxics* **2022**, *10*, 591, doi:10.3390/toxics10100591 . . . . **141**

Athina Stavroulaki, Manolis N. Tzatzarakis, Vasiliki Karzi, Ioanna Katsikantami, Elisavet Renieri and Elena Vakonaki et al.
Antibiotics in Raw Meat Samples: Estimation of Dietary Exposure and Risk Assessment
Reprinted from: *Toxics* **2022**, *10*, 456, doi:10.3390/toxics10080456 . . . . **167**

Claire Vignault, Véronique Cadoret, Peggy Jarrier-Gaillard, Pascal Papillier, Ophélie Téteau and Alice Desmarchais et al.
Bisphenol S Impairs Oestradiol Secretion during In Vitro Basal Folliculogenesis in a Mono-Ovulatory Species Model
Reprinted from: *Toxics* **2022**, *10*, 437, doi:10.3390/toxics10080437 . . . . **183**

Preface to "Environmental Exposure to Toxic Chemicals and Human Health"

It was recently reported that pollution was responsible for 9 million premature deaths in 2015, making it the world's largest environmental risk factor for disease and premature death. Throughout life, people are exposed to both naturally occurring and human-made chemicals. Human health can be influenced by many factors, including exposure to physical, chemical, biological, and radiological contaminants in the environment. These exposures are a root cause of a significant disease burden that could be prevented by reducing or removing chemical exposure. In recent decades, the awareness of toxic chemicals among citizens has been a topic of interest, particularly concerning national and international policy decision makers, expert/scientific platforms, and health protection organizations (WHO, UNEP, CDC, EFSA, IPEN, etc.).

As a complex field, researchers continue to wrestle with important issues, which require an integrative and multidisciplinary research approach to this problem, resorting to complementary methodologies to measure human exposure to environmental chemicals and assess their health effects.

Biomonitoring studies are a good example of this complementarity, encompassing the measurement of internal levels of chemicals/metabolites in easily accessible biological fluids or tissues, which help us to understand environmental health threats and to assist policy measures, namely in susceptible populations.

Preventing diseases arising from chemical environments requires the development of a consistent and rational approach to human biomonitoring as a complementary tool to assist in providing evidence-based public health and environmental measures, confirming the health effects of toxic chemical exposures, and validating regulatory actions and policies.

Virgínia Cruz Fernandes and Diogo Pestana
Editors

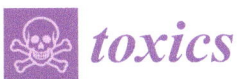

Editorial

Environmental Chemicals: Integrative Approach to Human Biomonitoring and Health Effects

Virgínia Cruz Fernandes [1,*] and Diogo Pestana [2,*]

1. REQUIMTE/LAQV, Instituto Superior de Engenharia do Porto, Instituto Politécnico do Porto, Rua Dr. António Bernardino de Almeida 431, 4249-015 Porto, Portugal
2. CINTESIS & NOVA Medical School | Faculdade de Ciências Médicas da Universidade Nova de Lisboa, Campo Mártires da Pátria 130, 1169-056 Lisboa, Portugal
* Correspondence: virginiacruz@graq.isep.ipp.pt (V.C.F.); diogopestana@nms.unl.pt (D.P.)

Citation: Fernandes, V.C.; Pestana, D. Environmental Chemicals: Integrative Approach to Human Biomonitoring and Health Effects. *Toxics* **2022**, *10*, 314. https://doi.org/10.3390/toxics10060314

Received: 2 June 2022
Accepted: 7 June 2022
Published: 10 June 2022

Publisher's Note: MDPI stays neutral with regard to jurisdictional claims in published maps and institutional affiliations.

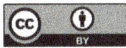

Copyright: © 2022 by the authors. Licensee MDPI, Basel, Switzerland. This article is an open access article distributed under the terms and conditions of the Creative Commons Attribution (CC BY) license (https://creativecommons.org/licenses/by/4.0/).

In recent decades, citizen awareness of toxic chemicals has been a topic of interest, particularly concerning national and international policy decision makers, expert/scientific platforms, and health protection organizations (WHO, UNEP, CDC, EFSA, IPEN, etc.). Even in a world of quick information access, synthesizing crucial scientific knowledge and evidence about environmental exposure and related health problems into readily understandable concepts and statistics remains a remarkable challenge.

Throughout life, people are exposed to both naturally occurring and human-made chemicals. These exposures are a root cause of a significant disease burden that could be prevented by reducing or removing chemical exposure. According to the WHO: in total, more than 2 million deaths and 53 million disability-adjusted life years (DALYs) were attributable to environmental exposure and management of selected chemicals, a higher estimate compared with those in 2016 and 2012 [1]. The largest contributors were cardiovascular diseases (42%, 848,778 deaths), chronic obstructive pulmonary disease (COPD, 26%, 517,734 deaths) and cancers (17%, 333,867 deaths). However, only a small number of chemical exposures, among the many chemicals we are exposed to, are considered in these analyses [1].

People are exposed to a wide range of environmental chemicals in their daily lives, in different contexts, and via multiple routes, including indoors and outdoors (e.g., air, soil, and water contamination; consumer products (e.g., cosmetics, cleaning agents, textiles, food, etc.); industrial chemicals; etc.) [2–7]. From this extensive exposure by several routes, the multiple contaminants to which we are exposed is exhausting and worrying. Some examples of the most reported toxic chemicals are pesticides [8–11], heavy metals [12] polycyclic aromatic hydrocarbon (PAH) [13,14], polychlorinated biphenyls (PCB) [15], pharmaceuticals [16], plastic-related chemicals (e.g., flame retardants, phthalates, etc.) [17,18], and microplastics [19–21]. Currently, it is impossible to escape exposure to environmental chemicals, namely those with endocrine-altering potential (endocrine-disrupting chemicals, EDCs).

Unintended exposure to pesticides can be extremely hazardous to humans and other living organisms as they are designed to be poisonous. Pesticide exposure is linked with various diseases including cancer, asthma, dermatitis, endocrine disorders, reproductive dysfunctions, immunotoxicity, neurobehavioral disorders, and congenital defects [22–24]. Data from a number of PAH occupational health studies suggest that there is an association between lung cancer and exposure to PAH compounds [25]. Studies in human and animals suggest a correlation between flame retardants exposure and adverse health outcomes, namely thyroid disorders; neurobehavior and development disorders; and reproductive, immunological, metabolic, oncological, and cardiovascular diseases [17,26]. Phthalate exposures were associated with all-cause and cardiovascular mortality, with societal costs approximating USD 39 billion/year or more in the USA [27]. Recently, microplastics that may cause inflammatory lesions, originating from the potential of their surface to interact with the tissues, have been reported. In addition, the increasing incidence of neurodegenerative diseases, immune disorders, and cancers may also be related to the increased exposure microplastics and their co-contaminants [19]. The effects of exposure in human health are influenced not only by the type and concentration of the chemicals but also by the effects and complexity of mixtures and, more importantly, by the timing of exposure. Indeed, there is an increased vulnerability to chemical exposure in windows of greater susceptibility, especially during childhood and pregnancy, which may impair lifetime health. Therefore, there is a need to biomonitor and evaluate all exposures across lifespans and its interaction with our own unique characteristics, the 'exposome'.

As a complex field, researchers continue to wrestle with important issues, which requires an integrative and multidisciplinary research approach to this problematic, resorting to complementary methodologies to measure human exposure to environmental chemicals and to assess their health effects. One can define three main pillars: (1) environmental chemical analysis and development of new detection methods, with the identification and quantification of biomarkers of exposure and/or effect and/or susceptibility and development of new analytical methodologies for the detection of biomarkers in several human matrices (e.g., blood, plasma, serum, urine, and adipose tissue); (2) evaluation of biological effects, through the assessment of exposure impact on human health (e.g., general population, and people with obesity or diabetes) and/or resorting to experimental and mechanistic approaches (in vitro/in vivo models); and (3) data management and statistical analysis, namely in study design and sampling in the human population.

Biomonitoring studies are a good example of this complementarity, encompassing the measurement of internal levels of chemicals/metabolites in easily accessible biological fluids or tissues, and aiming to understand environmental health threats and to assist policy measures, namely in susceptible populations such as children. It requires analytical methods of high selectivity and high sensitivity due to low concentrations and limited sample volumes. Toxic chemicals cover a wide range of chemical groups with different physical–chemical properties. Therefore, scientific literature presents several analytical methods even for the same substance groups. Depending on the chemical group, the human biomonitoring biomarkers are either parent compounds or metabolites. A large variety of matrices have been analyzed (blood, urine, adipose tissue, hair, nails, breast milk, etc.). This complexity calls for the urgent need to carry out further studies on the appropriate analytical methods for each group of compounds and matrices. Biomonitoring studies identify new chemicals in human tissues, monitor the distribution of exposures among the general population, and provide a measure of potential health risk.

Preventing diseases arising from chemical environments requires the development of a consistent and rational approach to human biomonitoring as a complementary tool to assist in providing evidence-based public health and environmental measures, confirming the health effects of toxic chemical exposures, and validating regulatory actions and policies.

Author Contributions: All authors contributed equally in all statements. All authors have read and agreed to the published version of the manuscript.

Funding: This work received financial support from projects UIDB/50006/2020, UIDP/50006/2020, and LA/P/0008/2020 by the Fundação para a Ciência e a Tecnologia (FCT)/Ministério da Ciência, Tecnologia e Ensino Superior (MCTES) through national funds. Virgínia Cruz Fernandes thanks FCT for the financial support through a postdoctoral fellowship (SFRH/BPD/109153/2015).

Informed Consent Statement: Not applicable.

Conflicts of Interest: The author declares that he has no known competing financial interests or personal relationships that could influence the work reported in this paper.

References

1. World Health Organization. *The Public Health Impact of Chemicals: Knowns and Unknowns-Data Addendum for 2016*; World Health Organization: Geneva, Switzerland, 2019.
2. Chen, L.; Wang, J.; Beiyuan, J.; Guo, X.; Wu, H.; Fang, L. Environmental and health risk assessment of potentially toxic trace elements in soils near uranium (U) mines: A global meta-analysis. *Sci. Total Environ.* **2021**, *816*, 151556. [CrossRef] [PubMed]
3. Saravanan, A.; Kumar, P.S.; Hemavathy, R.; Jeevanantham, S.; Harikumar, P.; Priyanka, G.; Devakirubai, D.R.A. A comprehensive review on sources, analysis and toxicity of environmental pollutants and its removal methods from water environment. *Sci. Total Environ.* **2021**, *812*, 152456. [CrossRef] [PubMed]
4. Guo, P.; Lin, E.Z.; Koelmel, J.P.; Ding, E.; Gao, Y.; Deng, F.; Dong, H.; Liu, Y.; Cha, Y.; Fang, J.; et al. Exploring personal chemical exposures in China with wearable air pollutant monitors: A repeated-measure study in healthy older adults in Jinan, China. *Environ. Int.* **2021**, *156*, 106709. [CrossRef] [PubMed]
5. Degrendele, C.; Klánová, J.; Prokeš, R.; Příbylová, P.; Šenk, P.; Šudoma, M.; Röösli, M.; Dalvie, M.A.; Fuhrimann, S. Current use pesticides in soil and air from two agricultural sites in South Africa: Implications for environmental fate and human exposure. *Sci. Total Environ.* **2021**, *807*, 150455. [CrossRef]
6. Crépet, A.; Luong, T.M.; Baines, J.; Boon, P.E.; Ennis, J.; Kennedy, M.; Massarelli, I.; Miller, D.; Nako, S.; Reuss, R.; et al. An international probabilistic risk assessment of acute dietary exposure to pesticide residues in relation to codex maximum residue limits for pesticides in food. *Food Control* **2020**, *121*, 107563. [CrossRef]
7. Sousa, S.; Maia, M.L.; Delerue-Matos, C.; Calhau, C.; Domingues, V.F. The role of adipose tissue analysis on Environmental Pollutants Biomonitoring in women: The European scenario. *Sci. Total Environ.* **2021**, *806*, 150922. [CrossRef]
8. Kim, K.-H.; Kabir, E.; Jahan, S.A. Exposure to pesticides and the associated human health effects. *Sci. Total Environ.* **2017**, *575*, 525–535. [CrossRef]
9. Dorosh, O.; Fernandes, V.C.; Moreira, M.M.; Delerue-Matos, C. Occurrence of pesticides and environmental contaminants in vineyards: Case study of Portuguese grapevine canes. *Sci. Total Environ.* **2021**, *791*, 148395. [CrossRef]
10. Lobato, A.; Fernandes, V.C.; Pacheco, J.G.; Delerue-Matos, C.; Gonçalves, L.M. Organochlorine pesticide analysis in milk by gas-diffusion microextraction with gas chromatography-electron capture detection and confirmation by mass spectrometry. *J. Chromatogr. A* **2020**, *1636*, 461797. [CrossRef]
11. Pestana, D.; Fernandes, V.; Teixeira, D.; Faria, A.; Monteiro, R.; Domingues, V.; Delerue-Matos, C.; Calhau, C. Accumulation of organochlorine pesticides in human visceral and subcutaneous adipose tissue—The Portuguese scenario. *Toxicol. Lett.* **2010**, *196*, S43. [CrossRef]
12. Zaynab, M.; Al-Yahyai, R.; Ameen, A.; Sharif, Y.; Ali, L.; Fatima, M.; Khan, K.A.; Li, S. Health and environmental effects of heavy metals. *J. King Saud Univ.-Sci.* **2021**, *34*, 101653. [CrossRef]
13. Sun, K.; Song, Y.; He, F.; Jing, M.; Tang, J.; Liu, R. A review of human and animals exposure to polycyclic aromatic hydrocarbons: Health risk and adverse effects, photo-induced toxicity and regulating effect of microplastics. *Sci. Total Environ.* **2021**, *773*, 145403. [CrossRef] [PubMed]
14. Oliveira, M.; Costa, S.; Vaz, J.; Fernandes, A.; Slezakova, K.; Delerue-Matos, C.; Teixeira, J.P.; Pereira, M.C.; Morais, S. Firefighters exposure to fire emissions: Impact on levels of biomarkers of exposure to polycyclic aromatic hydrocarbons and genotoxic/oxidative-effects. *J. Hazard. Mater.* **2019**, *383*, 121179. [CrossRef] [PubMed]
15. Heiger-Bernays, W.J.; Tomsho, K.S.; Basra, K.; Petropoulos, Z.E.; Crawford, K.; Martinez, A.; Hornbuckle, K.C.; Scammell, M.K. Human health risks due to airborne polychlorinated biphenyls are highest in New Bedford Harbor communities living closest to the harbor. *Sci. Total Environ.* **2019**, *710*, 135576. [CrossRef]
16. Semerjian, L.; Shanableh, A.; Semreen, M.H.; Samarai, M. Human health risk assessment of pharmaceuticals in treated wastewater reused for non-potable applications in Sharjah, United Arab Emirates. *Environ. Int.* **2018**, *121*, 325–331. [CrossRef]
17. Feiteiro, J.; Mariana, M.; Cairrão, E. Health toxicity effects of brominated flame retardants: From environmental to human exposure. *Environ. Pollut.* **2021**, *285*, 117475. [CrossRef]
18. Fernandes, V.C.; Luts, W.; Delerue-Matos, C.; Domingues, V.F. Improved QuEChERS for Analysis of Polybrominated Diphenyl Ethers and Novel Brominated Flame Retardants in Capsicum Cultivars Using Gas Chromatography. *J. Agric. Food Chem.* **2020**, *68*, 3260–3266. [CrossRef]
19. Prata, J.C.; da Costa, J.P.; Lopes, I.; Duarte, A.C.; Rocha-Santos, T. Environmental exposure to microplastics: An overview on possible human health effects. *Sci. Total Environ.* **2019**, *702*, 134455. [CrossRef]
20. Martinho, S.D.; Fernandes, V.C.; Figueiredo, S.A.; Delerue-Matos, C. Microplastic Pollution Focused on Sources, Distribution, Contaminant Interactions, Analytical Methods, and Wastewater Removal Strategies: A Review. *Int. J. Environ. Res. Public Health* **2022**, *19*, 5610. [CrossRef]
21. Selonen, S.; Dolar, A.; Kokalj, A.J.; Sackey, L.N.; Skalar, T.; Fernandes, V.C.; Rede, D.; Delerue-Matos, C.; Hurley, R.; Nizzetto, L.; et al. Exploring the impacts of microplastics and associated chemicals in the terrestrial environment–Exposure of soil invertebrates to tire particles. *Environ. Res.* **2021**, *201*, 111495. [CrossRef]
22. Kalyabina, V.P.; Esimbekova, E.N.; Kopylova, K.V.; Kratasyuk, V.A. Pesticides: Formulants, distribution pathways and effects on human health—A review. *Toxicol. Rep.* **2021**, *8*, 1179–1192. [CrossRef] [PubMed]

23. Pestana, D.; Teixeira, D.; Meireles, M.; Marques, C.; Norberto, S.; Sá, C.; Fernandes, V.C.; Correia-Sá, L.; Faria, A.; Guardão, L.; et al. Adipose tissue dysfunction as a central mechanism leading to dysmetabolic obesity triggered by chronic exposure to p,p′-DDE. *Sci. Rep.* **2017**, *7*, 2738. [CrossRef] [PubMed]
24. Pestana, D.; Faria, G.; Sá, C.; Fernandes, V.C.; Teixeira, D.; Norberto, S.; Faria, A.; Meireles, M.; Marques, C.; Correia-Sá, L.; et al. Persistent organic pollutant levels in human visceral and subcutaneous adipose tissue in obese individuals—Depot differences and dysmetabolism implications. *Environ. Res.* **2014**, *133*, 170–177. [CrossRef] [PubMed]
25. Kim, K.-H.; Jahan, S.A.; Kabir, E.; Brown, R.J.C. A review of airborne polycyclic aromatic hydrocarbons (PAHs) and their human health effects. *Environ. Int.* **2013**, *60*, 71–80. [CrossRef]
26. Maia, M.L.; Sousa, S.; Pestana, D.; Faria, A.; Teixeira, D.; Delerue-Matos, C.; Domingues, V.F.; Calhau, C. Impact of brominated flame retardants on lipid metabolism: An in vitro approach. *Environ. Pollut.* **2021**, *294*, 118639. [CrossRef]
27. Trasande, L.; Liu, B.; Bao, W. Phthalates and attributable mortality: A population-based longitudinal cohort study and cost analysis. *Environ. Pollut.* **2021**, *292*, 118021. [CrossRef]

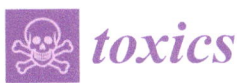

Article

Human Exposure to Pesticides in Dust from Two Agricultural Sites in South Africa

Céline Degrendele [1,2,*], Roman Prokeš [1,3], Petr Šenk [1], Simona Rozárka Jílková [1], Jiří Kohoutek [1], Lisa Melymuk [1], Petra Přibylová [1], Mohamed Aqiel Dalvie [4], Martin Röösli [5,6], Jana Klánová [1] and Samuel Fuhrimann [5,6,7]

1. RECETOX, Faculty of Science, Masaryk University, 625 00 Brno, Czech Republic
2. Aix-Marseille University, CNRS, LCE, 13003 Marseille, France
3. Global Change Research Institute of the Czech Academy of Sciences, 603 00 Brno, Czech Republic
4. Centre for Environmental and Occupational Health Research, School of Public Health and Family Medicine, University of Cape Town, Cape Town 7925, South Africa
5. University of Basel, 4002 Basel, Switzerland
6. Swiss Tropical and Public Health Institute (Swiss TPH), 4002 Basel, Switzerland
7. Institute for Risk Assessment Sciences (IRAS), Utrecht University, 3584 Utrecht, The Netherlands
* Correspondence: celine.degrendele@recetox.muni.cz

Abstract: Over the last decades, concern has arisen worldwide about the negative impacts of pesticides on the environment and human health. Exposure via dust ingestion is important for many chemicals but poorly characterized for pesticides, particularly in Africa. We investigated the spatial and temporal variations of 30 pesticides in dust and estimated the human exposure via dust ingestion, which was compared to inhalation and soil ingestion. Indoor dust samples were collected from thirty-eight households and two schools located in two agricultural regions in South Africa and were analyzed using high-performance liquid chromatography coupled to tandem mass spectrometry. We found 10 pesticides in dust, with chlorpyrifos, terbuthylazine, carbaryl, diazinon, carbendazim, and tebuconazole quantified in >50% of the samples. Over seven days, no significant temporal variations in the dust levels of individual pesticides were found. Significant spatial variations were observed for some pesticides, highlighting the importance of proximity to agricultural fields or of indoor pesticide use. For five out of the nineteen pesticides quantified in dust, air, or soil (i.e., carbendazim, chlorpyrifos, diazinon, diuron and propiconazole), human intake via dust ingestion was important (>10%) compared to inhalation or soil ingestion. Dust ingestion should therefore be considered in future human exposure assessment to pesticides.

Keywords: plant protection products; residential exposure; agriculture; Africa; exposure pathway; intake dose; temporal variations; spatial variations

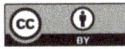

1. Introduction

Pesticides are the only chemicals that have been synthetized for about 70 years for their toxic properties. Their use has increased on a global scale, from 2.3 to 4.2 million tons between 1990 and 2019 [1]. In addition to their toxicity to target organisms, many pesticides cause a wide range of adverse effects for mammals, including humans [2,3]. For example, long-term exposure to some organophosphate insecticides has been associated with neurotoxic and developmental effects for chlorpyrifos [4], while diazinon exposure has induced oxidative stress, immune disorders, and gut microbiota dysbiosis [5], and exposure to several pesticides cause DNA damage [6,7]. Furthermore, there has been significant evidence of pesticide contamination of several environmental matrices, such as air, soil, or water [8–14]. Consequently, many concerns have arisen worldwide about the negative impacts of pesticides on the environment and human health. In particular, agricultural region residents are a highly exposed population, with higher quantification frequencies and levels of pesticides found in various environmental media from rural areas, such as air [15,16], dust [17–19], silicone wristbands [20,21], and human samples such as urine [22–24] and blood [25,26]. In addition, several epidemiological studies have found an association between residential proximity to agricultural fields and diseases such as autism [27,28], Parkinson's disease [29], childhood cancer [30,31], and also with neurobehavioral effects [32].

Humans are exposed to pesticides via three pathways: (i) ingestion of food, dust, and soil; (ii) inhalation; and (iii) dermal contact with products or materials containing pesticides [33]. For many legacy chemicals, food ingestion is generally the major contributor (>90%) to human exposure [34,35] although some studies have reported that inhalation [36] and dust ingestion [37] could also dominate the overall exposure. For pesticides that are currently used, the contribution of each pathway to the overall exposure is not well-understood, and contradictory results have been found [34,38–40]. However, a clear understanding of exposure pathways is crucial to assess the pesticide exposome [41,42], which has been a growing area of research in recent years [43].

The indoor environment, where humans spend about 90% of their time [44,45], is particularly important in terms of non-dietary exposure to pesticides or other pollutants [46,47]. Pesticides can penetrate indoors in four manners. Firstly, after their application to agricultural areas, depending on the meteorological conditions and the type of equipment used, up to 30% of pesticides do not reach their targets but are transported via the air to the surrounding environment [48], a phenomenon known as spray drift [49]. In addition, several weeks after outdoor application, pesticides can be transferred to the air (secondary drift) via volatilization from soils and plants [50,51] and wind erosion of soil particles on which pesticides are sorbed, followed by dispersion [42,52]. These pesticides present in outdoor air can then infiltrate into indoor spaces via ventilation. Secondly, agricultural workers (pesticide applicators, farm workers) can also bring pesticides indoors via shoes, clothes, skin, or hair, also known as the take-home exposure pathway [53–56]. Thirdly, pesticides can be directly applied indoors against insects (e.g., mosquitoes, fleas, ticks) [17,57]. Fourth, pesticides can volatilize from products present indoors containing pesticides (e.g., wooden furniture, textiles, carpets) [58]. Given this diversity of possible sources, it has often been difficult to identify the major source of pesticides present indoors [54,59].

Dust is considered a marker of indoor pollution by organic compounds [44,47]. The pesticides levels in indoor dust are affected by several factors, including their emissions (indoor), rates of air transport from outdoor to indoor, outdoor soil brought in by shoes, removal rates by ventilation and cleaning, indoor activities, and rates of degradation indoors [33,47]. However, infiltration from outdoors seems to be the most dominant source, as many studies have shown that humans living in proximity to agricultural fields had higher levels in household dust compared to non-agricultural residents [18,42,54,55,60]. On the global scale, the many studies performed earlier on pesticides in dust largely focused on insecticides and more particularly on organophosphates and pyrethroids, while data for fungicides and herbicides are still very limited [54]. In addition, the temporal variations of pesticide levels in dust have mainly been investigated from a seasonal perspective [61,62], while only two studies have focused on shorter time scales (i.e., days) [17,63]. In order to reduce human exposure to pesticides and the related health effects for the agricultural residents, it is therefore crucial to characterize the levels of pesticides in dust and to understand their spatio-temporal variabilities.

Information on pesticide exposure of agricultural residents is extremely limited in Africa [43] and particularly using dust samples [44]. Indeed, only one study has been done in South Africa [64]. With about 26,000 tons of pesticides used on a yearly basis and about 700 active ingredients registered for agricultural use [65], this country contributes to about one-third of all pesticides used in the African continent [1] and is therefore considered as a high-risk country for pesticide pollution [66]. Unfortunately, only a few pesticides were targeted (n = 8) in that study, and samples were only collected at a school. Therefore, there is a real need to characterize the levels of pesticides in household dust in South Africa.

Within the larger project "Child health Agricultural Pesticide cohort study in South Africa" (CapSA), assessing the health impacts of pesticide exposure of 1000 children in South Africa [67], we have previously highlighted the presence of many pesticides in air, soil, water, and silicone wristbands of two rural agricultural areas [20,68–70]. In this study, we present data on pesticides quantified in dust and assess the non-dietary exposure via dust ingestion of humans living in two intensive agricultural areas in South Africa. The specific aims of this study are to (i) assess the occurrence of pesticides in dust from two agricultural areas in South Africa and its spatial and temporal variations, (ii) compare the levels of pesticides in dust between children living on farms and those living in neighboring villages, (iii) determine the human uptake of pesticides due to dust ingestion, and (iv) assess the importance of exposure via dust ingestion compared to inhalation and soil ingestion.

2. Materials and Methods

2.1. Collection of Dust Samples

The sampling campaign occurred in Western Cape, South Africa, at two different agricultural sites: Hex River Valley (33°28′ S;19°38′ E) and Grabouw (34°12′ S;19°5′ E), located about 110 km from each other (Figure 1). These two sampling sites were selected due to their intensive monoculture. At Hex River Valley, 98% of the agricultural land consists of table grapes, while at Grabouw, pome fruits are the major (81%) crop [70]. In order to characterize the highest exposure to pesticides, the sampling campaign was performed during the main pesticide application season at both sites (22 October 2018–29 October 2018 at Hex River Valley and 30 October 2018–6 November 2018 at Grabouw).

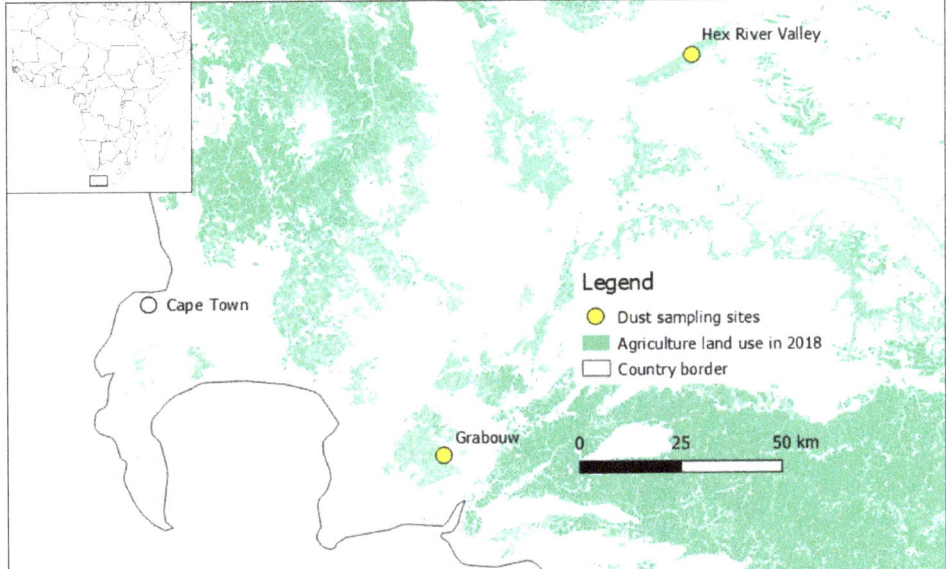

Figure 1. Map of the sampling sites.

At each site, dust samples were collected in 19 individual households representing different exposure scenarios and one school. Information on the recruitment of participants is available elsewhere [20]. For each site, half of the households were located on the farms, and half were located in the nearby village, within a distance to agricultural fields of <50 m and >0.5 km, respectively. Dust samples were taken on the floor of the child's bedroom for the households and of three classrooms for the two schools. Dust sampling was repeated after seven days at the same locations. A vacuum cleaner was used to collect dust samples, as this technique detects more compounds than wiped dust [58] or doormat dust [53]. The dust samples were collected on a quartz fiber filter (QFF, QMA, 101.6 mm, Whatman, UK) using a stainless steel inlet equipped with a pre-separation mesh sieving particles up to 1 mm connected to a conventional vacuum cleaner. This dust size fraction has been shown to contain most organic contaminants and to be relevant in terms of human exposure [71,72]. Ethanol was used to clean the sampling head of the vacuum cleaner prior to each use. The sampled surface varied from 1 to 8 m^2. After vacuuming, dust samples were immediately folded, wrapped in aluminum foil in order to avoid sunlight degradation, and placed into a zip-lock polyethylene bag. All the samples were carried to the University of Cape Town within a cooling box at 5 °C where they were stored in a freezer at −18 °C until shipment to RECETOX, Czech Republic.

2.2. Sample Preparation and Chemical Analysis

From the samples collected, all those from day 7 (n = 41) and only 13 from day 1 were analyzed for pesticides, resulting in a total amount of 54 dust samples. About 0.1 g of the dust samples were extracted with 10 mL of methanol using an ultrasonic bath, then centrifugated for 10 min at 10,000 rcf. This extraction was done for three cycles, and the final extract volume was 30 mL. The extracts were concentrated at 40 °C with a gentle stream of nitrogen and passed through Chromafil syringe filters (nylon membrane, 25 mm diameter, pore size 0.45 µm, Machery-Nagel, Düren, Germany) into mini vials. The extract volume was brought exactly to 0.5 mL by weight, and 0.5 mL of ultrapure water (Sartorius, Göttingen, Germany) was added to have the final volume 1 mL methanol:water 1:1. All samples were analyzed using a high-performance liquid chromatograph (Agilent 1290, Agilent, Santa Clara, CA, USA) with a Phenomenex Luna C-18 endcapped analytical column (100 mm × 2.0 mm × 3 µm). Analyte detection was performed by tandem mass spectrometry using an AB Sciex Qtrap 5500 (AB Sciex, Concord, ON, Canada), operating in positive electrospray ionization (ESI+). The isotope dilution method was used to quantify the analytes. The instrumental limits of detection (iLOD) and quantification (iLOQ) were defined as the quantity of an analyte with a signal-to-noise ratio of 3:1 and 10:1, respectively. Details on the analytical method used have been described elsewhere [68,69].

In total, thirty individual pesticides, including seventeen herbicides (i.e., acetochlor, alachlor, atrazine, chlorotoluron, chlorsulfuron, dimethachlor, diuron, fluroxypyr, isoproturon, metamitron, metazachlor, metribuzin, pendimethalin, pyrazon, simazine, S-metolachlor, and terbuthylazine); nine insecticides (i.e., azinphos methyl, carbaryl, chlorpyrifos, diazinon, dimethoate, fenitrothion, malathion, parathion methyl, and pirimicarb); and four fungicides (i.e., carbendazim, prochloraz, propiconazole, and tebuconazole) were analyzed in this study. Among these 30 pesticides, 27 are registered for agricultural use in South Africa [65]. In addition, 15 of the pesticides quantified in this study are widely used on the global scale [73], and 14 have been identified as highly hazardous or high-risk pesticides [74]. Even though the amount of pesticides investigated in this study is small compared to the almost 700 pesticides authorized for agricultural use in South Africa [65], it is more than most of the previous studies focused on the residential exposure to pesticides of agricultural residents, which looked at a median of seven pesticides [43].

2.3. Quality Assurance and Quality Control

In this study, six field blanks and seven solvent blanks were analyzed as per samples. None of the targeted pesticides were found in those blanks, suggesting that no contamination occurred during sampling, transport, sample preparation, and analysis. Recoveries of individual pesticides, determined from spiking experiments of QFFs, ranged from 42.5% ± 2.9 (acetochlor) to 120.1% ± 1.9 (chlorsulfuron) (Table S1 in the Supplementary Information).

2.4. Human Exposure via Dust Ingestion and Comparison with Inhalation and Soil Ingestion

The daily intakes of pesticides via dust ingestion ($DI_{ingestion\_dust}$, in pg day^{-1} kg^{-1}) were estimated for children (6 to 11 years) who are more sensitive to pesticide exposure [3] and adults (>21 years) using both the median and the maximum concentrations observed for each type of site as [75]:

$$DIingestion\_dust = \frac{C_{dust} \times IngR_{dust} \times AF}{BW} \quad (1)$$

where C_{dust} is the dust concentration (in pg g^{-1}), and $IngR_{dust}$ is the dust ingestion rate (in g day^{-1}), AF is the absorption factor via dust ingestion (unitless), and BW is the body weight (in kg). All the input parameters used [75] are provided in Table S2. Here, we assumed that the children spent 30% of their time at school and the remaining at home, while exposure for adults were estimated as if they spent all their time at home. Many studies have assumed that all pesticides present in dust were bioaccessible due to the lack of knowledge on bioaccessibility of pesticides ingested from indoor dust [47], leading to a possible overestimation of the health risks [76]. In a review, a bioaccessibility factor varying from 0.06 to 0.52 was reported for both legacy and current-use pesticides with a median of 0.14 [76], which we used in this study. We decided to not determine the human uptake via dermal contact with dust, as the exposure factors needed are associated with large uncertainties [47], and many studies for other organic pollutants have shown that this exposure pathway was several orders of magnitude lower than dust ingestion [47,77].

The pesticide daily intakes from dust ingestion from this study were compared with those from inhalation and soil ingestion previously reported from the same campaign [68]. In addition, we also estimated the health hazards due to the exposure via dust ingestion, inhalation, and soil ingestion of pesticides using (i) hazard quotients determined as the ratio of the daily intake to the acceptable daily intake via all routes of exposure obtained from European database [78], (ii) hazard index, and (iii) relative potency factors, as previously described [68].

2.5. Data analysis

Mann–Whitney tests were used to compare the differences between the two sampling days, the two studied areas, the two types of sites (farm vs. village), and the two population groups in terms of the dust concentrations of pesticides and human exposure. Significant differences were considered when p-value < 0.05. For these analysis, including summary statistics, the pesticides that were quantified in >50% of the samples were considered, and the values under LOQ were imputed with half LOQ. The software MATLAB® (version R2017a) was used to perform the data analysis and create all figures except for the map (Figure 1), which was done with the software QGIS (version 3.4 Madeira).

2.6. Ethical Statement

Informed consent was obtained from a member of each household. The study received ethical clearance from the University of Cape Town's Research Ethics Committee (HREC 637/2018).

3. Results

3.1. Quantification Frequency and Levels of Pesticides in Dust

Out of the 30 pesticides targeted, 10 were found in at least one dust sample (Table 1 and Tables S3–S5, Figure 2). Chlorpyrifos and terbuthylazine were the most frequently quantified pesticides (96% and 91%, respectively), followed by carbaryl, diazinon, carbendazim, and tebuconazole (59–74%). The remaining four pesticides were rarely found (<10%) either only at Grabouw (i.e., diuron, malathion, and S-metolachlor) or at both sites (i.e., propiconazole) and are not further discussed. All homes had at least three pesticides in dust, and a maximum of eight pesticides was found for one household and one school, both located in Grabouw. The median dust concentrations measured in households of individual pesticides spanned several orders of magnitude and ranged from 4.38 ng g^{-1} (tebuconazole) to 365 ng g^{-1} (chlorpyrifos) (Table 1). Besides chlorpyrifos, only carbaryl and diazinon had dust concentrations higher than 1 µg g^{-1}.

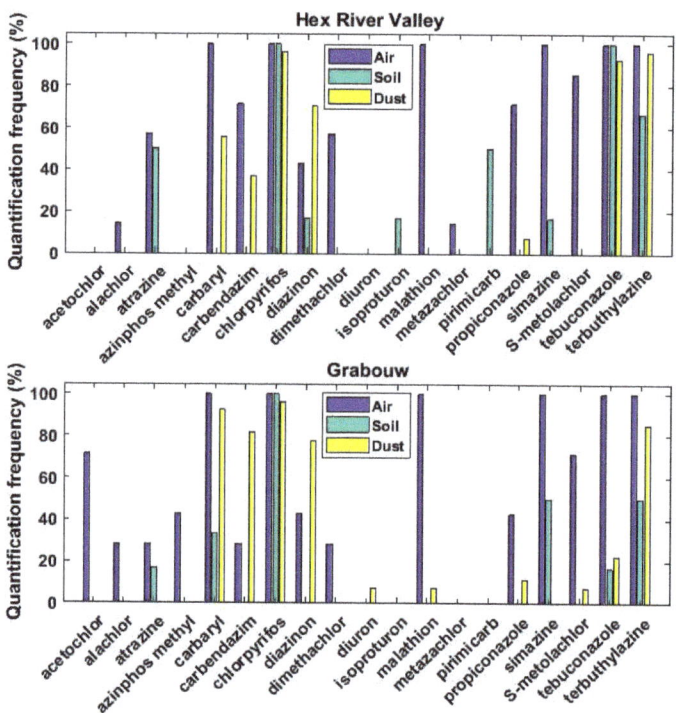

Figure 2. Quantification frequencies of the individual pesticides in air, soil, and dust. Data on pesticides in air and soil were obtained from [68].

Table 1. Summary of the concentrations (in ng g^{-1}) of individual pesticides found in the dust samples collected in households. QF indicates quantification frequency in percentage, IQR indicates interquartile range. For propiconazole, S-metolachlor, diuron, and malathion, only the concentrations above the quantification limits were considered, while for the remaining pesticides, imputed data were considered for statistics.

		Chlorpyrifos	Terbuthylazine	Carbaryl	Diazinon	Carbendazim	Tebuconazole	Propiconazole	S-Metolachlor	Diuron	Malathion
All $n = 50$	QF	96	90	76	72	60	58	8	4	2	4
	Mean	1250	9.30	1020	122	16.3	13.6				
	Median	365	4.54	247	9.29	7.02	4.38				
	Min	0.19	0.05	5	0.29	0.14	0.19	3.63	10.3	26.8	43.9
	Max	19,500	90.8	17,200	2210	257	99.0	12.5	46.6	26.8	150
	IQR25	135	2.76	64	0.30	0.15	0.20				
	IQR75	986	9.25	544	31.2	14.2	15.8				
Hex River Valley $n = 25$	QF	96	96	60	68	36	92	8	0	0	0
	Mean	1810	5.38	292	136	17.5	25.1				
	Median	398	4.47	102	6.41	0.15	15.7				
	Min	0.19	0.05	5	0.29	0.14	0.20	3.63			
	Max	19,500	11.0	1980	1680	257	99.0	9.60			
	IQR25	142	3.04	5	0.29	0.15	7.96				
	IQR75	1850	7.70	266	15.5	7.45	35.4				
Grabouw $n = 25$	QF	96	84	92	76	84	24	8	8	4	8
	Mean	690	13.2	1740	109	15.1	2.04				
	Median	268	4.62	525	11.2	11.0	0.20				
	Min	0.20	0.05	5	0.29	0.14	0.19	3.63	10.3	26.8	43.9
	Max	4700	90.8	17,200	2210	64.1	19.6	12.5	46.6	26.8	150
	IQR25	133	2.70	207	4.37	5.94	0.19				
	IQR75	948	13.6	1660	37.4	17.8	0.20				

3.2. Temporal and Spatial Variations in Pesticide Levels in Dust

For those twelve households and one school for which dust samples were analyzed, on both day 1 and day 7, no significant temporal variations ($p > 0.05$, Mann–Whitney test) were observed for none of the pesticides investigated (Figures 3 and S1). Indeed, for about two-third of all the pairs ($n = 78$) investigated, the dust concentrations of the individual pesticides measured on day 1 and day 7 were within 25% of each other, while large differences (up to a factor of 100) were found in the remaining cases (Figures 3 and S1).

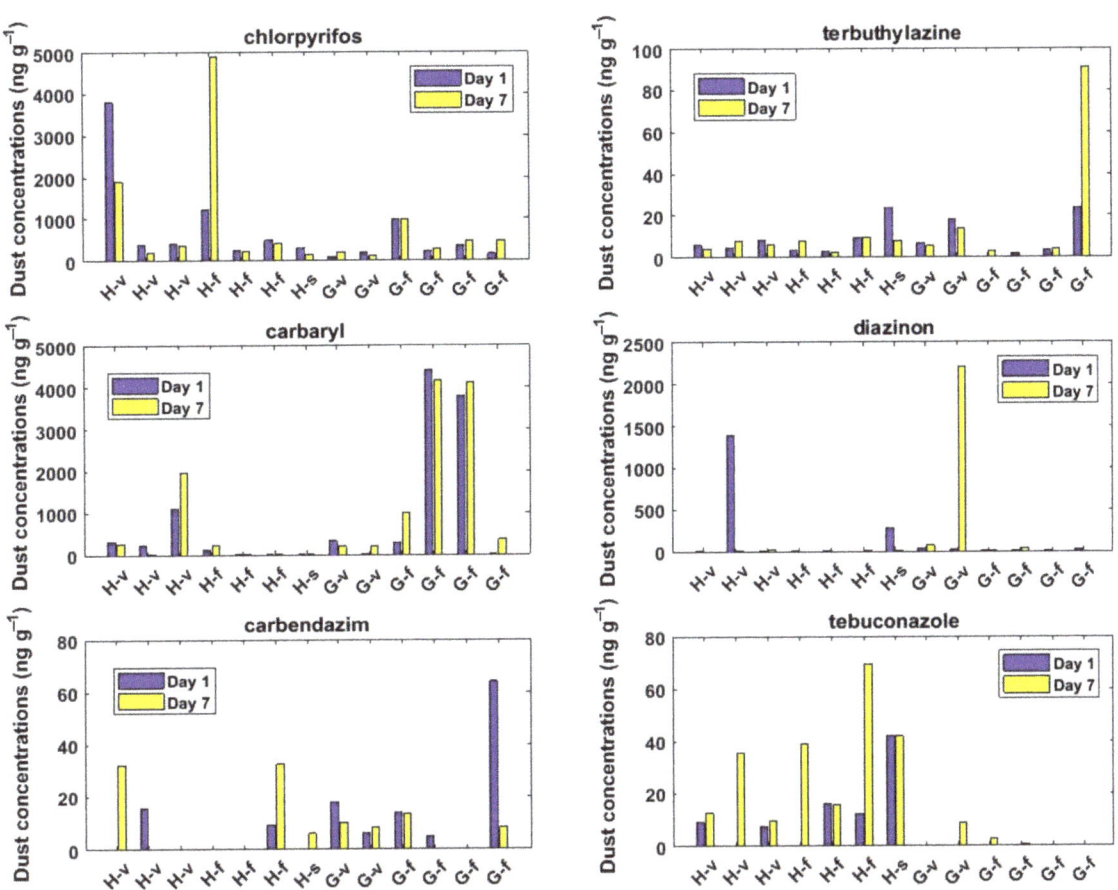

Figure 3. Temporal variations of pesticide levels in dust samples (in ng g^{-1}) collected at Hex River Valley (H) or Grabouw (G) at households living in farms (f), village (v), or at the school (s).

Significant differences in the levels of pesticides in dust were found between the areas (i.e., Hex River Valley and Grabouw) and the locations (village, farm, school). Indeed, when considering all samples (i.e., households, school, day 1, and day 7), the dust levels of carbaryl and carbendazim were significantly higher at Grabouw compared to Hex River Valley, while the opposite was found for tebuconazole (Figure S2). In addition, when focusing only on those samples collected on day 7, differences were observed between the different locations (farm, village, school) for some pesticides. Indeed, the concentrations of chlorpyrifos at Grabouw and tebuconazole at Hex River Valley on the farm were on average 6.16 and 2.22 times higher, respectively, than those in the village (Figure 4). On the other hand, at Grabouw, diazinon and tebuconazole had, respectively, 35.8 and 11.4 times higher levels in dust collected in village than those from the farm (Figure 4). Finally, at

Grabouw, the two samples collected at the school had on average 12.2 times higher levels of carbendazim than those collected in households (farm or village).

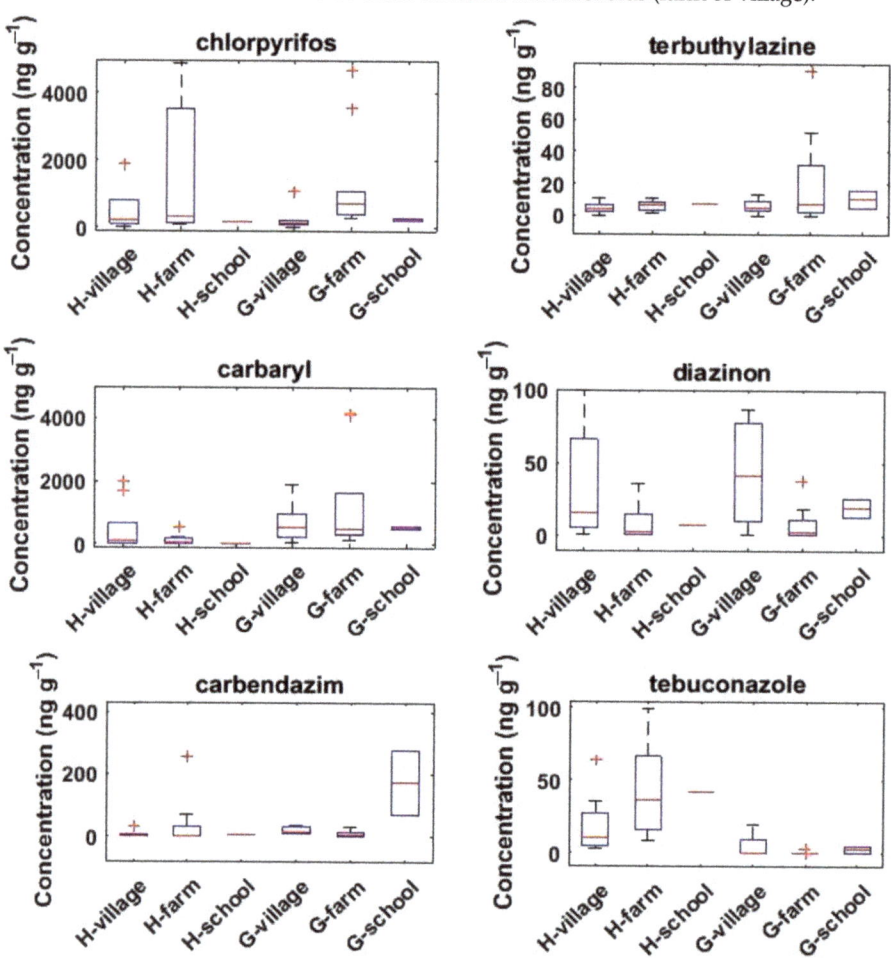

Figure 4. Spatial variations in dust levels of pesticides (in ng g^{-1}) among the different sites and areas from the samples collected on day 7 only (n = 41). H and G denote Hex River Valley and Grabouw, respectively. Some outliers are not shown for better visibility. Boxplots represent the 25–75th percentile, whiskers represent the minimum and maximum values (excluding outliers which are shown as the red crosses) and the line within the box represents the median value.

3.3. Daily Intakes of Pesticides via Dust Ingestion

The daily intakes of individual pesticides via dust ingestion for children (estimated using the median concentrations measured in dust and the median ingestion rate) ranged from 0.16 (tebuconazole) to 100 (chlorpyrifos) pg kg^{-1} day^{-1} (Table S6). The other cases considered (i.e., adults, maximum concentrations, and high ingestion rate) are presented in Tables S6 and S7 and will be discussed only when the findings differ. Chlorpyrifos and carbaryl dominated the pesticide exposure via dust ingestion, as they contributed respectively for 64–76% and 11–22% at Hex River Valley and 19–50% and 43–68% at Grabouw, of the daily intakes (Figure 5). The total daily pesticides intakes of children were about three times higher in Grabouw compared to Hex River Valley when the median or maximum concentrations were used (Tables S6 and S7). Except for carbendazim at

Grabouw, the children had daily intakes on average 4.4 times higher than adults. For carbendazim at Grabouw, the children-to-adult ratios of daily intake via dust ingestion were 22 and 38 for village and farm, respectively. When using the higher ingestion rate, the daily intakes of all individual pesticides were three times higher (Tables S6 and S7).

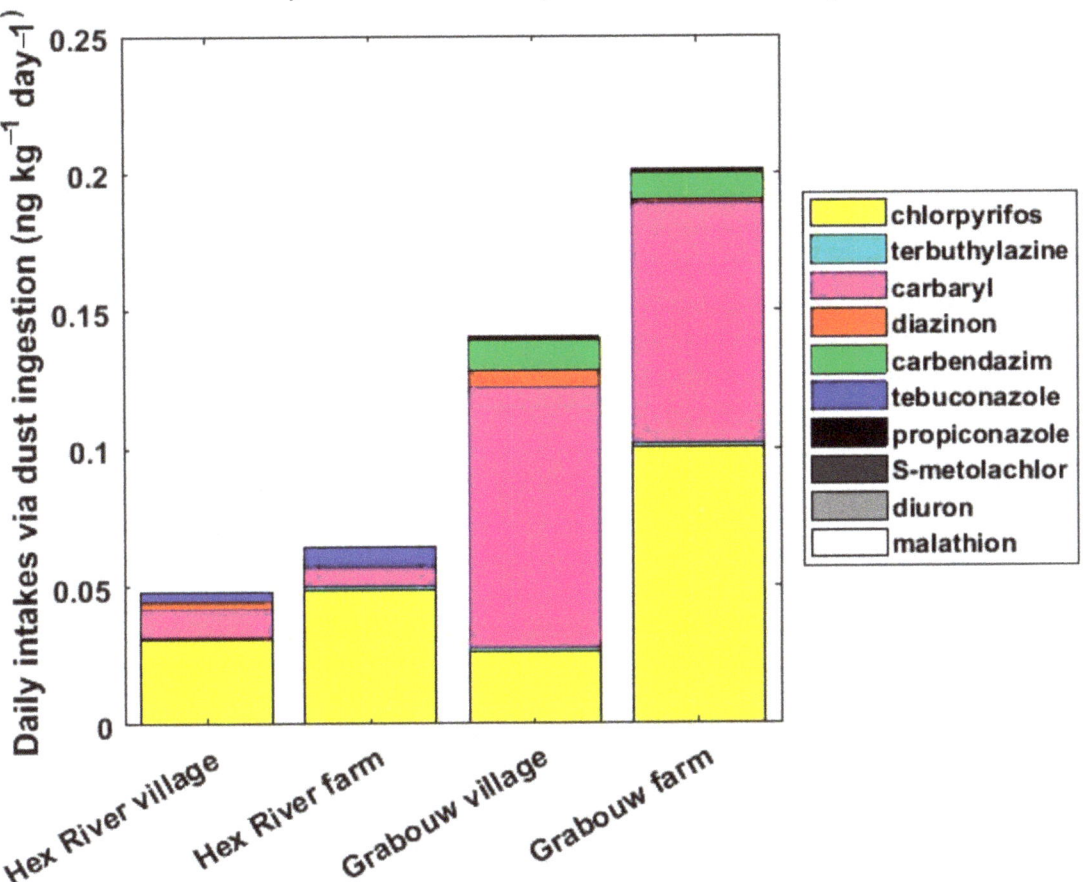

Figure 5. Daily intake of pesticides (in pg kg^{-1} day^{-1}) via dust ingestion for children using the median concentrations measured and the median ingestion rate.

3.4. Comparison of Daily Intakes from Dust Ingestion with Inhalation and Soil Ingestion

In addition to dust, the same pesticides were also quantified in air and soil samples collected from this field campaign [68]. In total, 19 individual pesticides were found in at least one of these three environmental media investigated. Among these, six (i.e., acetochlor, alachlor, azinphos methyl, dimethachlor, malathion, and metazachlor) were found only in air, two (i.e., isoproturon and pirimicarb) only in soil, and one (i.e., diuron) only in dust. Therefore, their dominant routes of exposure were, respectively, inhalation, soil ingestion, and dust ingestion. For the remaining pesticides, the results discussed here are for the children using the median concentrations and ingestion rate (Figure 6), while those for adults, maximum concentrations and high ingestion rate are shown in Figures S3–S7. For these ten pesticides that were found in at least two environmental matrices, six (i.e., atrazine, carbaryl, simazine, S-metolachlor, tebuconazole, and terbuthylazine) had inhalation as the major route (>90%) of exposure via the three studied pathways (i.e., inhalation, soil ingestion, and dust ingestion) at both sites. This was observed with all possible scenarios

(Figures S3–S7), except for carbaryl. On the other hand, for diazinon, it was dust ingestion (contributing for 62–94% depending on the site considered). For carbendazim, inhalation was the major route at Hex River Valley (>90%), but at Grabouw, it was dust ingestion (>97%). For propiconazole, inhalation was the major route at both sites, with dust ingestion being significant (37%) at Grabouw. For chlorpyrifos, inhalation dominated exposure at Hex River Valley (81% and 73% for the village and farm, respectively), while at Grabouw, there were pronounced differences between the two types of locations, with a contribution of inhalation, soil ingestion, and dust ingestion of 52%, 30%, and 18% at the village and 35%, 20%, and 45% at the farm. Using the high ingestion rate, the maximum concentrations or the input parameters for adults do not substantially modify the contribution of each exposure pathway for most of the pesticides investigated (Figure 6 and Figures S3–S7). However, for carbaryl at Hex River Valley and tebuconazole at Grabouw, using the high dust ingestion rate or the maximum concentrations led to a significant increase of the contribution of dust ingestion, reaching about 20–30% of the overall daily intake.

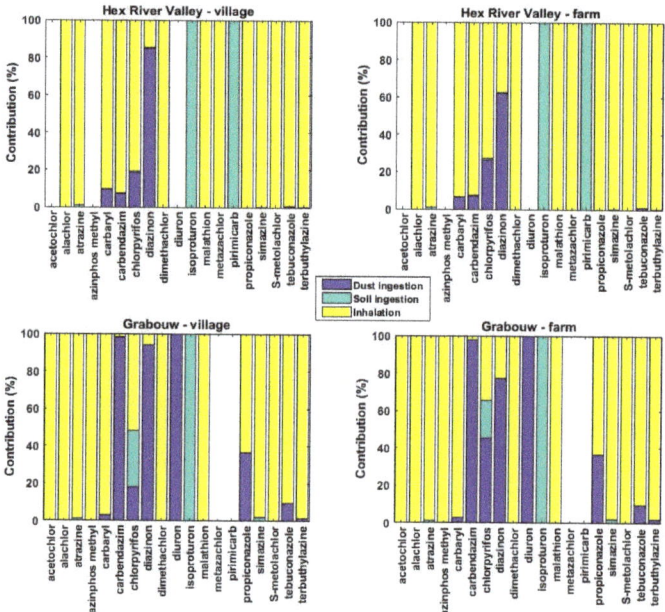

Figure 6. Contribution of three exposure pathways (dust ingestion, soil ingestion, and inhalation) on the daily uptake of pesticides of children living at farm and village locations at Hex River Valley and Grabouw using the median concentrations. Blank columns corresponds to the cases when a pesticide was not quantified in air, soil, and dust.

In this study, all hazard quotients estimated using the daily intakes from the three exposure pathways were three to twelve orders of magnitude lower than one (Tables S8 and S9), suggesting minor risks. Carbaryl, chlorpyrifos, and tebuconazole were the compounds having the highest hazard quotients, up to 1.33×10^{-3} (Tables S8 and S9). Similarly, the cumulative exposures (data not shown) were at least three orders of magnitude lower than one, suggesting negligible risks.

4. Discussion

4.1. Quantification Frequency and Levels of Pesticides Found

In this work, ten pesticides were quantified in dust samples collected from thirty-eight households and two schools located in two agricultural areas in South Africa. The ratio of quantified-to-targeted pesticides in this study (i.e., 0.33) was smaller than in others done in the Northern Hemisphere (i.e., 0.50–1.00) [53,60,63,79]. The presence of pesticides in indoor dust is mainly affected by (i) the amount of pesticides applied in the vicinity (outdoors and indoors), (ii) the application technique used, (iii) the physico-chemical properties of individual pesticides and their degradation half-lives in air, dust and soil, and (iv) the meteorological conditions [42,80]. The low amount of pesticides quantified in this study could be related to the fact that pesticides are usually sprayed manually for these two crops (i.e., pome fruits and table grapes), which could limit the distribution of pesticides beyond the cropland in comparison to mechanical pesticide applications [81].

More specifically, chlorpyrifos, terbuthylazine, carbaryl, diazinon, carbendazim, and tebuconazole were frequently quantified (in 59–96% of the samples). In particular, chlorpyrifos, which is associated with neurotoxic and developmental effects [4,82], was the most frequently quantified pesticide in dust, similarly to what has been found in the USA [17,19,38,83], Pakistan [84], or Taiwan [81]. Its widespread occurrence in the two studied areas in environmental media (dust, air, soil, and water [64,68–70]) and human samples [64,82] is related to its common agricultural use, which was previously reported [70]. However, this pesticide, which is a candidate for the Stockholm Convention on Persistent Organic Pollutants [85], is prone to long-range atmospheric transport [86], and some fraction could have also been transported from other agricultural areas. Diazinon and carbaryl have also frequently been reported in other studies [17,38,79,87,88]. The presence of carbendazim and tebuconazole in dust samples has been only studied once from an agricultural region in the Netherlands, where they were also frequently found (>50%) [53].

The analysis of the presence of these pesticides in dust in comparison to air and soil that was previously reported [68] can provide valuable information. Among the 30 targeted pesticides, more were found in air (n = 16) [68] than in dust (n = 10) or in soil (n = 9) at these two sampling sites (Figure 2). In particular, carbaryl, chlorpyrifos, tebuconazole, and terbuthylazine were the pesticides found the most frequently in these three environmental matrices (Figure 2), which highlights their widespread occurrence in these two agricultural areas. Besides diuron, every pesticide found in dust was also present in air, and except diazinon (at both sites) and carbendazim (at Grabouw), their quantification frequencies in air were always higher than in dust. In addition, many pesticides never found in soils were often quantified (>20%) in air samples but never or rarely (<10%) in dust samples (e.g., malathion, propiconazole, S-metolachlor, acetochlor, alachlor, azinphos methyl, and dimethachlor). This could suggest some influence from medium- to long-range atmospheric transport and indicates that they do not penetrate the indoor environment or that the concentrations in dust were too low to be quantified. Atrazine and simazine, two relatively persistent triazines [78], were quantified only in soil and air but not in dust, which likely reflects their past agricultural use and volatilization from soils enhanced by higher temperatures [50]. Diuron was only quantified in dust in one household, which likely reflects its use at the domestic level. Overall, these results highlight the importance of air in the transport of pesticides from the outdoor environment to the indoors. Due to the significant correlations observed between the levels in dust and air of many organic compounds [79,89], several researchers have concluded that one matrix could be used as a surrogate for the other one using partitioning models [33,90]. This approach has been validated for many legacy pollutants [33,91,92] but showed rather poor performance for predicting the levels of chlorpyrifos in dust [79]. For pesticides, the lack of accurate data on their physico-chemical properties and the possible lack of equilibrium between dust and air for compounds that have a high octanol–air partitioning coefficient or that are currently used [33,79,93] limits our capacity to use these models [92]. However, as more pesticides were quantified in air than in dust, the validity of these partitioning models that were developed for more persistent substances is questionable.

The levels of individual pesticides reported here varied over several orders of magnitude (Table 1). For chlorpyrifos, for which the most data are available in the literature, the dust concentrations observed in this study were similar to those found in Taiwan [94], North Carolina [38], and Australia [89] but lower than in Pakistan [84] and higher than in Spain [95]. To the best of our knowledge, only one study done in the Netherlands investigated the levels of terbuthylazine, carbendazim, and tebuconazole in dust [53], in which terbuthylazine was rarely found, while the levels of carbendazim were higher, and those of tebuconazole were similar to the present study. Similar dust levels of diazinon (e.g., 10–200 ng g^{-1}) were reported by previous studies [38,63,88].

4.2. Temporal and Spatial Differences in Pesticide Levels

For all pesticides investigated, no significant temporal differences in the dust levels measured at day 1 and day 7 were found for the 13 pairs investigated. This suggests that within short time scales (i.e., one week), one dust measurement provides a reliable estimate of human exposure. This finding is consistent with the findings from various field and laboratory studies. Indeed, the only two field studies existing on short temporal variations of pesticide levels in dust reported that within 5–8 days, measurements were relatively stable indicators of potential indoor exposure to pesticides [17,63]. Additionally, under laboratory conditions, the levels of cypermethrin and beta-cyfluthrin in dust samples remained constant for 56 days, with a significant decrease only observed 112 days after application [96]. This persistence in indoor dust could be due to limited solar radiation, constant indoor temperatures, lower microbial population, and moisture [21,47,96].

In terms of spatial variations, significant differences in the dust levels of some pesticides were found between the areas (i.e., Hex River Valley and Grabouw) and the locations (village, farm, school), which can help to identify the sources of these pesticides. Regarding the areas, three pesticides (i.e., carbaryl, carbendazim, and tebuconazole) showed significant differences in their dust levels, with carbaryl and carbendazim being the highest at Grabouw and tebuconazole at Hex River Valley. Interestingly, similar spatial variations were also found with soil and air samples for carbaryl and tebuconazole but not for carbendazim [68]. These consistent spatial variations observed in the three studied environmental matrices for carbaryl and tebuconazole suggests that agricultural activities control their environmental levels. On the other hand, significant differences between the two areas in the levels of terbuthylazine were found in air but not in soil or dust. This suggests that these three environmental matrices do not necessarily react in the same manner to point sources, further supported by the large spatial heterogeneity in levels of organic chemicals observed in soil [50] or dust [47].

Significant differences in pesticide dust levels were also found between the two locations (farm, village) studied. Indeed, the highest levels found in samples collected on farms for chlorpyrifos at Grabouw and for tebuconazole at Hex River Valley confirm that agricultural activities were the main source of pollution and that distance to agricultural fields is an important factor determining the levels of these pesticides in indoor dust. However, it is unclear whether these differences are due to spray drift and subsequent partitioning to dust, to take home exposures, or brought in via shoes, as it is known that indoor dust is composed of about 35% outdoor soil [97]. Negative associations between the levels of pesticides in house dust and the distance from the farms have also previously been reported in some studies [42,43,53,54,59,98] as well as positive ones between the levels of pesticides in house dust and agricultural acreages around the house [99], but this trend was not found in other studies [55,80,81]. In the present work, this was observed only for two pesticides out of the ten found. Therefore, further epidemiological studies should be cautious when using only geographic information systems (GIS) based on the distance to agricultural lands to predict human exposure to a large number of pesticides [43]. On the other hand, for diazinon and tebuconazole at Grabouw, the significantly higher levels found in dust collected from village compared to farm suggest these pesticides were used at the household level. Unfortunately, although questionnaires were deployed in this study [20], they failed to identify the specific active ingredients used at the domestic household level. Several studies have also shown the importance of residential use of pesticides on their dust levels for imidacloprid, malathion, chlorpyrifos, diazinon, carbaryl, or prallethrin [53,54,57,59,63,81,87]. It is interesting to note that tebuconazole showed a distinct behavior between the two sites, which shows that generalization about the influence of proximity to agricultural fields on the levels of pesticides in dust is not accurate, and site-specific differences should be considered in further exposure assessment to pesticides. Finally, at Grabouw, the significantly higher levels of carbendazim found at the school, for which existing data are scarce [44,58], compared to the households suggests its use in the close vicinity or within the school during the sampling campaign.

4.3. Daily Uptakes of Pesticides via Dust Ingestion

Chlorpyrifos and carbaryl, which are known for their toxic effects on humans [4,100], had the highest daily intakes at both sites showing the importance of these two pesticides in terms of human exposure for the agricultural residents of these two sites. Except for carbendazim, children had daily intakes of pesticides about four times higher than adults. This is similar to previous studies [89,95] and is due to their higher ingestion rate and lower weight (Table S2). Considering that young children are a particularly vulnerable group due to the well-documented detrimental effects of pesticide exposure on child neurodevelopment [101,102], the higher exposure levels reported in this and other studies require further attention. For carbendazim, the children-to-adult ratio of daily intake via dust ingestion was much higher (i.e., 22–38 at Grabouw) due to the significantly higher levels of carbendazim measured in the two dust samples collected at schools where adults are not exposed. This highlights the importance of having several micro-environments investigated when assessing human exposure to organic chemicals via dust ingestion, particularly for children. In addition to the micro-environment frequented, the dust ingestion rate is an important factor that can lead to uncertainties within a factor of three and should therefore be better characterized.

4.4. Comparison of Daily Intakes from Dust Ingestion with Inhalation and Soil Ingestion

Daily uptakes of pesticides via dust ingestion were compared with those from inhalation and soil ingestion previously reported [68]. Inhalation was generally the major route of exposure (>90%) for 13 out of the 19 pesticides quantified in at least one of the three environmental matrices investigated. For the remaining six pesticides, the major pathway was soil ingestion for isoproturon and pirimicarb and dust ingestion for diuron and diazinon, while chlorpyrifos and carbendazim differed depending on the site considered (Figure 6). Considering that the air concentrations were obtained from the outdoor environment where concentrations of organic compounds such as pesticides are several orders of magnitude lower than indoors [92], this highlights the importance of inhalation in non-dietary exposure to pesticides. This is similar to what has been found for North Carolina children, who were about 10 times more exposed to chlorpyrifos via inhalation than via both soil and dust ingestion [38]. Similarly, it was estimated that dust was contributing less than 15% of the levels of dialkyphosphates metabolites measured in urine [55]. One can notice the important role of input parameters such as the ingestion rate or the concentrations used (median or maximum) in the contribution of dust ingestion for carbaryl and tebuconazole, which increased by a factor of three. For other semi-volatile organic compounds, several studies have found that uptake via inhalation was higher than via dust ingestion and dermal contact with dust for compounds that are volatile, while the opposite was found for the non-volatile compounds [36,79]. However, this influence of physico-chemical properties on the contribution of different exposure pathways was not observed in our study.

The health risks estimated in this study were negligible, both for individual pesticides or cumulative exposure. This was also found by several other studies (focusing only on dust ingestion) [63,89,95]. However, we should keep in mind that the risks estimated in this study from several environmental matrices do not take into account dietary ingestion, which can dominate human exposure [38,103–105]. Carbaryl, chlorpyrifos, and terbuthylazine, which were the pesticides the most frequently found in all the three matrices investigated, had the highest hazard quotients. Therefore, further studies could investigate the health risks due to their transformation products, as many of them could have significant health effects [106].

4.5. Limitations and Strengths

The main strengths of this study are: (i) the characterization of the levels of several herbicides and fungicides that have been poorly characterized worldwide in dust, (ii) the first characterization of daily intakes via dust ingestion of multiple pesticides in Africa, and (iii) the improvement of our understanding on the contribution of several non-dietary exposure pathways. This study has three main limitations. The first concerns the characteristics of the sampling campaign, which was short (seven days at each site) and involved a limited amount of samples (n = 54). In addition, dust is associated with large spatial heterogeneity of the levels of contaminants [92,107], particularly before and after pesticide use [39]. Therefore, the spot samples collected might not be representative of the entire room. Secondly, there are high uncertainties associated with the input parameters of the model used to characterize human exposure via the three pathways. Indeed, the data on the bioaccessibility of pesticides or dust ingestion rates are highly uncertain [47], which could contribute to a 20-fold variability in the daily doses estimates [108]. In addition, outdoor and not indoor air levels of pesticides were used. However, we expect this to have a minor effect, as several studies have found a significant correlation between these [19,98], and levels indoors are usually higher than outdoors [92,109,110]. Finally, the outcome of the health impact assessment is limited by the fact that it considers only a limited amount of active ingredients and does not take into account synergistic effects [111]. Additionally, some mechanisms of toxicity (e.g., suppressed expression of serotonin transporter genes) are not considered in the definition of the reference dose [63].

5. Conclusions

In this study, the spatial and temporal variations of 30 pesticides in dust and the human exposure via dust ingestion in comparison to inhalation and soil ingestion were investigated at two agricultural sites in South Africa. Within seven days, no significant temporal variations in the dust levels of individual pesticides were found. On the other hand, significant spatial variations were observed for some pesticides, highlighting either the importance of proximity to agricultural fields (chlorpyrifos at Grabouw and tebuconazole at Hex River Valley) or use at the domestic level (diazinon at Grabouw and tebuconazole at Grabouw) or applied at or in the vicinity of the school (carbendazim at Grabouw). The agricultural residents of the two sites investigated were exposed to 10 pesticides via dust ingestion. However, this exposure pathway was found negligible (<10%) compared to inhalation or soil ingestion for 14 out of the 19 pesticides found in dust, air, or soil. Further studies should confirm this finding by characterizing the levels of pesticides in several environmental matrices and the contribution of several non-dietary exposure pathways in both spraying and non-spraying seasons.

Supplementary Materials: The following supporting information can be downloaded at: https://www.mdpi.com/article/10.3390/toxics10100629/s1, Table S1: Average recoveries and their standard deviations determined from spiking experiments; Table S2: Input parameters used for the assessment of daily intakes from dust ingestion; Table S3: Basic statistics of pesticide levels found in all dust samples; Table S4: Basic statistics of pesticide levels found in all household dust samples collected at Hex River Valley; Table S5: Basic statistics of pesticide levels found in all household dust samples collected at Grabouw; Table S6: Daily intake (in pg kg^{-1} day^{-1}) of individual pesticides via dust ingestion for a child; Table S7: Daily intake (in pg kg^{-1} day^{-1}) of individual pesticides via dust ingestion for an adult; Table S8: Hazard quotients of children due to the exposure to individual pesticides via dust ingestion, inhalation, and soil ingestion found in this study; Table S9: Hazard quotients of adults due to the exposure to individual pesticides via dust ingestion, inhalation, and soil ingestion found in this study; Figure S1: Dust levels of individual pesticides in 12 households and one school measured at day 1 and day 7; Figure S2: Boxplots of concentrations of individual pesticides in dust samples; Figure S3: Contribution of three exposure pathways on the daily uptake of pesticides of a children living at farm and village locations at Hex River Valley and Grabouw using the maximum concentrations; Figure S4: Contribution of three exposure pathways on the daily uptake of pesticides of a children living at farm and village locations at Hex River Valley and Grabouw using the median concentrations and high ingestion rate; Figure S5: Contribution of three exposure pathways on the daily uptake of pesticides of an adult living at farm and village locations at Hex River Valley and Grabouw using median concentrations; Figure S6: Contribution of three exposure pathways on the daily uptake of pesticides of an adult living at farm and village locations at Hex River Valley and Grabouw using the maximum concentrations; Figure S7: Contribution of three exposure pathways on the daily uptake of pesticides of an adult living at farm and village locations at Hex River Valley and Grabouw using the median concentrations and the high ingestion rate of dust.

Author Contributions: Conceptualization, C.D. and S.F.; methodology, C.D., R.P., P.Š., S.R.J., L.M., P.P., J.K. (Jiří Kohoutek) and S.F.; investigation, C.D.; writing original draft, C.D.; writing—review and editing, all; project administration, C.D., S.F., M.A.D., M.R. and J.K. (Jana Klánová); funding acquisition, C.D., S.F., M.A.D., M.R. and J.K. (Jana Klánová). All authors have read and agreed to the published version of the manuscript.

Funding: This work has received funding from the European Union's Horizon 2020 research and innovation programme under grant agreement No 857340 and No 857560, the Swiss National Science Foundation (P4P4PM_199228); the South Africa National Research Foundation (NRF) SARChI Programme (grant number 94883); and the Swiss State Secretariat for Education, Research and Innovation, the University of Basel, and the Swiss TPH. This publication reflects only the author's view, and the European Commission is not responsible for any use that may be made of the information it contains.

Institutional Review Board Statement: Informed consent was obtained from a member of each household. The study received ethical clearance from the University of Cape Town's Research Ethics Committee (HREC 637/2018).

Informed Consent Statement: Informed consent was obtained from all subjects involved in the study.

Data Availability Statement: Data available on request.

Acknowledgments: The authors are thankful for the contribution of Barblin Michelson, Keith Van Aarde, Neville Peterson, and Kharan Van Mali for their help during sampling and of Adriana Fernandes Veludo for support. The authors thank also the RECETOX Research Infrastructure (No LM2018121) and ACTRIS-CZ (LM2018122) research infrastructure financed by the Ministry of Education, Youth and Sports, and the Operational Programme Research, Development and Education (the CETOCOEN EXCELLENCE project No. CZ.02.1.01/0.0/0.0/17_043/0009632) for supportive background.

Conflicts of Interest: The authors declare no conflict of interest. The funders had no role in the design of the study; in the collection, analyses, or interpretation of data; in the writing of the manuscript; or in the decision to publish the results.

References

1. FAO. FAOSTAT-Pesticides Use/Crops. Available online: http://www.fao.org/faostat/en/#data/RP/visualize (accessed on 10 December 2019).
2. Mostafalou, S.; Abdollahi, M. Pesticides: An update of human exposure and toxicity. *Arch. Toxicol.* **2017**, *91*, 549–599. [CrossRef] [PubMed]
3. Kim, K.; Kabir, E.; Ara, S. Exposure to pesticides and the associated human health effects. *Sci. Total Environ.* **2017**, *575*, 525–535. [CrossRef] [PubMed]
4. Burke, R.D.; Todd, S.W.; Lumsden, E.; Mullins, R.J.; Mamczarz, J.; Fawcett, W.P.; Gullapalli, R.P.; Randall, W.R.; Pereira, E.F.R.; Albuquerque, E.X. Developmental neurotoxicity of the organophosphorus insecticide chlorpyrifos: From clinical findings to preclinical models and potential mechanisms. *J. Neurochem.* **2017**, *142*, 162–177. [CrossRef] [PubMed]
5. Tang, J.; Wang, W.; Jiang, Y.; Chu, W. Diazinon exposure produces histological damage, oxidative stress, immune disorders and gut microbiota dysbiosis in crucian carp (*Carassius auratus gibelio*). *Environ. Pollut.* **2021**, *269*, 116129. [CrossRef] [PubMed]
6. Bagchi, D.; Bagchi, M.; Hassoun, E.A.; Stohs, S.J. In vitro and in vivo generation of reactive oxygen species, DNA damage and lactate dehydrogenase leakage by selected pesticides. *Toxicology* **1995**, *104*, 129–140. [CrossRef]
7. Ledda, C.; Cannizzaro, E.; Cinà, D.; Filetti, V.; Vitale, E.; Paravizzini, G.; Di Naso, C.; Iavicoli, I.; Rapisarda, V. Oxidative stress and DNA damage in agricultural workers after exposure to pesticides. *J. Occup. Med. Toxicol.* **2021**, *16*, 1. [CrossRef]

8. Désert, M.; Ravier, S.; Gille, G.; Quinapallo, A.; Armengaud, A.; Pochet, G.; Savelli, J.L.; Wortham, H.; Quivet, E. Spatial and temporal distribution of current-use pesticides in ambient air of Provence-Alpes-Côte-d'Azur Region and Corsica, France. *Atmos. Environ.* **2018**, *192*, 241–256. [CrossRef]
9. Silva, V.; Mol, H.G.J.; Zomer, P.; Tienstra, M.; Ritsema, C.J.; Geissen, V. Pesticide residues in European agricultural soils—A hidden reality unfolded. *Sci. Total Environ.* **2019**, *653*, 1532–1545. [CrossRef] [PubMed]
10. Syafrudin, M.; Kristanti, R.A.; Yuniarto, A.; Hadibarata, T.; Rhee, J. Pesticides in Drinking Water—A Review. *Int. J. Environ. Res. Public Health* **2021**, *18*, 468. [CrossRef]
11. Degrendele, C.; Okonski, K.; Melymuk, L.; Landlová, L.; Kukučka, P.; Audy, O.; Kohoutek, J.; Čupr, P.; Klánová, J. Pesticides in the atmosphere: A comparison of gas-particle partitioning and particle size distribution of legacy and current-use pesticides. *Atmos. Chem. Phys.* **2016**, *16*, 1531–1544. [CrossRef]
12. Pérez-Indoval, R.; Rodrigo-Ilarri, J.; Cassiraga, E.; Rodrigo-Clavero, M.E. Numerical modeling of groundwater pollution by chlorpyrifos, bromacil and terbuthylazine. Application to the buñol-cheste aquifer (spain). *Int. J. Environ. Res. Public Health* **2021**, *18*, 3511. [CrossRef] [PubMed]
13. Pérez-Indoval, R.; Rodrigo-Ilarri, J.; Cassiraga, E.; Rodrigo-Clavero, M.E. PWC-based evaluation of groundwater pesticide pollution in the Júcar River Basin. *Sci. Total Environ.* **2022**, *847*, 157386. [CrossRef] [PubMed]
14. Rodrigo-Ilarri, J.; Rodrigo-Clavero, M.E.; Cassiraga, E.; Ballesteros-Almonacid, L. Assessment of groundwater contamination by terbuthylazine using vadose zone numerical models. Case study of valencia province (spain). *Int. J. Environ. Res. Public Health* **2020**, *17*, 3280. [CrossRef]
15. Coscollà, C.; López, A.; Yahyaoui, A.; Colin, P.; Robin, C.; Poinsignon, Q.; Yusà, V. Human exposure and risk assessment to airborne pesticides in a rural French community. *Sci. Total Environ.* **2017**, *584–585*, 856–868. [CrossRef]
16. Fuhrimann, S.; Klánová, J.; Přibylová, P.; Kohoutek, J.; Dalvie, M.A.; Röösli, M.; Degrendele, C. Qualitative assessment of 27 current-use pesticides in air at 20 sampling sites across Africa. *Chemosphere* **2020**, *258*, 127333. [CrossRef]
17. Quirós-Alcalá, L.; Bradman, A.; Smith, K.; Weerasekera, G.; Odetokun, M.; Barr, D.B.; Nishioka, M.; Castorina, R.; Hubbard, A.E.; Nicas, M.; et al. Organophosphorous pesticide breakdown products in house dust and children's urine. *J. Expo. Sci. Environ. Epidemiol.* **2012**, *22*, 559–568. [CrossRef] [PubMed]
18. Trunnelle, K.J.; Bennett, D.H.; Tancredi, D.J.; Gee, S.J.; Stoecklin-Marois, M.T.; Hennessy-Burt, T.E.; Hammock, B.D.; Schenker, M.B. Pyrethroids in house dust from the homes of farm worker families in the MICASA study. *Environ. Int.* **2013**, *61*, 57–63. [CrossRef]
19. Bradman, A.; Whitaker, D.; Quirós, L.; Castorina, R.; Henn, B.C.; Nishioka, M.; Morgan, J.; Barr, D.B.; Harnly, M.; Brisbin, J.A.; et al. Pesticides and their metabolites in the homes and urine of farmworker children living in the Salinas Valley, CA. *J. Expo. Sci. Environ. Epidemiol.* **2007**, *17*, 331–349. [CrossRef]
20. Fuhrimann, S.; Mol, H.G.J.; Dias, J.; Dalvie, M.A.; Röösli, M.; Degrendele, C.; Figueiredo, D.M.; Huss, A.; Portengen, L.; Vermeulen, R. Quantitative assessment of multiple pesticides in silicone wristbands of children/guardian pairs living in agricultural areas in South Africa. *Sci. Total Environ.* **2022**, *812*, 152330. [CrossRef]
21. Arcury, T.A.; Chen, H.; Quandt, S.A.; Talton, J.W.; Anderson, K.A.; Scott, R.P.; Jensen, A.; Laurienti, P.J. Pesticide exposure among Latinx children: Comparison of children in rural, farmworker and urban, non-farmworker communities. *Sci. Total Environ.* **2021**, *763*, 144233. [CrossRef]
22. Fišerová, P.S.; Kohoutek, J.; Degrendele, C.; Dalvie, M.A.; Klánová, J. New sample preparation method to analyse 15 specific and non-specific pesticide metabolites in human urine using LC-MS/MS. *J. Chromatogr. B Anal. Technol. Biomed. Life Sci.* **2021**, *1166*, 122542. [CrossRef] [PubMed]
23. Bravo, N.; Grimalt, J.O.; Mazej, D.; Tratnik, J.S.; Sarigiannis, D.A.; Horvat, M. Mother/child organophosphate and pyrethroid distributions. *Environ. Int.* **2020**, *134*, 105264. [CrossRef] [PubMed]
24. Molomo, R.N.; Basera, W.; Chetty-Mhlanga, S.; Fuhrimann, S.; Mugari, M.; Wiesner, L.; Röösli, M.; Dalvie, M.A. Relation between organophosphate pesticide metabolite concentrations with pesticide exposures, socio-economic factors and lifestyles: A cross-sectional study among school boys in the rural western cape, South Africa. *Environ. Pollut.* **2021**, *275*, 116660. [CrossRef] [PubMed]
25. Huen, K.; Bradman, A.; Harley, K.; Yousefi, P.; Boyd Barr, D.; Eskenazi, B.; Holland, N. Organophosphate pesticide levels in blood and urine of women and newborns living in an agricultural community. *Environ. Res.* **2012**, *117*, 8–16. [CrossRef]
26. Afata, T.N.; Mekonen, S.; Tucho, G.T. Evaluating the Level of Pesticides in the Blood of Small-Scale Farmers and Its Associated Risk Factors in Western Ethiopia. *Environ. Health Insights* **2021**, *15*, 11786302211043660. [CrossRef]
27. Von Ehrenstein, O.S.; Ling, C.; Cui, X.; Cockburn, M.; Park, A.S.; Yu, F.; Wu, J.; Ritz, B. Prenatal and infant exposure to ambient pesticides and autism spectrum disorder in children: Population based case-control study. *BMJ* **2019**, *364*, l962. [CrossRef]
28. Roberts, E.M.; English, P.B.; Grether, J.K.; Windham, G.C.; Somberg, L.; Wolff, C. Maternal residence near agricultural pesticide applications and autism spectrum disorders among children in the California Central Valley. *Environ. Health Perspect.* **2007**, *115*, 1482–1489. [CrossRef]
29. Yitshak Sade, M.; Zlotnik, Y.; Kloog, I.; Novack, V.; Peretz, C.; Ifergane, G. Parkinson's disease prevalence and proximity to agricultural cultivated fields. *Parkinsons. Dis.* **2015**, *2015*, 576564. [CrossRef]

30. Patel, D.M.; Gyldenkærne, S.; Jones, R.R.; Olsen, S.F.; Tikellis, G.; Granström, C.; Dwyer, T.; Stayner, L.T.; Ward, M.H. Residential proximity to agriculture and risk of childhood leukemia and central nervous system tumors in the Danish national birth cohort. *Environ. Int.* **2020**, *143*, 105955. [CrossRef]
31. Gómez-Barroso, D.; García-Pérez, J.; López-Abente, G.; Tamayo-Uria, I.; Morales-Piga, A.; Pardo Romaguera, E.; Ramis, R. Agricultural crop exposure and risk of childhood cancer: New findings from a case-control study in Spain. *Int. J. Health Geogr.* **2016**, *15*, 18. [CrossRef]
32. Chetty-Mhlanga, S.; Fuhrimann, S.; Basera, W.; Eeftens, M.; Röösli, M.; Dalvie, M.A. Association of activities related to pesticide exposure on headache severity and neurodevelopment of school-children in the rural agricultural farmlands of the Western Cape of South Africa. *Environ. Int.* **2021**, *146*, 106237. [CrossRef] [PubMed]
33. Weschler, C.J.; Nazaroff, W.W. Semivolatile organic compounds in indoor environments. *Atmos. Environ.* **2008**, *42*, 9018–9040. [CrossRef]
34. Glorennec, P.; Serrano, T.; Fravallo, M.; Warembourg, C.; Monfort, C.; Cordier, S.; Viel, J.F.; Le Gléau, F.; Le Bot, B.; Chevrier, C. Determinants of children's exposure to pyrethroid insecticides in western France. *Environ. Int.* **2017**, *104*, 76–82. [CrossRef] [PubMed]
35. Yu, Y.; Li, C.; Zhang, X.; Zhang, X.; Pang, Y.; Zhang, S.; Fu, J. Route-specific daily uptake of organochlorine pesticides in food, dust, and air by Shanghai residents, China. *Environ. Int.* **2012**, *50*, 31–37. [CrossRef] [PubMed]
36. Li, L.; Arnot, J.A.; Wania, F. How are Humans Exposed to Organic Chemicals Released to Indoor Air? *Environ. Sci. Technol.* **2019**, *53*, 11276–11284. [CrossRef]
37. Fischer, D.; Hooper, K.; Athanasiadou, M.; Athanassiadis, I.; Bergman, Å. Children show highest levels of polybrominated diphenyl ethers in a California family of four: A case study. *Environ. Health Perspect.* **2006**, *114*, 1581–1584. [CrossRef]
38. Morgan, M.K.; Wilson, N.K.; Chuang, J.C. Exposures of 129 preschool children to organochlorines, organophosphates, pyrethroids, and acid herbicides at their homes and daycares in North Carolina. *Int. J. Environ. Res. Public Health* **2014**, *11*, 3743–3764. [CrossRef]
39. Morgan, M.K. Children's exposures to pyrethroid insecticides at home: A review of data collected in published exposure measurement studies conducted in the United States. *Int. J. Environ. Res. Public Health* **2012**, *9*, 2964–2985. [CrossRef]
40. Deziel, N.; Friesen, M.; Hoppin, J.; Hines, C.; Thomas, K.; Beane Freeman, L. Exposition non professionnelle des femmes aux pesticides en milieu rural: État des lieux des connaissances. *Environ. Risques Sante* **2015**, *14*, 473–475.
41. Shaffer, R.M.; Smith, M.N.; Faustman, E.M. Developing the regulatory utility of the exposome: Mapping exposures for risk assessment through lifestage exposome snapshots (LEnS). *Environ. Health Perspect.* **2017**, *125*, 085003. [CrossRef]
42. Teysseire, R.; Manangama, G.; Baldi, I.; Carles, C.; Brochard, P.; Bedos, C.; Delva, F. Determinants of non-dietary exposure to agricultural pesticides in populations living close to fields: A systematic review. *Sci. Total Environ.* **2021**, *761*. [CrossRef] [PubMed]
43. Teysseire, R.; Manangama, G.; Baldi, I.; Carles, C.; Brochard, P.; Bedos, C.; Delva, F. Assessment of residential exposures to agricultural pesticides: A scoping review. *PLoS ONE* **2020**, *15*, e0232258. [CrossRef] [PubMed]
44. Lucattini, L.; Poma, G.; Covaci, A.; de Boer, J.; Lamoree, M.H.; Leonards, P.E.G. A review of semi-volatile organic compounds (SVOCs) in the indoor environment: Occurrence in consumer products, indoor air and dust. *Chemosphere* **2018**, *201*, 466–482. [CrossRef]
45. Schweizer, C.; Edwards, R.D.; Bayer-Oglesby, L.; Gauderman, W.J.; Ilacqua, V.; Juhani Jantunen, M.; Lai, H.K.; Nieuwenhuijsen, M.; Künzli, N. Indoor time-microenvironment-activity patterns in seven regions of Europe. *J. Expo. Sci. Environ. Epidemiol.* **2007**, *17*, 170–181. [CrossRef]
46. Salthammer, T.; Zhang, Y.; Mo, J.; Koch, H.M.; Weschler, C.J. Assessing Human Exposure to Organic Pollutants in the Indoor Environment. *Angew. Chem.* **2018**, *130*, 12406–12443. [CrossRef]
47. Melymuk, L.; Demirtepe, H.; Jílková, S.R. Indoor dust and associated chemical exposures. *Curr. Opin. Environ. Sci. Health* **2020**, *15*, 1–6. [CrossRef]
48. Van den Berg, F.; Kubiak, R.; Benjey, W.G.; Majewski, M.S.; Yates, S.R.; Reeves, G.L.; Smelt, J.H.; van der Linden, A.M.A. Emission of pesticides into the air. *Water. Air. Soil Pollut.* **1999**, *115*, 195–218. [CrossRef]
49. Das, S.; Hageman, K.J.; Taylor, M.; Michelsen-Heath, S.; Stewart, I. Fate of the organophosphate insecticide, chlorpyrifos, in leaves, soil, and air following application. *Chemosphere* **2020**, *243*, 125194. [CrossRef]
50. Degrendele, C.; Audy, O.; Hofman, J.; Kučerik, J.; Kukučka, P.; Mulder, M.D.; Přibylová, P.; Prokeš, R.; Šáňka, M.; Schaumann, G.E.; et al. Diurnal variations of air-soil exchange of semivolatile organic compounds (PAHs, PCBs, OCPs, and PBDEs) in a Central European receptor area. *Environ. Sci. Technol.* **2016**, *50*, 4278–4288. [CrossRef]
51. Davie-Martin, C.L.; Hageman, K.J.; Chin, Y.-P.P.; Rougé, V.; Fujita, Y. Influence of temperature, relative humidity, and soil properties on the soil-air partitioning of semivolatile pesticides: Laboratory measurements and predictive models. *Environ. Sci. Technol.* **2015**, *49*, 10431–10439. [CrossRef]
52. FOCUS Air Group. FOCUS Pesticides in Air: Considerations for Exposure Assessment. *Rep. Focus Work. Gr. Pestic. Air* **2008**, *327*, 12–74.
53. Figueiredo, D.M.; Nijssen, R.; Krop, E.J.M.; Buijtenhuijs, D.; Gooijer, Y.; Lageschaar, L.; Duyzer, J.; Huss, A.; Mol, H.; Vermeulen, R.C.H. Pesticides in doormat and floor dust from homes close to treated fields: Spatio-temporal variance and determinants of occurrence and concentrations. *Environ. Pollut.* **2022**, *301*, 119024. [CrossRef] [PubMed]
54. Deziel, N.C.; Friesen, M.C.; Hoppin, J.A.; Hines, C.J.; Thomas, K.; Beane Freeman, L.E. A Review of Nonoccupational Pathways for Pesticide Exposure in Women Living in Agricultural Areas. *Environ. Health Perspect.* **2015**, *123*, 515–524. [CrossRef] [PubMed]

55. Curl, C.L.; Fenske, R.A.; Kissel, J.C.; Shirai, J.H.; Moate, T.F.; Griffith, W.; Coronado, G.; Thompson, B. Evaluation of Take-Home Organophosphorus Pesticide Exposure among Agricultural Workers and Their Children. *Environ. Health Perspect.* **2002**, *110*, A787–A792. [CrossRef]
56. Lu, C.; Fenske, R.A.; Simcox, N.J.; Kalman, D. Pesticide exposure of children in an agricultural community: Evidence of household proximity to farmland and take home exposure pathways. In *Proceedings of the Environmental Research*; Academic Press Inc.: New York, NY, USA, 2000; Volume 84, pp. 290–302.
57. Gunier, R.B.; Ward, M.H.; Airola, M.; Bell, E.M.; Colt, J.; Nishioka, M.; Buffler, P.A.; Reynolds, P.; Rull, R.P.; Hertz, A.; et al. Determinants of agricultural pesticide concentrations in carpet dust. *Environ. Health Perspect.* **2011**, *119*, 970–976. [CrossRef]
58. Raffy, G.; Mercier, F.; Blanchard, O.; Derbez, M.; Dassonville, C.; Bonvallot, N.; Glorennec, P.; Le Bot, B. Semi-volatile organic compounds in the air and dust of 30 French schools: A pilot study. *Indoor Air* **2017**, *27*, 114–127. [CrossRef]
59. Deziel, N.C.; Beane Freeman, L.E.; Graubard, B.I.; Jones, R.R.; Hoppin, J.A.; Thomas, K.; Hines, C.J.; Blair, A.; Sandler, D.P.; Chen, H.; et al. Relative contributions of agricultural drift, para-occupational, and residential use exposure pathways to house dust pesticide concentrations: Meta-regression of published data. *Environ. Health Perspect.* **2017**, *125*, 296–305. [CrossRef]
60. Bennett, B.; Workman, T.; Smith, M.N.; Griffith, W.C.; Thompson, B.; Faustman, E.M. Longitudinal, seasonal, and occupational trends of multiple pesticides in house dust. *Environ. Health Perspect.* **2019**, *127*, 017003. [CrossRef]
61. Li, H.; Ma, H.; Lydy, M.J.; You, J. Occurrence, seasonal variation and inhalation exposure of atmospheric organophosphate and pyrethroid pesticides in an urban community in South China. *Chemosphere* **2014**, *95*, 363–369. [CrossRef]
62. Jiang, W.; Conkle, J.L.; Luo, Y.; Li, J.; Xu, K.; Gan, J. Occurrence, distribution, and accumulation of pesticides in exterior residential areas. *Environ. Sci. Technol.* **2016**, *50*, 12592–12601. [CrossRef]
63. Quirós-Alcalá, L.; Bradman, A.; Nishioka, M.; Harnly, M.E.; Hubbard, A.; McKone, T.E.; Ferber, J.; Eskenazi, B. Pesticides in house dust from urban and farmworker households in California: An observational measurement study. *Environ. Health Glob. Access Sci. Source* **2011**, *10*, 19. [CrossRef] [PubMed]
64. Dalvie, M.A.; Sosan, M.B.; Africa, A.; Cairncross, E.; London, L. Environmental monitoring of pesticide residues from farms at a neighbouring primary and pre-school in the Western Cape in South Africa. *Sci. Total Environ.* **2014**, *466–467*, 1078–1084. [CrossRef] [PubMed]
65. AVCASA. Croplife South Africa Agricultural Remedies Database. Available online: https://www.croplife.co.za/images/croplife/home/CROPLIFESOUTHAFRICAAGRICULTURALREMEDIESDATABASEINTRODUCTION.pdf (accessed on 30 August 2022).
66. Tang, F.H.M.; Lenzen, M.; McBratney, A.; Maggi, F. Risk of pesticide pollution at the global scale. *Nat. Geosci.* **2021**, *14*, 206–210. [CrossRef]
67. Chetty-Mhlanga, S.; Basera, W.; Fuhrimann, S.; Probst-Hensch, N.; Delport, S.; Mugari, M.; Van Wyk, J.; Roosli, M.; Dalvie, M.A.; Röösli, M.; et al. A prospective cohort study of school-going children investigating reproductive and neurobehavioral health effects due to environmental pesticide exposure in the Western Cape, South Africa: Study protocol. *BMC Public Health* **2018**, *18*, 857. [CrossRef]
68. Degrendele, C.; Klánová, J.; Prokeš, R.; Příbylová, P.; Šenk, P.; Šudoma, M.; Röösli, M.; Dalvie, M.A.; Fuhrimann, S. Current use pesticides in soil and air from two agricultural sites in South Africa: Implications for environmental fate and human exposure. *Sci. Total Environ.* **2022**, *807*, 150455. [CrossRef]
69. Veludo, A.F.; Martins Figueiredo, D.; Degrendele, C.; Masinyana, L.; Curchod, L.; Kohoutek, J.; Kukučka, P.; Martiník, J.; Přibylová, P.; Klánová, J.; et al. Seasonal variations in air concentrations of 27 organochlorine pesticides (OCPs) and 25 current-use pesticides (CUPs) across three agricultural areas of South Africa. *Chemosphere* **2022**, *289*, 133162. [CrossRef]
70. Curchod, L.; Oltramare, C.; Junghans, M.; Stamm, C.; Dalvie, M.A.; Röösli, M.; Fuhrimann, S. Temporal variation of pesticide mixtures in rivers of three agricultural watersheds during a major drought in the Western Cape, South Africa. *Water Res. X* **2020**, *6*, 100039. [CrossRef]
71. Cao, Z.G.; Yu, G.; Chen, Y.S.; Cao, Q.M.; Fiedler, H.; Deng, S.B.; Huang, J.; Wang, B. Particle size: A missing factor in risk assessment of human exposure to toxic chemicals in settled indoor dust. *Environ. Int.* **2012**, *49*, 24–30. [CrossRef]
72. Mercier, F.; Glorennec, P.; Thomas, O.; Bot, B. Le Organic contamination of settled house dust, a review for exposure assessment purposes. *Environ. Sci. Technol.* **2011**, *45*, 6716–6727. [CrossRef]
73. Maggi, F.; Tang, F.H.M.; la Cecilia, D.; McBratney, A. PEST-CHEMGRIDS, global gridded maps of the top 20 crop-specific pesticide application rates from 2015 to 2025. *Sci. Data* **2019**, *6*, 170. [CrossRef]
74. Jepson, P.C.; Murray, K.; Bach, O.; Bonilla, M.A.; Neumeister, L. Selection of pesticides to reduce human and environmental health risks: A global guideline and minimum pesticides list. *Lancet Planet. Health* **2020**, *4*, e56–e63. [CrossRef]
75. U.S. Environmental Protection Agency (EPA). *Exposure Factors Handbook: 2011 Edition*; EPA/600/R-09/052F; U.S. Environmental Protection Agency (EPA): Washington, DC, USA,, 2011.
76. Raffy, G.; Mercier, F.; Glorennec, P.; Mandin, C.; Le Bot, B. Oral bioaccessibility of semi-volatile organic compounds (SVOCs) in settled dust: A review of measurement methods, data and influencing factors. *J. Hazard. Mater.* **2018**, *352*, 215–227. [CrossRef] [PubMed]
77. Besis, A.; Botsaropoulou, E.; Balla, D.; Voutsa, D.; Samara, C. Toxic organic pollutants in Greek house dust: Implications for human exposure and health risk. *Chemosphere* **2021**, *284*, 131318. [CrossRef] [PubMed]
78. Lewis, K.A.; Tzilivakis, J.; Warner, D.J.; Green, A. An international database for pesticide risk assessments and management. *Hum. Ecol. Risk Assess.* **2016**, *22*, 1050–1064. [CrossRef]

79. Dodson, R.E.; Camann, D.E.; Morello-Frosch, R.; Brody, J.G.; Rudel, R.A. Semivolatile organic compounds in homes: Strategies for efficient and systematic exposure measurement based on empirical and theoretical factors. *Environ. Sci. Technol.* **2015**, *49*, 113–122. [CrossRef]
80. Coronado, G.D.; Holte, S.; Vigoren, E.; Griffith, W.C.; Barr, D.B.; Faustman, E.; Thompson, B. Organophosphate pesticide exposure and residential proximity to nearby fields: Evidence for the drift pathway. *J. Occup. Environ. Med.* **2011**, *53*, 884–891. [CrossRef]
81. Simaremare, S.R.S.; Hung, C.C.; Yu, T.H.; Hsieh, C.J.; Yiin, L.M. Association between pesticides in house dust and residential proximity to farmland in a rural region of taiwan. *Toxics* **2021**, *9*, 180. [CrossRef]
82. Motsoeneng, P.M.; Dalvie, M.A. Relationship between urinary pesticide residue levels and neurotoxic symptoms among women on farms in the Western Cape, South Africa. *Int. J. Environ. Res. Public Health* **2015**, *12*, 6281–6299. [CrossRef]
83. Fenske, R.A.; Lu, C.; Barr, D.; Needham, L. Children's Exposure to Chlorpyrifos and Parathion in an Agricultural Community in Central Washington State. *Environ. Health Perspect.* **2002**, *110*, 549–553. [CrossRef]
84. Waheed, S.; Halsall, C.; Sweetman, A.J.; Jones, K.C.; Malik, R.N. Pesticides contaminated dust exposure, risk diagnosis and exposure markers in occupational and residential settings of Lahore, Pakistan. *Environ. Toxicol. Pharmacol.* **2017**, *56*, 375–382. [CrossRef]
85. UNEP Stockholm Convention. Available online: http://chm.pops.int (accessed on 31 August 2022).
86. Balmer, J.E.; Morris, A.D.; Hung, H.; Jantunen, L.; Vorkamp, K.; Rigét, F.; Evans, M.; Houde, M.; Muir, D.C.G. Levels and trends of current-use pesticides (CUPs) in the arctic: An updated review, 2010–2018. *Emerg. Contam.* **2019**, *5*, 70–88. [CrossRef]
87. Colt, J.S.; Lubin, J.; Camann, D.; Davis, S.; Cerhan, J.; Severson, R.K.; Cozen, W.; Hartge, P. Comparison of pesticide levels in carpet dust and self-reported pest treatment practices in four US sites. *J. Expo. Anal. Environ. Epidemiol.* **2004**, *14*, 74–83. [CrossRef] [PubMed]
88. Julien, R.; Adamkiewicz, G.; Levy, J.I.; Bennett, D.; Nishioka, M.; Spengler, J.D. Pesticide loadings of select organophosphate and pyrethroid pesticides in urban public housing. *J. Expo. Sci. Environ. Epidemiol.* **2008**, *18*, 167–174. [CrossRef] [PubMed]
89. Wang, X.; Banks, A.P.W.; He, C.; Drage, D.S.; Gallen, C.L.; Li, Y.; Li, Q.; Thai, P.K.; Mueller, J.F. Polycyclic aromatic hydrocarbons, polychlorinated biphenyls and legacy and current pesticides in indoor environment in Australia–occurrence, sources and exposure risks. *Sci. Total Environ.* **2019**, *693*, 133588. [CrossRef] [PubMed]
90. Wei, W.; Ramalho, O.; Mandin, C. A long-term dynamic model for predicting the concentration of semivolatile organic compounds in indoor environments: Application to phthalates. *Build. Environ.* **2019**, *148*, 11–19. [CrossRef]
91. Wei, W.; Mandin, C.; Blanchard, O.; Mercier, F.; Pelletier, M.; Le Bot, B.; Glorennec, P.; Ramalho, O. Semi-volatile organic compounds in French dwellings: An estimation of concentrations in the gas phase and particulate phase from settled dust. *Sci. Total Environ.* **2019**, *650*, 2742–2750. [CrossRef]
92. Melymuk, L.; Bohlin-Nizzetto, P.; Kukučka, P.; Vojta, Š.; Kalina, J.; Čupr, P.; Klánová, J. Seasonality and indoor/outdoor relationships of flame retardants and PCBs in residential air. *Environ. Pollut.* **2016**, *218*, 392–401. [CrossRef]
93. Mackay, D.; Celsie, A.K.D.; Parnis, J.M. Kinetic Delay in Partitioning and Parallel Particle Pathways: Underappreciated Aspects of Environmental Transport. *Environ. Sci. Technol.* **2019**, *53*, 234–241. [CrossRef]
94. Hung, C.C.; Huang, F.J.; Yang, Y.Q.; Hsieh, C.J.; Tseng, C.C.; Yiin, L.M. Pesticides in indoor and outdoor residential dust: A pilot study in a rural county of Taiwan. *Environ. Sci. Pollut. Res.* **2018**, *25*, 23349–23356. [CrossRef]
95. Velázquez-Gómez, M.; Hurtado-Fernández, E.; Lacorte, S. Differential occurrence, profiles and uptake of dust contaminants in the Barcelona urban area. *Sci. Total Environ.* **2019**, *648*, 1354–1370. [CrossRef]
96. Nakagawa, L.E.; Costa, A.R.; Polatto, R.; Nascimento, C.M.d.; Papini, S. Pyrethroid concentrations and persistence following indoor application. *Environ. Toxicol. Chem.* **2017**, *36*, 2895–2898. [CrossRef] [PubMed]
97. Calabrese, E.J.; Stanek, E.J. What proportion of household dust is derived from outdoor soil? *J. Soil Contam.* **1992**, *1*, 253–263. [CrossRef]
98. Simcox, N.J.; Fenske, R.A.; Wolz, S.A.; Lee, I.-C.; Kalman, D.A. Pesticides in Household Dust and Soil: Exposure Pathways for Children of Agricultural Families. *Environ. Health Perspect.* **1995**, *103*, 1126–1134. [CrossRef] [PubMed]
99. Ward, M.H.; Lubin, J.; Giglierano, J.; Colt, J.S.; Wolter, C.; Bekiroglu, N.; Camann, D.; Hartge, P.; Nuckols, J.R. Proximity to crops and residential to agricultural herbicides in Iowa. *Environ. Health Perspect.* **2006**, *114*, 893–897. [CrossRef] [PubMed]
100. Branch, R.; Jacqz, E. Is carbaryl as safe as its reputation? *Am. J. Med.* **1986**, *81*, 1124–1125.
101. Rosas, L.G.; Eskenazi, B. Pesticides and child neurodevelopment. *Curr. Opin. Pediatr.* **2008**, *20*, 191–197. [CrossRef]
102. van Wendel de Joode, B.; Mora, A.M.; Lindh, C.H.; Hernández-Bonilla, D.; Córdoba, L.; Wesseling, C.; Hoppin, J.A.; Mergler, D. Pesticide exposure and neurodevelopment in children aged 6–9 years from Talamanca, Costa Rica. *Cortex* **2016**, *85*, 137–150. [CrossRef]
103. Clayton, C.A.; Pellizzari, E.D.; Whitmore, R.W.; Quackenboss, J.J.; Adgate, J.; Sefton, K. Distributions, associations, and partial ag-gregate exposure of pesticides and polynuclear aromatic hydrocarbons in the Minnesota Children's Pesticide Exposure Study (MNCPES). *J. Expo. Anal. Environ. Epidemiol.* **2003**, *13*, 100–111. [CrossRef]
104. Lu, C.; Toepel, K.; Irish, R.; Fenske, R.A.; Barr, D.B.; Bravo, R. Organic diets significantly lower children's dietary exposure to organophosphorus pesticides. *Environ. Health Perspect.* **2006**, *114*, 260–263. [CrossRef]
105. Wilson, N.K.; Chuang, J.C.; Lyu, C.; Menton, R.; Morgan, M.K. Aggregate exposures of nine preschool children to persistent organic pollutants at day care and at home. *J. Expo. Anal. Environ. Epidemiol.* **2003**, *13*, 187–202. [CrossRef]

106. Fenner, K.; Canonica, S.; Wackett, L.P.; Elsner, M. Evaluating pesticide degradation in the environment: Blind spots and emerging opportunities. *Science* **2013**, *341*, 752–758. [CrossRef] [PubMed]
107. Jílková, S.; Melymuk, L.; Vojta, Š.; Vykoukalová, M.; Bohlin-Nizzetto, P.; Klánová, J. Small-scale spatial variability of flame retardants in indoor dust and implications for dust sampling. *Chemosphere* **2018**, *206*, 132–141. [CrossRef] [PubMed]
108. Wason, S.C.; Julien, R.; Perry, M.J.; Smith, T.J.; Levy, J.I. Modeling exposures to organophosphates and pyrethroids for children living in an urban low-income environment. *Environ. Res.* **2013**, *124*, 13–22. [CrossRef]
109. Goldstein, A.H.; Nazaroff, W.W.; Weschler, C.J.; Williams, J. How Do Indoor Environments Affect Air Pollution Exposure? *Environ. Sci. Technol.* **2021**, *55*, 100–108. [CrossRef] [PubMed]
110. Salthammer, T. Emerging indoor pollutants. *Int. J. Hyg. Environ. Health* **2020**, *224*. [CrossRef]
111. Zhou, Y.; Guo, J.; Wang, Z.; Zhang, B.; Sun, Z.; Yun, X.; Zhang, J. Levels and inhalation health risk of neonicotinoid insecticides in fine particulate matter (PM2.5) in urban and rural areas of China. *Environ. Int.* **2020**, *142*, 105822. [CrossRef]

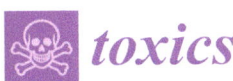

Article

Evaluation of Health Economic Loss Due to Particulate Matter Pollution in the Seoul Subway, South Korea

Prakash Thangavel [1], Kyoung Youb Kim [2], Duckshin Park [3,*] and Young-Chul Lee [1,*]

1. Department of BioNano Technology, Gachon University, 1342 Seongnam-daero, Sujeong-gu, Seongnam-si 13120, Gyeonggi-do, Republic of Korea
2. Department of Mobile IoT, Osan University, 45 Cheonghak-ro, Osan-si 18119, Gyeonggi-do, Republic of Korea
3. Korea Railroad Research Institute (KRRI), 176 Cheoldobakmulkwan-ro, Uiwang-si 16105, Gyeonggi-do, Republic of Korea

* Correspondence: dspark@krri.re.kr (D.P.); dreamdbs@gachon.ac.kr (Y.-C.L.); Tel.: +82-10-3343-2862 (D.P.); +82-31-750-8751 (Y.-C.L.); Fax: +82-31-460-5367 (D.P.); +82-31-750-4748 (Y.-C.L.)

Abstract: Evaluating an illness's economic impact is critical for developing and executing appropriate policies. South Korea has mandatory national health insurance in the form of NHIS that provides propitious conditions for assessing the national financial burden of illnesses. The purpose of our study is to provide a comprehensive assessment of the economic impact of $PM_{2.5}$ exposure in the subway and a comparative analysis of cause-specific mortality outcomes based on the prevalent health-risk assessment of the health effect endpoints (chronic obstructive pulmonary disease (COPD), asthma, and ischemic heart disease (IHD)). We used the National Health Insurance database to calculate the healthcare services provided to health-effect endpoints, with at least one primary diagnosis in 2019. Direct costs associated with health aid or medicine, treatment, and indirect costs (calculated based on the productivity loss in health effect endpoint patients, transportation, and caregivers, including morbidity and mortality costs) were both considered. The total cost for the exposed population for these endpoints was estimated to be USD 437 million per year. Medical costs were the largest component (22.08%), followed by loss of productivity and premature death (15.93%) and other costs such as transport and caregiver costs (11.46%). The total incurred costs (per 1000 persons) were accounted to be USD 0.1771 million, USD 0.42 million, and USD 0.8678 million for COPD, Asthma, and IHD, respectively. Given that the economic burden will rise as the prevalence of these diseases rises, it is vital to adopt effective preventative and management methods strategies aimed at the appropriate population.

Keywords: economic loss; subway PM exposure; health burden; long-term mortality; morbidity

1. Introduction

Exposure to pollution has short- and long-term effects on humans and poses a greater risk to public health than other forms of pollution, such as groundwater contamination or sludge contamination, because it affects more people. Particulate matter (PM) is a complex aerosolized substance produced primarily by vehicle exhausts and road dust. As a result, PM can have a wide range of particle sizes (2.5–10 μM), elemental compositions, and surface areas, producing a variety of health effects on humans [1].

With over eight million daily passengers utilizing the Seoul Metropolitan Subway, subway rail commuting is a major means of transportation in South Korea. However, subway commuters are frequently exposed to indoor $PM_{2.5}$ pollution which is generated inside the subway stations and accumulates in subway platforms, waiting rooms, and train cabins [2]. Elevated $PM_{2.5}$ concentration levels have been reported in subway platforms around the world, including in Los Angeles [3], London [4], Stockholm [5], Budapest [6], and South Korea [1]. $PM_{2.5}$ is a major air pollutant in Seoul's subway system and has been directly linked to several comorbidities in human health [7,8]. Furthermore, $PM_{2.5}$-bound metals and polycyclic aromatic hydrocarbons (PAHs) have been related to major health effects such as lung cancer and reduced immunological function [9]. Furthermore, because of their high teratogenicity (pre- and early-pregnancy $PM_{2.5}$ exposure has been linked to a higher occurrence of congenital anomalies, exposure to air pollution during pregnancy has, in particular, been linked to the development of congenital abnormalities, low birth weight, stillbirth, and newborn respiratory illnesses) and carcinogenicity [10,11]. Many countries, including the United States, China, the European Union, and India, have included benzo[a]pyrene (B[a]P) and metals in their air quality monitoring standards [12,13]. Because of the subway's intrinsic characteristics, such as its compact size, airtight atmosphere, and higher passenger density per unit area, great attention has been paid to the interior air quality in subways or subterranean metro stations. Although passengers only spend a brief time in subway stations, repeated exposure to everyday commuters, as well as short-term exposure to excessive levels of air pollutants, can result in severe or acute health impacts. Furthermore, personnel working in subterranean metro stations are exposed to high levels of air pollution for extended periods of time, which might have long-term health repercussions. Although subterranean metro stations have greatly reduced ambient air pollution, internal air quality concerns may be more serious than outside air quality concerns [14–16].

South Korean legislation requires the surveillance of varied types of air pollutants, including PM with diameters of 10 µm or less (PM_{10}) and 2.5 µm or less ($PM_{2.5}$), nitrogen dioxide (NO_2), carbon monoxide (CO), sulfur dioxide (SO_2), and ozone [17]. Particle exposure has been linked to a variety of health issues, including premature death in people with respiratory disease, fatal and non-fatal heart attacks, heart palpitations, asthma, decreased lung function, and increased respiratory symptoms like airway irritation, shortness of breath, or breathing difficulties. In addition to increased cardiovascular morbidity and mortality, recent large-population epidemiological studies have found that $PM_{2.5}$ exposure can contribute to the initiation and progression of diabetes mellitus (DM) as well as adverse birth outcomes [18–24]. Air pollution causes alteration of the airway epithelial barrier and signal transduction pathways, parenchymal damage, oxidative stress, phagocytosis impairment, inflammatory cell infiltration, dysregulated cell immunity, epigenetic changes, and autophagy [25]. Asthma prevalence, onset, symptoms, and treatment response can all be influenced by air pollution [26]. Air quality is important in the early development of asthma and as a cause of later-life asthma exacerbations. NO2 exposure throughout childhood increases the risk of getting asthma. Exposure to traffic-related air pollution during infancy has been linked to reduced lung function and long-term respiratory consequences in susceptible newborns [27]. PM exposure may produce physiologic changes in the respiratory system. PM suspensions increased cholinergic hyperresponsiveness while decreasing host defense in mice, resulting in neutrophil influx, bronchoalveolar lavage protein, and cytokine release in lung tissues. Ambient air particles may produce reactive oxygen species and inflammatory factors in alveolar macrophages and polymorphonuclear granulocytes [20], and bronchial epithelial cells. Reactive oxygen species, inflammatory factor production, and respiratory inflammation all played important roles in lung tissue destruction and the increased risk of COPD [28–30]. The amount of research addressing the processes behind the influence of air pollution on CVD has expanded dramatically over the last decade. The three most common starting mechanisms are (1) oxidative stress and inflammation, (2) autonomic nerve imbalance, and (3) direct particle translocation. These pathways may activate secondary pathways such as endothelial dysfunction, thrombotic pathways, hypothalamic-pituitary-adrenal axis (HPA) activation, and epigenomic changes. The pathways are distinct and occur at different times and locations throughout the body, but they are highly interconnected, with effects that may converge at some point to increase the risk of CVD outcomes [31–33]. In 2010, $PM_{2.5}$ was responsible for approximately 7.1% of global mortality. Ambient air pollution is widely established to have a variety of acute and long-term consequences on human health. Several epidemiological studies have found that the amount of particulate matter ($PM_{2.5}$) or NO_2 in the air is linked to daily mortality, primarily from cardiovascular and respiratory disorders [34–37]. An epidemiological study by Kim et al. 2017, found considerable deleterious consequences of pollution that endure over the long term. The study discovered that men and the elderly are the most affected, whereas children appear to recover entirely from the early shocks [38]. Kim et al. 2020 and Kim et al. 2022, in a study on the Indonesian population, present evidence of large and long-term harmful consequences of air pollution on mental health. Using a natural experiment in Indonesia, the study discovered that exposure to severe air pollution considerably increases the prevalence of depressive symptoms in both men and women, as well as the incidence of clinical depression in women, even 10 years later. The study also discovered robust substantial effects of pollution on the intensity of moderate symptoms of depression that persist over time in both sexes [39,40]. A study by Jayachandran 2009 on air pollution due to wildfire in Indonesia in late 1997 found that the air pollution led to over 15,500 child, infant, and fetal deaths. The study presented evidence of the most detrimental timing of exposure to pollution in utero that has the greatest influence on survival. Particulate matter has a significant influence on early-life mortality at levels that are common both indoors and outdoors in many poor nations [41].

In 2016, $PM_{2.5}$ was responsible for 4.09 million premature deaths, with chronic obstructive pulmonary disease (COPD), lower respiratory infections, lung cancer, and ischemic heart disease (IHD) accounting for 19.23, 15.97, 6.83, and 38.51% of fatalities, respectively. The health repercussions of $PM_{2.5}$ have a direct influence on economic activity as measured by national accounts and GDP (GDP). Researchers have calculated the economic cost of extra illness and death caused by PM_{10} and 2.5 [42–46]. Kim et al. (2017) evaluated the impact of air pollution on labor supply in the short and long run. Using the 1997 Indonesian forest fires as a natural experiment, the researchers concluded that pollution had long-term detrimental effects on hours worked. Based on their estimates, average pollution levels in 1997, labor force participation rates, and Indonesian minimum wages, a conservative value of roughly USD 10 billion was lost as a result of this pollution incident in the year 2000 alone [47]. The quantification of the impacts of air pollution is becoming an important component in policy formulation. The effects of health on the economy can be seen from the perspectives of the people and the country [48]. As a result, there are two techniques to assess the health costs associated with air pollution: the economic burden of illness assessment and the macroeconomic approach. The former is further subdivided into the human capital approach and the willingness-to-pay technique, whilst the latter is further subdivided into the macro-econometric approach and the general equilibrium approach [49,50]. Several studies link PM exposures to exacerbated chronic illnesses such as COPD and asthma and ischemic heart disease. In this study, we specifically focus on $PM_{2.5}$-associated long-term illnesses, such as ischemic heart disease, and respiratory disorders, such as asthma and COPD [33]. One of the primary goals of this research is to give a complete assessment of the economic impact of $PM_{2.5}$ exposure in the subway, as well as a comparative analysis of cause-specific death outcomes based on the widespread health-risk assessment of the health effect endpoint. The study is based on newly accessible subway $PM_{2.5}$ concentration data as well as an economic assessment of individual health-related expenditures.

2. Data and Methodology
2.1. Overview

As a prevalence-based technique that calculates the economic cost of all cases in a particular time, we computed the yearly costs related to the health impact endpoints of COPD, asthma, and IHD. The major source for cost estimates was the NHIS claims database, which contained virtually all of Korea's claim records [51,52]. A person was considered a patient if they had at least one inpatient or outpatient claim that included a diagnosis. We evaluated both direct and indirect expenses in our analyses. Direct costs were those related to diagnosis and medication, whereas indirect costs were those associated with patient and caregiver productivity loss associated with inpatient and outpatient treatment methods. All costs are approximated in USD. The entire population exposed to $PM_{2.5}$ from subway pollution was evaluated to determine the theoretical number of fatalities in the human risk assessment.

2.2. Study Area

The Beomgye subway station in Seoul, South Korea, was chosen for the study and was analyzed to determine the PM concentration and human economic loss due to $PM_{2.5}$-induced health damage. The PM levels of Beomgye subway station were obtained from the Korean Railway Research Institute (KRRI).

2.3. Data Sources

$PM_{10\&2.5}$ levels of Beomgye station for the period January to March 2019 were obtained from the KRRI. The average or mean concentration of PM_{10}, $PM_{2.5}$, and the average number of passengers have been obtained from the KRRI. The 2019 GDP per capita data and total GDP and mortality due to respiratory and circulatory system data were obtained from the Korean Statistical Information Service (KOSIS) [53,54].

Daily PM levels of the platform, waiting room, and train cabin, and the number of passengers boarding and getting off the train at Beomgye station, Seoul, South Korea were obtained from the KRRI from January to March 2019 (Table 1). The 24 h data were averaged for all values. The variations in PM_{10} and $PM_{2.5}$ concentrations on the platform and the waiting room are shown in Figure 1.

Table 1. Average concentrations of PM_{10} and $PM_{2.5}$ and average number of patients traveled.

Platform µg/m³		Waiting Room µg/m³		Cabin µg/m³		Avg. No. of People Travelling per Day	
PM_{10}	$PM_{2.5}$	PM_{10}	$PM_{2.5}$	PM_{10}	$PM_{2.5}$	Boarding	Alighting
42.18	21.00	8.74	5.01	20.69	13.13	5478	5364
83.90	23.72	56.14	18.17	32.64	24.40	8331.6	8388
92.04	22.46	72.84	21.17	49.82	41.05	7306.2	7089
72.70	22.38	49.9	14.23	34.383	26.19	7038.6	6947

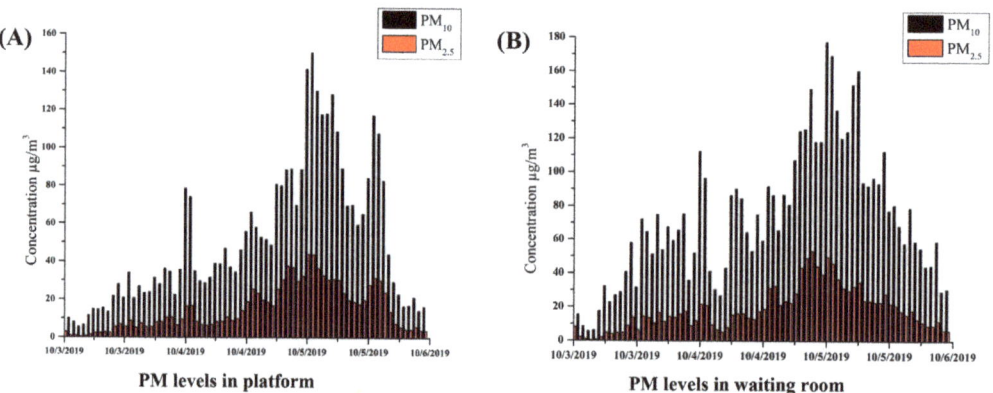

Figure 1. (**A**) PM_{10} and $PM_{2.5}$ concentrations on the platform, (**B**) PM_{10} and $PM_{2.5}$ concentrations in the waiting room.

2.4. Exposed Population

Given that air quality is highly connected to the degree of modernization of the transportation system, everyday commuters who utilize the subway are the most likely population exposed to air pollution. As a result, conventional epidemiology considers commuters to be the primary population susceptible to $PM_{2.5}$.

The cabin data of passengers boarding and getting off trains and the data on the total number of people and morbidity and mortality costs (sourced from NHIS) [54–56] of each health effect endpoint passengers developing or at risk of $PM_{2.5}$-associated health risks reveal that an average of 30% of passengers will develop $PM_{2.5}$-associated health problems (Table 2). We further normalized to 30% (1000 commuters, 166.6 commuters in a cabin) based on the obtained values of $PM_{2.5}$ concentration and inhaled dose in a cabin linked with $PM_{2.5}$-associated comorbidities, assuming that this 30% of commuters are at risk of developing PM-associated comorbidities.

Table 2. Burden of $PM_{2.5}$ per 1000 persons for each health effect endpoint.

Disease	Risk/Prevalence/Development of a Disease per 1000 Patients (Morbidity)	Mortality-Associated Costs (Million USD) per 1000 Persons	Average Median $PM_{2.5}$ Exposure Concentration (µg)
COPD	373	9.3	1.05
Asthma	44	1.1	1.03
IHD	19	0.4	1.07

The GDP per capita, average per capita disposable income, and mortality due to respiratory and circulatory system diseases in Korea in 2019 were sourced from KOSIS and NHIS and were found to be USD 31,846.2, USD 21,882, 36,655, and 60,252, respectively. Moreover, the highest concentrations of PM_{10} and $PM_{2.5}$ were much more than the minimum exposure concentration. The concentrations of PM observed in the subway platforms exceeded the WHO-defined daily values of 50 and 35 µg/m³ for PM_{10} and $PM_{2.5}$ [55,56] (Figure 2).

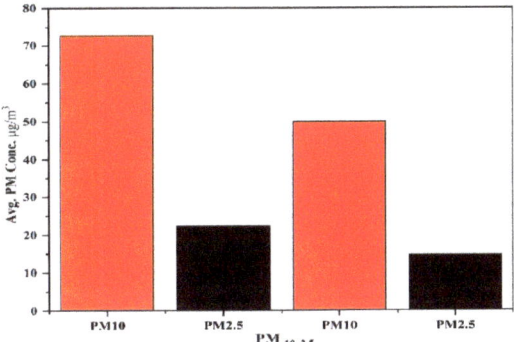

Figure 2. Average concentrations of PM_{10} and $PM_{2.5}$ on the platform and in the waiting room (the two bars on the left represent the values observed in the subway PM and the two bars on the right represent the value defined by WHO.

2.5. Exposure Route

The human body can be exposed to $PM_{2.5}$ in two ways: through inhalation and eating. $PM_{2.5}$ can directly harm human health by allowing fine particles from the atmosphere to enter the human body through the respiratory tract and travel through the bronchi, disrupting gas exchange in the lungs. Fine dust in the environment can also fall into or settle on food or drink, affecting human health when consumed. To estimate the inhalational or ingested dose of $PM_{2.5}$, we adopted an equation from a study by Manojkumar et al., 2021 [55].

$$ID = C \times MV \times T \tag{1}$$

where ID is the Inhaled dose per trip (μg), C is the exposure concentration (μg/m^3), MV is minute ventilation (m^3 min^{-1}), and T is the trip duration (min).

The equation has been widely adopted in previous studies [56–58]. In this study, the per-minute ventilation rates recommended by the United States Environmental Protection Agency's Exposure Factors Handbook, EPA 2011 [59,60] were used and the per-minute ventilation rate for active commuters was set as 0.015 m^3 min^{-1}. Earlier studies adopted similar values for estimating inhaled doses [61,62]. The data are provided in Table 3.

Table 3. Average dose inhaled per trip at different time intervals.

Average Time Spent by a Commuter in the Subway (min)	30	60	90
Average exposure concentration $PM_{2.5}$ (μg/m^3)	16.22	16.22	16.22
Average minute ventilation rate by commuter (m^3 min^{-1})	0.015	0.015	0.015
Inhaled dose per trip (μg) $PM_{2.5}$	7.299	14.598	21.895

2.6. Health-Effect Endpoint

It has been proven that $PM_{2.5}$ can cause severe health risks such as damage to the lungs, respiratory system, and cardiovascular system, increased rates of premature death, and increased risks of cancers, chronic bronchitis, emphysema, and asthma. Based on this causation, we evaluated the economic loss due to $PM_{2.5}$ on the following health effect endpoints:

- COPD (Chronic Obstructive Pulmonary Disease).
- Asthma.
- Cardiovascular diseases.

3. Health Economic Accounting

3.1. Poisson Regression Model

The likelihood of any endpoint for health effects in the context of the overall population is low, making them low-likelihood events. The actual distribution of endpoints is consistent with the Poisson distribution statistics as a time-series model. The relative risk model of Poisson regression is currently used in health-risk assessments of $PM_{2.5}$ pollution. This works by quantifying the health effect caused by increases in $PM_{2.5}$ concentration by calculating the corresponding health loss. We employed the Poisson regression model since it has been widely adopted by other studies [57].

The formula is as follows:

$$E = \exp[\beta(C - C_0)] E_0 \tag{2}$$

$$\Delta E = E - E_0 \tag{3}$$

where E is the population health effect under the actual concentration of $PM_{2.5}$, E_0 is the population health effect under the $PM_{2.5}$ threshold concentration, β is the exposure-response relationship coefficient of a health-effect endpoint, C is the mean $PM_{2.5}$ concentration (Mean concentration of platform and waiting room 48.5 μg/m^3), and C_0 is the threshold concentration of $PM_{2.5}$ (35 μg/m^3) [53,63]. ΔE is the excess health effect—that is, the difference in health effects between the mean concentration and the threshold concentration.

3.2. Measurement of Direct and Indirect Cost

3.2.1. Direct Cost

The formal expenses for the diagnosis and treatment of asthma in the official health system were described as direct medical costs and included the costs for inpatient and outpatient care, as well as the costs for any prescription. The care costs assumed by the insurance company were calculated based on the NHIS claims records and KOSIS statistics [63–66].

3.2.2. Indirect Cost

In general, indirect costs are described as "loss of productivity owing to discontinuation or reduction in productivity due to sickness or death" [59]. In this study, indirect costs were assessed using the human capital method, which assesses human output in terms of market gains and includes sickness costs, death costs, and caregiver time costs (average daily caregiver cost). In the case of patients with severe asthma, the indirect cost was computed by multiplying the number of visits by age and gender, particular average daily income, and employment rates for the age group 20 to 69 years. However, Loss of productivity at work was not considered since the human capital approach is used. Instead, we calculated the total loss of productivity based on (mortality and morbidity) in terms of market gains (GDP). Mortality costs, defined as the loss of potential future income up to the age of 69 due to early death, were calculated by multiplying the amount of associated health effect endpoint by the amount of related health effect endpoint. Deaths in 2019 with gender- and age-specific average yearly earnings and employment rates for each death were used to calculate the present value of future admissions using a 3% discount rate. The expenses of caregiving time were calculated using literature studies and NHIS claims. In Korea, a family member, generally a middle-aged woman, provides practically all care for each health effect endpoint. To measure both direct and indirect costs, we employed the scheme of Lee et al., 2011 [63].

The scheme for estimating indirect costs was as follows:

- Morbidity costs
- Mortality costs
- Caregivers' time costs
- Methods used to determine the health care costs are given in Table 4

Table 4. Methods used to determine health care costs.

Health Care Costs	Outpatient	Inpatient	Formula
Direct medical costs	✓	✓	The NHIS database was used to get hospital expenses covered by co-payment plans in Korea for inpatients and outpatient visits, including Emergency Department visits.
Nonmedical costs Transportation	✓	✓	Total transportation expenses were determined by multiplying transportation costs by the number of outpatient visits and hospitalizations based on NHIS claims for each kind of hospital treatment.
Caregiving		✓	The overall caregiving expenses were estimated by dividing the average daily caregiving cost by the total days of hospital admissions obtained from the NHIS.
Indirect costs	✓	✓	Using the human capital method, productivity costs for patients under 70 and over 60 years old were assessed.

Morbidity Costs

$$= \sum_j \{(I_{ij} + 1/3 O_{ij})\} D_{ij} E_{ij} \quad (4)$$

where I is the age, j is the gender, I is the total number of inpatient days, O is the number of outpatient visits, D is the average daily earnings, and E is the employment rate.

Mortality Costs

$$= \sum_i \sum_j \sum_t \left[\frac{F_{ij} r_{ij}^{t+k} E_{ij}}{(1+r)^k} \right] \quad (5)$$

where I is the age, j is the gender, t is the age of death, F is the number of deaths, γ is the average yearly productivity at t k (The exponent "$t + k$ denotes the adjusted years of productivity loss due to premature death before the age of 70), E is the employment rate, k is the number of years after death until the age of 70 (average years of life lost before the age of 70), and r is the discount rate. For each health effect endpoint, the number of years of life lost correlates with productivity loss.

Caregivers' Time Costs

$$\frac{\sum_i \sum_j (N_{ij} \times IC)}{E_j \sum_{i \geq 10} (O_{ij} \times IC) 1/3} \quad (6)$$

where I is the age, j is the gender, N_{ij} is the number of days spent in the hospital, O_{ij} is the number of outpatient visits, and IC is the average daily informal care expenditures. The caregiving expenses were determined by dividing the average daily caregiving cost by the total days of hospital admissions obtained from the NHIS [42].

4. Results and Discussion

The changes in PM concentrations are characterized by the tallest column in Figure 1. The highest concentrations of PM_{10} and $PM_{2.5}$ on the platform and in the waiting room were 150.38 and 43.24 µg/m^3, and 177.27 and 53.24 µg/m^3, respectively, and the lowest were 20.34 and 4.32 µg/m^3, and 5.55 and 0.34 µg/m^3, respectively (Figure 1A,B). The concentrations also peaked from midday to midnight, indicating that temperature, ventilation, and seasonal variation might play a major role in PM concentrations inside the subway. As shown in Table 3, the inhaled doses estimated using the above formula were 7.2, 14.5, and 21.8 µg for $PM_{2.5}$ for 30, 60, and 90 min trips, respectively. Total costs were calculated according to each component of direct and indirect costs. We applied the Poisson regression model to estimate the risk of each health effect endpoint. To calculate a per capita cost, the anticipated total expenditures were divided by the number of commuters at risk of acquiring $PM_{2.5}$ comorbidities for each health consequence endpoint. The data collected were then statistically analyzed. The economic cost of each health effect endpoint was measured using Equations (1)–(6). Using mortality and morbidity estimations and the economic costs for each health effect endpoint, we calculated the total economic loss for the exposed population developing $PM_{2.5}$-related health effects (Table 5).

Table 5. Direct and indirect costs of each disease.

Disease	Direct Cost (Million USD; per 1000 Persons)	Indirect Cost (Million USD; per 1000 Persons)	Total Cost (Million USD; per 1000 Persons)
COPD	0.10591	0.0718	0.17771
ASTHMA	0.55	0.07	0.42
IHD	0.57478	0.294	0.86878

In this study, we analyzed the $PM_{2.5}$ levels over a period of 3 months (January-March) in Beomgye station, Seoul, Korea. The $PM_{2.5}$ levels found in the subway, on the platform, and in the waiting room exceed the defined values set by WHO, which in turn poses a great risk to the commuters and the operators. People with chronic disease of the lung, COPD, and asthma, and the aged are at higher risk of developing further complications. On our comprehensive health risk assessment of each health effect endpoint, we estimated that 373 (COPD), 44 (Asthma), and 19 (IHD) commuters (per trip in a train) were at risk of developing $PM_{2.5}$-mediated comorbidities for each health effect endpoint. The total cost incurred by these comorbidities was estimated to be USD 437 million annually (Table 5). Medical costs were the largest component (22.08%), followed by lost productivity and premature deaths (15.93%) and nonmedical costs such as transportation and caregiver costs (11.46%) (Table 6). The total costs incurred by health effect endpoints (per 1000 persons) were estimated to be USD 0.1771 million (COPD; Table 6), USD 0.42 million (Asthma; Table 6), and USD 0.8678 million (IHD; Table 6). The finding that medical charges (direct costs) accounted for the majority of the overall cost suggests that $PM_{2.5}$-induced health consequences are burdensome chronic conditions that need extensive outpatient monitoring. This pattern, which has been observed in other developed nations, might be considered an indirect indicator of a health consequence endpoint being adequately managed at the outpatient level and not progressing to the emergency or hospitalization level [67]. The lost productivity, premature deaths, and transportation and caregiver cost ranked second due to subjective assumptions, such as children needing medical attention for $PM_{2.5}$-induced health effects, as other studies have established [68,69]. The heaviest economic burden is for commuters aged above 60 because of their high mortality and morbidity and this burden is mainly driven by the high proportion of hospitalization and inpatient treatment. Nonetheless, to evaluate the true indirect costs, productivity loss in any form must be considered [70–73]. As a result, the true socioeconomic burden in South Korea, including the low productivity due to health effect endpoints, will be much higher than our estimates. In addition, a previous study determined that workplace inactivity accounted for 50% of total productivity losses; as this factor was considered based on the KOSIS statistics, we have not considered actual productivity loss at the workplace in our study, and the real socioeconomic costs of each health endpoint may be more substantial than those reported in this study. Our findings indicated that the health burden and economic losses associated with short-term air pollution exposure are significant [74]. To date, only a few studies on the health burden caused by short-term exposure to air pollutants have been conducted in China, Korea, and other countries. The exposure-response coefficients of short-term exposure to air pollutants are likely to be much lower than those of long-term exposure [4,75,76].

Table 6. Economic loss due to COPD, asthma, and IHD.

Category	Costs (Million USD; per 1000 Persons)					
	COPD	Contribution (%)	Asthma	Contribution (%)	IHD	Contribution (%)
Direct						
Medical						
Formal (Treatment)	0.029	16.6	0.2	54.8	0.302	34.76
Informal (Medical Equipment)	0.00631	3.5	0.02	7.4	0.16	18.41
Non-Medical						
Transportation	0.0006	0.3	0.08	2.4	0.07	8.066
Nursing	0.070	39	0.05	14.1	0.04278	4.92
Indirect						3.33
Loss of Work	0.0588	32.7	0.04	12.4	0.029	30.5
Premature deaths	0.013	7.7	0.03	9	0.265	100
Total	0.17771	100	0.42	100	0.86878	

In recent years, $PM_{2.5}$ has been widely regarded as the primary air pollutant with the greatest health impact. Several studies have reported that the concentrations of $PM_{2.5}$ inside trains are generally lower than in subway stations, which suggests that time spent on the platform and in the waiting room can be a better predictor of personal exposure [76,77]. However, commuters who travel every day are repeatedly exposed, which can lead to chronic health effects. Nonetheless, even short periods spent in underground environments can exacerbate health risks for vulnerable groups such as children, the elderly, and individuals with pre-existing health conditions. Train operators and other employees who spend many hours in the subway each day are more likely to be exposed to $PM_{2.5}$ levels than the public and are thus at a potentially greater health risk.

A number of studies have revealed that high traffic counts are connected with an increased incidence of respiratory disease [78]. One large British assessment on traffic-related pollution discovered a risk gradient that rose significantly with day-to-day exposure [79]. A large study in southern California found an increased incidence of asthma and wheezing among children who commute on a daily basis [80]. Another study, conducted by Jerrett et al. using data from the same southern California cohort, found a connection between the incidence of asthma and other illnesses and exposure to traffic-related pollution [81]. Much remains unknown about which contaminants cause the majority of respiratory impacts and which signaling pathways are important for exacerbating chronic respiratory disorders. The processes underlying the induction of respiratory aggravation and ischemic heart disease by subway particles require further exploration, as do the interactions of coarse subway particles with major pollutants in provoking oncogenesis.

5. Limitations and Conclusions

The limitation of our approach to study was that work engagement was not taken into account when evaluating indirect costs, and because we utilized GDP per capita, the loss of work engagement cannot be depended upon. Cost-of-illness studies, including this one, fail to account for job involvement because existing report sets do not gather this information on a regular basis; instead, such information is often collected through self-reporting [82]. Implied speculations regarding lost production, productive time, and caretaker qualities may compromise the accuracy of projected indirect costs. The methodology for evaluating indirect costs in cost-of-illness research studies is organically based on various assumptions about human and productivity values; it is crucial to compare research with similar assumptions and methodologies [83]. The findings of this study come from a relatively small proportion of the population (1000); this may have led to an underestimation of outcomes. Another limitation of this study is that there is disagreement over the validity of NHIS claims data in terms of diagnostic accuracy. According to one research, only 70% of discharged diagnoses in NHIS claims data were concordant with medical records [84,85]. By using the direct costs of inpatient and outpatient care and indirect costs composed of morbidity and mortality costs based on NHIS claims and KOSIS, the outcomes may vary from those of other similar studies [86,87].

Furthermore, the results provided here are based on $PM_{2.5}$, but no correlation is made between more toxic particles, such as those with high levels of sorbed toxic components. The study ignores the effects of exposure to ultrafine particles, which are implicated in numerous diseases, but for which measurements are lacking.

Altogether, the study found that the economic burden of COPD, Asthma, and IHD caused by commuter subway exposure to $PM_{2.5}$ is large, with significant shares of overall expenditures ascribed to direct and indirect expenses. Given that the burden would increase in tandem with increases in these illnesses, effective preventive and management measures targeting the right population are necessary.

Author Contributions: All authors made significant contributions to the study's conception and design. P.T. and Y.-C.L.; prepared the materials, collected the data, and analyzed it. P.T. and Y.-C.L.; did formal and statistical analyses. P.T., Y.-C.L. and K.Y.K.; wrote the original draft of the manuscript. Y.-C.L. and D.P.; thoroughly reviewed the book for essential intellectual substance. The manuscript version for publication has been approved by all authors. The final manuscript was reviewed and approved by all writers. All authors have read and agreed to the published version of the manuscript.

Funding: This research was funded by a grant from the Ministry of Land Infrastructure and Transport of the Republic of Korea (21QPPW-B152306-03) and the Basic Science Research Capacity Enhancement Project through a Korea Basic Science Institute (National Research Facilities and Equipment Center) grant funded by the Ministry of Education of the Republic of Korea (2019R1A6C1010016).

Institutional Review Board Statement: Not applicable.

Informed Consent Statement: Not applicable.

Data Availability Statement: Not applicable.

Conflicts of Interest: The authors state that they have no financial or non-financial conflict of interest to report.

References

1. Lee, Y.; Yang, J.; Lim, Y.; Kim, C. Economic damage cost of premature death due to fine particulate matter in Seoul, Korea. *Environ. Sci. Pollut. Res.* **2021**, *28*, 51702–51713. [CrossRef] [PubMed]
2. Kwon, S.B.; Jeong, W.; Park, D.; Kim, K.T.; Cho, K.H. A multivariate study for characterizing particulate matter (PM_{10}, $PM_{2.5}$, and PM1) in Seoul metropolitan subway stations, Korea. *J. Hazard. Mater.* **2015**, *297*, 295–303. [PubMed]
3. Kam, W.; Cheung, K.; Daher, N.; Sioutas, C. Particulate matter (PM) concentrations in underground and ground-level rail systems of the Los Angeles Metro. *Atmos. Environ.* **2011**, *45*, 1506–1516.
4. Seaton, A.; Cherrie, J.; Dennekamp, M.; Donaldson, K.; Hurley, J.F.; Tran, C.L. The London Underground: Dust and hazards to health. *Occup. Environ. Med.* **2005**, *62*, 355–362. [CrossRef] [PubMed]
5. Johansson, C.; Johansson, P.Å. Particulate matter in the underground of Stockholm. *Atmos. Environ.* **2003**, *37*, 3–9.
6. Salma, I.; Pósfai, M.; Kovács, K.; Kuzmann, E.; Homonnay, Z.; Posta, J. Properties and sources of individual particles and some chemical species in the aerosol of a metropolitan underground railway station. *Atmos. Environ.* **2009**, *43*, 3460–3466.
7. Chuang, K.J.; Yan, Y.H.; Chiu, S.Y.; Cheng, T.J. Long-term air pollution exposure and risk factors for cardiovascular diseases among the elderly in Taiwan. *Occup. Environ. Med.* **2011**, *68*, 64–68.
8. Shah, A.S.; Langrish, J.P.; Nair, H.; McAllister, D.A.; Hunter, A.L.; Donaldson, K.; Newby, D.E.; Mills, N.L. Global association of air pollution and heart failure: A systematic review and meta-analysis. *Lancet* **2013**, *382*, 1039–1048.
9. Behera, D.; Balamugesh, T. Lung cancer in India. *Indian J. Chest Dis. Allied Sci.* **2004**, *46*, 269–281.
10. Koo, E.J.; Bae, J.G.; Kim, E.J.; Cho, Y.H. Correlation between Exposure to Fine Particulate Matter ($PM_{2.5}$) during Pregnancy and Congenital Anomalies: Its Surgical Perspectives. *J. Korean Med. Sci.* **2021**, *36*, e236.
11. Seeni, I.; Ha, S.; Nobles, C.; Liu, D.; Sherman, S.; Mendola, P. Air pollution exposure during pregnancy: Maternal asthma and neonatal respiratory outcomes. *Ann. Epidemiol.* **2018**, *28*, 612–618. [CrossRef] [PubMed]
12. Ravindra, K.; Sokhi, R.; Van Grieken, R. Atmospheric polycyclic aromatic hydrocarbons: Source attribution, emission factors and regulation. *Atmos. Environ.* **2008**, *42*, 2895–2921.
13. Sin, D.W.; Wong, Y.C.; Choi, Y.Y.; Lam, C.H.; Louie, P.K. Distribution of polycyclic aromatic hydrocarbons in the atmosphere of Hong Kong. *J. Environ. Monit.* **2003**, *5*, 989–996. [CrossRef] [PubMed]
14. Passi, A.; Nagendra, S.S.; Maiya, M.P. Characteristics of indoor air quality in underground metro stations: A critical review. *Build. Environ.* **2021**, *198*, 107907.
15. Carrer, P.; Wolkoff, P. Assessment of indoor air quality problems in office-like environments: Role of occupational health services. *Int. J. Environ. Res. Public Health* **2018**, *15*, 741. [PubMed]
16. Bernstein, J.A.; Alexis, N.; Bacchus, H.; Bernstein, I.L.; Fritz, P.; Horner, E.; Li, N.; Mason, S.; Nel, A.; Oullette, J.; et al. The health effects of non-industrial indoor air pollution. *J. Allergy Clin. Immunol.* **2008**, *121*, 585–591. [CrossRef] [PubMed]
17. Park, W.M.; Park, D.U.; Hwang, S.H. Factors affecting ambient endotoxin and particulate matter concentrations around air vents of subway sta-tions in South Korea. *Chemosphere* **2018**, *205*, 45–51. [CrossRef]
18. Atkinson, R.W.; Fuller, G.W.; Anderson, H.R.; Harrison, R.M.; Armstrong, B. Urban ambient particle metrics and health: A time-series analysis. *Epidemiology* **2010**, *21*, 501–511.
19. Cadelis, G.; Tourres, R.; Molinie, J. Short-term effects of the particulate pollutants contained in Saharan dust on the visits of children to the emergency department due to asthmatic conditions in Guadeloupe (French Archipelago of the Caribbean). *PLoS ONE* **2014**, *9*, e91136. [CrossRef]
20. Correia, A.W.; Pope, C.A., III; Dockery, D.W.; Wang, Y.; Ezzati, M.; Dominici, F. The effect of air pollution control on life expectancy in the United States: An analysis of 545 US counties for the period 2000 to 2007. *Epidemiology* **2013**, *24*, 23.
21. Fang, Y.; Naik, V.; Horowitz, L.W.; Mauzerall, D.L. Air pollution and associated human mortality: The role of air pollutant emissions, climate change and methane concentration increases from the preindustrial period to present. *Atmos. Chem. Phys.* **2013**, *13*, 1377–1394.
22. Meister, K.; Johansson, C.; Forsberg, B. Estimated short-term effects of coarse particles on daily mortality in Stockholm, Sweden. *Environ. Health Perspect.* **2012**, *120*, 431–436. [CrossRef]
23. Ting, G.; Guoxing, L.; Meimei, X.; Xuying, W.; Fengchao, L.; Qiang, Z.; Xiaochuan, P. Evaluation of atmospheric $PM_{2.5}$ health economic loss based on willingness to pay. *J. Environ. Health* **2015**, *32*, 697–700.
24. Zhao, X.; Yu, X.; Wang, Y.; Fan, C. Economic evaluation of health losses from air pollution in Beijing, China. *Environ. Sci. Pollut. Res.* **2016**, *23*, 11716–11728. [CrossRef] [PubMed]
25. Jiang, X.Q.; Mei, X.D.; Feng, D. Air pollution and chronic airway diseases: What should people know and do? *J. Thorac. Dis.* **2016**, *8*, E31.
26. Zheng, T.; Niu, S.; Lu, B.; Fan, X.E.; Sun, F.; Wang, J.; Zhang, Y.; Zhang, B.; Owens, P.; Hao, L.; et al. Childhood asthma in Beijing, China: A population-based case-control study. *Am. J. Epidemiol.* **2002**, *156*, 977–983.
27. Liu, F.; Zhao, Y.; Liu, Y.Q.; Liu, Y.; Sun, J.; Huang, M.M.; Liu, Y.; Dong, G.H. Asthma and asthma related symptoms in 23,326 Chinese children in relation to indoor and outdoor environmental factors: The Seven Northeastern Cities (SNEC) Study. *Sci. Total Environ.* **2014**, *497*, 10–17.

28. Song, Q.; Christiani, D.C.; Wang, X.; Ren, J. The global contribution of outdoor air pollution to the incidence, prevalence, mortality and hospital admission for chronic obstructive pulmonary disease: A systematic review and meta-analysis. *Int. J. Environ. Res. Public Health* **2014**, *11*, 11822–11832.
29. Zhou, Y.; Zou, Y.; Li, X.; Chen, S.; Zhao, Z.; He, F.; Zou, W.; Luo, Q.; Li, W.; Pan, Y.; et al. Lung function and incidence of chronic obstructive pulmonary disease after improved cooking fuels and kitchen ventilation: A 9-year prospective cohort study. *PLoS Med.* **2014**, *11*, e1001621. [CrossRef]
30. Hwang, Y.I. Reducing chronic obstructive pulmonary disease mortality in Korea: Early diagnosis matters. *Korean J. Intern. Med.* **2019**, *34*, 1212. [CrossRef]
31. Hamanaka, R.B.; Mutlu, G.M. Particulate matter air pollution: Effects on the cardiovascular system. *Front. Endocrinol.* **2018**, *9*, 680. [CrossRef] [PubMed]
32. Wold, L.E.; Ying, Z.; Hutchinson, K.R.; Velten, M.; Gorr, M.W.; Velten, C.; Youtz, D.J.; Wang, A.; Lucchesi, P.A.; Sun, Q.; et al. Cardiovascular remodeling in response to long-term exposure to fine particulate matter air pollution. *Circ. Heart Fail.* **2012**, *5*, 452–461. [CrossRef] [PubMed]
33. Thangavel, P.; Park, D.; Lee, Y.C. Recent insights into particulate matter ($PM_{2.5}$)-mediated toxicity in humans: An overview. *Int. J. Environ. Res. Public Health* **2022**, *19*, 7511. [PubMed]
34. Alexeeff, S.E.; Liao, N.S.; Liu, X.; Van Den Eeden, S.K.; Sidney, S. Long-term $PM_{2.5}$ exposure and risks of ischemic heart disease and stroke events: Review and meta-analysis. *J. Am. Heart Assoc.* **2021**, *10*, e016890.
35. Kyung, S.Y.; Jeong, S.H. Particulate-matter related respiratory diseases. *Tuberc. Respir. Dis.* **2020**, *83*, 116. [CrossRef]
36. Liu, C.; Chen, R.; Sera, F.; Vicedo-Cabrera, A.M.; Guo, Y.; Tong, S.; Coelho, M.S.; Saldiva, P.H.; Lavigne, E.; Matus, P.; et al. Ambient particulate air pollution and daily mortality in 652 cities. *N. Engl. J. Med.* **2019**, *381*, 705–715.
37. Schikowski, T.; Mills, I.C.; Anderson, H.R.; Cohen, A.; Hansell, A.; Kauffmann, F.; Krämer, U.; Marcon, A.; Perez, L.; Sunyer, J.; et al. Ambient air pollution: A cause of COPD? *Eur. Respir. J.* **2014**, *43*, 250–263. [CrossRef]
38. Kim, Y.; Manley, J.; Radoias, V. Air pollution and long term mental health. *Atmosphere* **2020**, *11*, 1355. [CrossRef]
39. Kim, Y.; Radoias, V. Severe Air Pollution Exposure and Long-Term Health Outcomes. *Int. J. Environ. Res. Public Health* **2022**, *19*, 14019.
40. Jayachandran, S. Air quality and early-life mortality evidence from Indonesia's wildfires. *J. Hum. Resour.* **2009**, *44*, 916–954. [CrossRef]
41. Takizawa, H. Impacts of particulate air pollution on asthma: Current understanding and future perspectives. *Recent Pat. Inflamm. Allergy Drug Discov.* **2015**, *9*, 128–135. [CrossRef] [PubMed]
42. Hanna, R.; Oliva, P. The effect of pollution on labor supply: Evidence from a natural experiment in Mexico City. *J. Public Econ.* **2015**, *122*, 68–79.
43. Lanzi, E.; Dellink, R.; Chateau, J. The sectoral and regional economic consequences of outdoor air pollution to 2060. *Energy Econ.* **2018**, *71*, 89–113. [CrossRef]
44. Li, L.; Lei, Y.; Pan, D.; Yu, C.; Si, C. Economic evaluation of the air pollution effect on public health in China's 74 cities. *SpringerPlus* **2016**, *5*, 402.
45. Li, S.; Williams, G.; Guo, Y. Health benefits from improved outdoor air quality and intervention in China. *Environ. Pollut.* **2016**, *214*, 17–25.
46. Kim, Y.; Manley, J.; Radoias, V. Medium-and long-term consequences of pollution on labor supply: Evidence from Indonesia. *IZA J. Labor Econ.* **2017**, *6*, 5.
47. Wan, Y.; Yang, H.W.; Masui, T. Considerations in applying the general equilibrium approach to environmental health assessment. *Biomed. Environ. Sci.* **2005**, *18*, 356.
48. Wong, C.M.; Lai, H.K.; Tsang, H.; Thach, T.Q.; Thomas, G.N.; Lam, K.B.; Chan, K.P.; Yang, L.; Lau, A.K.; Ayres, J.G.; et al. Satellite-based estimates of long-term exposure to fine particles and association with mortality in elderly Hong Kong residents. *Environ. Health Perspect.* **2015**, *123*, 1167–1172.
49. Wan, Y.U.; Yang, H.O.; Masui, T. Air pollution-induced health impacts on the national economy of China: Demonstration of a computable general equilibrium approach. *Rev. Environ. Health* **2005**, *20*, 119–140.
50. Kang, H.Y.; Yang, K.H.; Kim, Y.N.; Moon, S.H.; Choi, W.J.; Kang, D.R.; Park, S.E. Incidence and mortality of hip fracture among the elderly population in South Korea: A population-based study using the national health insurance claims data. *BMC Public Health* **2010**, *10*, 230. [CrossRef]
51. Choi, S.; Park, J.H.; Bae, S.Y.; Kim, S.Y.; Byun, H.; Kwak, H.; Hwang, S.; Park, J.; Park, H.; Lee, K.H.; et al. Characteristics of PM_{10} levels monitored for more than a decade in subway stations in South Korea. *Aerosol Air Qual. Res.* **2019**, *19*, 2746–2756.
52. Korea Ministry of Environment (KMOE). *2018 White Paper of Environment*; Publication No. 11-1480000-000586-10; Ministry of Environment, Republic of Korea: Sejong, Republic of Korea, 2018.
53. Korean Statistical Information Service. Available online: http://www.me.go.kr/ (accessed on 16 November 2021).
54. Manojkumar, N.; Monishraj, M.; Srimuruganandam, B. Commuter exposure concentrations and inhalation doses in traffic and residential routes of Vellore city, India. *Atmos. Pollut. Res.* **2021**, *12*, 219–230.
55. Betancourt, R.M.; Galvis, B.; Balachandran, S.; Ramos-Bonilla, J.P.; Sarmiento, O.L.; Gallo-Murcia, S.M.; Contreras, Y. Exposure to fine particulate, black carbon, and particle number concentration in transportation microenvironments. *Atmos. Environ.* **2017**, *157*, 135–145.

56. Ham, W.; Vijayan, A.; Schulte, N.; Herner, J.D. Commuter exposure to $PM_{2.5}$, BC, and UFP in six common transport microenvironments in Sacramento, California. *Atmos. Environ.* **2017**, *167*, 335–345. [CrossRef]
57. Ramos, C.A.; Silva, J.R.; Faria, T.; Wolterbeek, T.H.; Almeida, S.M. Exposure assessment of a cyclist to particles and chemical elements. *Environ. Sci. Pollut. Res.* **2017**, *24*, 11879–11889.
58. Shang, Y.; Sun, Z.; Cao, J.; Wang, X.; Zhong, L.; Bi, X.; Li, H.; Liu, W.; Zhu, T.; Huang, W. Systematic review of Chinese studies of short-term expo-sure to air pollution and daily mortality. *Environ. Int.* **2013**, *54*, 100–111. [CrossRef] [PubMed]
59. US Environmental Protection Agency. *Exposure Factors Handbook 2011 Edition (Final)*; US EPA: Washington, DC, USA, 2011.
60. Toelle, B.G.; Ng, K.K.; Crisafulli, D.; Belousova, E.G.; Almqvist, C.; Webb, K.; Tovey, E.R.; Kemp, A.S.; Mellis, C.M.; Leeder, S.R.; et al. Eight-year outcomes of the childhood asthma prevention study. *J. Allergy Clin. Immunol.* **2010**, *126*, 388–389.
61. Sullivan, P.W.; Ghushchyan, V.H.; Slejko, J.F.; Belozeroff, V.; Globe, D.R.; Lin, S.L. The burden of adult asthma in the United States: Evidence from the Medical Expenditure Panel Survey. *J. Allergy Clin. Immunol.* **2011**, *127*, 363–369. [CrossRef]
62. Lee, Y.H.; Yoon, S.J.; Kim, E.J.; Kim, Y.A.; Seo, H.Y.; Oh, I.H. Economic burden of asthma in Korea. *Allergy Asthma Proc.* **2011**, *32*, 35.
63. National Health Insurance Service. Available online: https://www.nhis.or.kr/ (accessed on 16 November 2021).
64. Available online: http://kosis.kr/eng/ (accessed on 12 December 2021).
65. Available online: https://kosis.kr/statHtml/ (accessed on 10 August 2021).
66. Yu, G.; Wang, F.; Hu, J.; Liao, Y.; Liu, X. Value assessment of health losses caused by $PM_{2.5}$ in Changsha City, China. *Int. J. Environ. Res. Public Health* **2019**, *16*, 2063.
67. Arshad, S.H. Environmental control for secondary prevention of asthma. *Clin. Exp. Allergy* **2010**, *40*, 2–4. [PubMed]
68. Rachelefsky, G.S. From the page to the clinic: Implementing new National Asthma Education and Prevention Program guidelines. *Clin. Cornerstone* **2009**, *9*, 9–19. [PubMed]
69. Chen, X.; Wang, X.; Huang, J.J.; Zhang, L.W.; Song, F.J.; Mao, H.J.; Chen, K.X.; Chen, J.; Liu, Y.M.; Jiang, G.H.; et al. Nonmalignant respiratory mortality and long-term exposure to PM_{10} and SO2: A 12-year cohort study in northern China. *Environ. Pollut.* **2017**, *231*, 761–767. [CrossRef] [PubMed]
70. Chillrud, S.N.; Epstein, D.; Ross, J.M.; Sax, S.N.; Pederson, D.; Spengler, J.D.; Kinney, P.L. Elevated airborne exposures of teenagers to manganese, chromium, and iron from steel dust and New York City's subway system. *Environ. Sci. Technol.* **2004**, *38*, 732–737. [CrossRef]
71. Goel, R.; Gani, S.; Guttikunda, S.K.; Wilson, D.; Tiwari, G. On-road $PM_{2.5}$ pollution exposure in multiple transport microenvironments in Delhi. *Atmos. Environ.* **2015**, *123*, 129–138.
72. Qiu, H.; Yu, H.; Wang, L.; Zhu, X.; Chen, M.; Zhou, L.; Deng, R.; Zhang, Y.; Pu, X.; Pan, J. The burden of overall and cause-specific respiratory mor-bidity due to ambient air pollution in Sichuan Basin, China: A multi-city time-series analysis. *Environ. Res.* **2018**, *167*, 428–436. [CrossRef]
73. Aarnio, P.; Yli-Tuomi, T.; Kousa, A.; Mäkelä, T.; Hirsikko, A.; Hämeri, K.; Räisänen, M.; Hillamo, R.; Koskentalo, T.; Jantunen, M. The concentrations and composition of and exposure to fine particles ($PM_{2.5}$) in the Helsinki subway system. *Atmos. Environ.* **2005**, *39*, 5059–5066.
74. Martins, V.; Moreno, T.; Minguillón, M.C.; Amato, F.; de Miguel, E.; Capdevila, M.; Querol, X. Exposure to airborne particulate matter in the sub-way system. *Sci. Total Environ.* **2015**, *511*, 711–722.
75. Salma, I.; Weidinger, T.; Maenhaut, W. Time-resolved mass concentration, composition and sources of aerosol particles in a metropolitan under-ground railway station. *Atmos. Environ.* **2007**, *41*, 8391–8405. [CrossRef]
76. Minguillón, M.C.; Schembari, A.; Triguero-Mas, M.; de Nazelle, A.; Dadvand, P.; Figueras, F.; Salvado, J.A.; Grimalt, J.O.; Nieuwenhuijsen, M.; Querol, X. Source apportionment of indoor, outdoor and personal $PM_{2.5}$ exposure of pregnant women in Barcelona, Spain. *Atmos. Environ.* **2012**, *59*, 426–436.
77. Morris, S.E.; Sale, R.C.; Wakefield, J.C.; Falconer, S.; Elliott, P.; Boucher, B.J. Hospital admissions for asthma and chronic obstructive airways disease in east London hospitals and proximity of residence to main roads. *J. Epidemiol. Community Health* **2000**, *54*, 75–76.
78. Venn, A.J.; Lewis, S.A.; Cooper, M.; Hubbard, R.; Britton, J. Living near a main road and the risk of wheezing illness in children. *Am. J. Respir. Crit. Care Med.* **2001**, *164*, 2177–2180. [CrossRef] [PubMed]
79. McConnell, R.; Berhane, K.; Yao, L.; Jerrett, M.; Lurmann, F.; Gilliland, F.; Künzli, N.; Gauderman, J.; Avol, E.D.; Thomas, D.; et al. Traffic, susceptibility, and childhood asthma. *Environ. Health Perspect.* **2006**, *114*, 766–772. [PubMed]
80. Jerrett, M.; Shankardass, K.; Berhane, K.; Gauderman, W.J.; Künzli, N.; Avol, E.; Gilliland, F.; Lurmann, F.; Molitor, J.N.; Molitor, J.T.; et al. Traffic-related air pollution and asthma onset in children: A prospective cohort study with individual exposure measurement. *Environ. Health Perspect.* **2008**, *116*, 1433–1438. [CrossRef] [PubMed]
81. Gergen, P.J. Understanding the economic burden of asthma. *J. Allergy Clin. Immunol.* **2001**, *107*, S445–S448. [CrossRef]
82. Thanh, N.X.; Ohinmaa, A.; Yan, C. Asthma-related productivity losses in Alberta, Canada. *J. Asthma Allergy* **2009**, *2*, 43. [CrossRef]
83. Lamb, C.E.; Ratner, P.H.; Johnson, C.E.; Ambegaonkar, A.J.; Joshi, A.V.; Day, D.; Sampson, N.; Eng, B. Economic impact of workplace productivity losses due to allergic rhinitis compared with select medical conditions in the United States from an employer perspective. *Curr. Med. Res. Opin.* **2006**, *22*, 1203–1210.
84. Rice, D.P. Cost of illness studies: What is good about them? *Inj. Prev.* **2000**, *6*, 177–179. [CrossRef]
85. Shin, H.S.; Lee, S.H.; Kim, J.S.; Kim, J.S.; Han, K.H. Socioeconomic costs of food-borne disease using the cost-of-illness model: Applying the QALY method. *J. Prev. Med. Public Health* **2010**, *43*, 352–361. [CrossRef]

86. Pak, H.Y.; Pak, Y.S. The effects of PM_{10} on the hospital admission of patients with respiratory disease in Seoul, Korea. *J. Converg. Inf. Technol.* **2019**, *9*, 194–201.
87. Ban, J.; Wang, Q.; Ma, R.; Zhang, Y.; Shi, W.; Zhang, Y.; Chen, C.; Sun, Q.; Wang, Y.; Guo, X.; et al. Associations between short-term exposure to $PM_{2.5}$ and stroke incidence and mortality in China: A case-crossover study and estimation of the burden. *Environ. Pollut.* **2021**, *268*, 115743. [PubMed]

Disclaimer/Publisher's Note: The statements, opinions and data contained in all publications are solely those of the individual author(s) and contributor(s) and not of MDPI and/or the editor(s). MDPI and/or the editor(s) disclaim responsibility for any injury to people or property resulting from any ideas, methods, instructions or products referred to in the content.

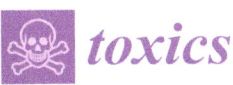

Article

TDP-43 CSF Concentrations Increase Exponentially with Age in Metropolitan Mexico City Young Urbanites Highly Exposed to PM$_{2.5}$ and Ultrafine Particles and Historically Showing Alzheimer and Parkinson's Hallmarks. Brain TDP-43 Pathology in MMC Residents Is Associated with High Cisternal CSF TDP-43 Concentrations

Lilian Calderón-Garcidueñas [1,2,*], Elijah W. Stommel [3], Ingolf Lachmann [4], Katharina Waniek [4], Chih-Kai Chao [1], Angélica González-Maciel [5], Edgar García-Rojas [2], Ricardo Torres-Jardón [6], Ricardo Delgado-Chávez [7] and Partha S. Mukherjee [8]

1 College of Health, The University of Montana, Missoula, MT 59812, USA
2 Universidad del Valle de México, Mexico City 14370, Mexico
3 Department of Neurology, Geisel School of Medicine at Dartmouth, Hanover, NH 03755, USA
4 Roboscreen GmbH, 04129 Leipzig, Germany
5 Instituto Nacional de Pediatría, Mexico City 04530, Mexico
6 Instituto de Ciencias de la Atmósfera y Cambio Climático, Universidad Nacional Autónoma de México, Mexico City 04510, Mexico
7 Independent Researcher, Mexico City 04310, Mexico
8 Interdisciplinary Statistical Research Unit, Indian Statistical Institute, Kolkata 700108, India
* Correspondence: lilian.calderon-garciduenas@umontana.edu

Abstract: Environmental exposures to fine particulate matter (PM$_{2.5}$) and ultrafine particle matter (UFPM) are associated with overlapping Alzheimer's, Parkinson's and TAR DNA-binding protein 43 (TDP-43) hallmark protein pathologies in young Metropolitan Mexico City (MMC) urbanites. We measured CSF concentrations of TDP-43 in 194 urban residents, including 92 MMC children aged 10.2 ± 4.7 y exposed to PM$_{2.5}$ levels above the USEPA annual standard and to high UFPM and 26 low pollution controls (11.5 ± 4.4 y); 43 MMC adults (42.3 ± 15.9 y) and 14 low pollution adult controls (33.1 ± 12.0 y); and 19 amyotrophic lateral sclerosis (ALS) patients (52.4 ± 14.1 y). TDP-43 neuropathology and cisternal CSF data from 20 subjects—15 MMC (41.1 ± 18.9 y) and 5 low pollution controls (46 ± 16.01 y)—were included. CSF TDP-43 exponentially increased with age ($p < 0.0001$) and it was higher for MMC residents. TDP-43 cisternal CSF levels of 572 ± 208 pg/mL in 6/15 MMC autopsy cases forecasted TDP-43 in the olfactory bulb, medulla and pons, reticular formation and motor nuclei neurons. A 16 y old with TDP-43 cisternal levels of 1030 pg/mL exhibited TDP-43 pathology and all 15 MMC autopsy cases exhibited AD and PD hallmarks. Overlapping TDP-43, AD and PD pathologies start in childhood in urbanites with high exposures to PM$_{2.5}$ and UFPM. Early, sustained exposures to PM air pollution represent a high risk for developing brains and MMC UFPM emissions sources ought to be clearly identified, regulated, monitored and controlled. Prevention of deadly neurologic diseases associated with air pollution ought to be a public health priority and preventive medicine is key.

Keywords: ALS; air pollution; Alzheimer's; Aβ1–42; α synuclein; children; cerebrospinal fluid; cisternal CSF; fronto-temporal dementia; Metropolitan Mexico City; nanoparticles; olfactory bulb granule cells; PM$_{2.5}$; Parkinson's; hyperphosphorylated tau; TDP-43

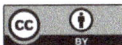

1. Introduction

Neurodegenerative disorders with complex environmental and genetic pathogenesis start decades before clinical symptomatology is present [1–3]. Quadruple aberrant neural pathology starting in childhood and environmental damage to fetal brains in utero likely have short- and long-term neuropsychiatric and neuropathological outcomes [2–4]. Air pollution has been associated with neuroinflammation and oxidative stress, and fine particulate matter ($PM_{2.5}$), ozone (O_3), and nitrogen dioxide (NO_2) are strongly associated with higher risks of several types of dementia and Parkinson's disease (PD) [5–11]. Psychiatric outcomes, including depression and suicide, are reported in association with air pollution exposures [12–15]. The pediatric impact of traffic pollution includes cognitive deficits, altered neurobehavioral performance, structural brain changes and increased risk of attention deficit/hyperactivity and autistic spectrum disorders, and maternal exposures to traffic air pollution during late pregnancy contribute to oxidative stress and inflammation in newborn children [16–23]. A key component of $PM_{2.5}$ is the ≤ 100 nm fraction: ultrafine PM (UFPM) and nanoparticles (NPs). Anthropogenic UFPM are primarily generated via combustion (e.g., vehicular sources) and subsequent processes of particle nucleation, coagulation and vapor condensation, while NPs are frequently referred to as engineered or manufactured because they are designed and generated for a particular purpose; e.g., medical [24]. Anthropogenic UFPM and industrial NPs are ubiquitous and have detrimental neural impacts [25–29].

We have previously shown that cerebrospinal fluid (CSF) concentrations of cytokines and chemokines, cellular prion protein (PrPc), total tau (T-tau), tau phosphorylated at threonine 181 (P-Tau), amyloid Aβ1-42, α-synuclein (t-α-syn and d-α-synuclein), brain-derived neurotrophic factor (BDNF), insulin and leptin can be used to distinguish MMC children from low pollution controls [30–33]. Moreover, CSF myelin basic protein autoantibodies and nickel concentrations, as well as Mn, Ni and Cr concentrations in frontal tissues, are higher in MMC cases vs. low pollution controls [34,35]. Of particular relevance to this work are the significantly lower amyloid Aβ1-42 and BDNF concentrations in MMC children versus low pollution controls ($p = 0.005$ and 0.02, respectively) and the fact that non-P-Tau cases showed significantly faster increases in MMC residents versus controls ($p = 0.005$) [31–33].

The overlap of several aberrant CSF proteins in children and young MMC adults, including hyperphosphorylated tau, beta amyloid, alpha synuclein and TDP 43 [1,2,4], drove our current investigation of MMC children and adults with TDP-43 in CSF and brain tissues versus low pollution controls, and we selected hospital-diagnosed amyotrophic lateral sclerosis (ALS) as an example of patients with a clinical syndrome with complex biological determinants characterized by TDP-43 pathology and high TDP-43 lumbar CSF concentrations. Moreover, our 203 forensic autopsy MMC data cases for residents ≤ 40 y, with 18% showing TDP-43 pathology, drove our interest in the relationship between cisterna magna TDP-43 concentrations and brain pathology.

Two research groups were critical in defining the relationship and the interpretation of protein concentrations in cisternal versus lumbar CSF; the work by Reiber [36,37] and by Peyron et al. [38]. More specifically, Reiber states that *"nonlinearly increasing protein concentrations between ventricular and lumbar CSF are fitting to a Gaussian error function, the differential of the nonlinear concentration distribution function between blood and CSF"* [36] and that the relationship between blood-CSF and blood–brain barrier (BBB) dysfunction is an expression of reduced CSF, or CSF flow rate, and CSF protein gradients [37]. These conclusions support the positive relationship between cisterna magna TDP-43 concentrations and our 3 ± 1.2 h after death autopsy findings [38].

TDP-43 nuclear depletion and aggregation are hallmarks of ALS and frontotemporal dementia (FTD) [39–42]. TDP-43 immunocytochemical profiles in children and young MMC adults have shown loss of nuclear expression and powdery cytoplasmic particles in the substantia nigrae pars compacta and non-motor neurons, as well as significant involvement of mesencephalic, pontine and medullary reticular formation [2,41–44]. Of particular concern, we have reported sleep disorders in MMC residents [45] along key brainstem sleep and arousal hubs, showing solid UFPM from anthropogenic combustion, mainly diesel exhaust, as well as non-exhaust sources coming from tire and brake wearing and from engineered NPs [46–48]. Although FTD and ALS epidemiological data are not extensively studied in Mexico [49,50], the presence of overlapping quadruple pathologies in MMC children and young adults [2,45,46] raises the question of why such diagnoses are missing in our populations. Providing an early ALS diagnosis is clinically difficult [51], and development of research criteria for the diagnosis of prodromal behavioral variant frontotemporal dementia (bvFTD) is ongoing [52]. Given the current challenges in defining mechanisms underlying the development of TDP-43 pathology and the early identification of individuals at risk for FTD and ALS, we hypothesized that CSF TDP-43 quantification from air pollution-exposed residents is highly relevant. Our rationale is summarized as follows: (i) even at the earliest age examined, CSF TDP-43 shows significant differences from contrasting polluted environments; (ii) the measurement of cisterna magna CSF TDP-43 and its correlative relationship with TDP43 pathology in the brain tissue of children and young adults is crucial; and (iii) The contribution of UFPM and NP exposures to changes in CSF TDP-43 levels in highly exposed residents versus clean air controls supports the hypothesis that UFPM fractions [53–55] are highly neurotoxic and lead to TDP-43 pathology.

In sum, the purpose of the present study was to assess, in MMC versus lower pollution age-matched subjects, the impact of lifetime exposures to highly polluted environments on CSF TDP-43 burden. Our results identify lumbar CSF TDP-43 increasing exponentially with age in young urbanites with high exposures to PM pollution and TDP-43 cisternal CSF levels of 572 ± 208 pg/mL forecasting TDP-43 pathology in young MMC residents.

There is a strong association between TAR DNA-binding protein 43, frontotemporal lobar degeneration (FTLD) and amyotrophic lateral sclerosis (ALS) [39–44,51,52]; thus, our findings in young, highly PM-exposed megacity residents are highly relevant for the global medical community, from both the neuropathology and clinical viewpoints.

2. Materials and Methods

2.1. Study Cities and Air Quality

MMC residents have been chronically exposed to significant concentrations of fine particulate matter ($PM_{2.5}$) and O_3 for the last three decades [56–59]. Figure 1 shows the time series trend of annual mean 24 h $PM_{2.5}$ concentrations, averaged over 3 years, for representative MMC monitoring stations in the period between 1990 to April 2020 and their comparison with $PM_{2.5}$ from the US EPA NAAQS.

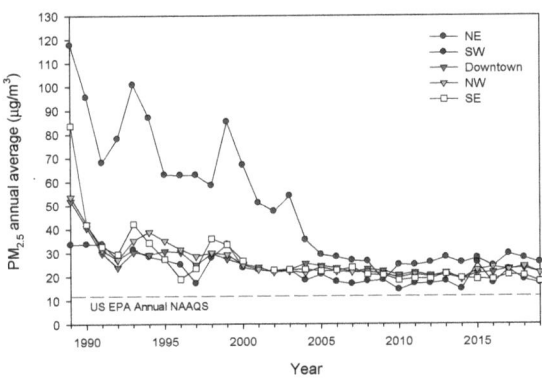

Figure 1. Time series trends showing annual mean 24 h $PM_{2.5}$ concentrations, averaged over 3 years, for five representative MMC monitoring stations from 1990 to April 2020 and their comparison with the respective annual US EPA NAAQS. Annual means from the years before 2004 were estimated from available information of PM_{10} since 1990 and the mean slope of the correlation PM_{10} vs. $PM_{2.5}$ between 2004 and 2007. Data from: http://www.aire.cdmx.gob.mx/default.php# (accessed on 4 June 2022).

UFPM and NPs have a very low mass compared with larger diameter particles; therefore, the PM fraction <100 nm in MMC was evaluated through measurements of particle number concentration (PNC) [60–63]. The expected PNC trend in MMC was estimated using CO and $PM_{2.5}$ measurements integrated in a nonlinear regression by our laboratory (CO and $PM_{2.5}$ are tracers of vehicular emissions) [46]. The estimated PNC for the 1990s was around 300,000 cm^{-3}. Given that catalytic converters in cars and unleaded gasoline were not enforced in Mexico until the year 2000, MMC CO and $PM_{2.5}$ levels before 2000 were among the highest levels of criteria pollutants registered in North America [57]. MMC residents born before 2002 were exposed to PNCs in the range of 300,000 cm^{-3} and, given that the PNC trend decreased to the overall average of 44,000 cm^{-3} after 2003, exposures of MMC residents reached the average PNC for 40 urban areas across Asia, North America, Europe and Australia precisely after 2003 [63]. Figure 2 shows the annual PNC trends calculated for MMC from 1989 to 2019. The symbols in the figure correspond to the median PNCs and the dates of measurement reported by Dunn et al. [60]—commercial with median industry and heavy traffic site, size of measured UFPMs between 3–15 nm; Caudillo et al. [53]—residential with low traffic site, size of measured UFPMs between 20–100 nm; Velasco et al. [54]—commercial with moderate to heavy traffic, size of measured UFPMs < 50 nm; Kleinman et al. [61]—PNC urban background estimated from the extrapolation down to surface of the average UFPMs with sizes < 100 nm measured by aircraft across the MMC at an average altitude level of 350 m above surface.

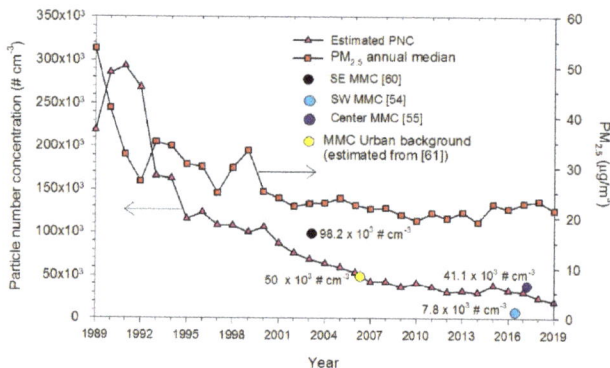

Figure 2. Annual PNC trends estimated from the medians of annual measured levels of CO and estimated (before 2004) and measured (after 2004) $PM_{2.5}$ registered in the MMC from 1989 to 2019. Source of $PM_{2.5}$ data was: http://www.aire.cdmx.gob.mx/default.php# (accessed on 4 June 2022).

MMC is an example of uncontrolled urban growth and environmental pollution [53–64]; the area of MMC is over 2000 km^2, and it lies in an elevated basin 7400 feet above sea level. MMC has nearly 22 million inhabitants, over 50,000 industries and over 5 million vehicles consuming more than 50 million liters of petroleum fuels per day. In this megacity, MMC motor vehicles release abundant amounts of primary $PM_{2.5}$, elemental carbon, particle-bound polycyclic aromatic hydrocarbons, carbon monoxide, nitrogen oxides and a wide range of air toxins and other toxics, including formaldehyde, acetaldehyde, benzene, toluene and xylenes [55,57–59,64]. The high altitude and tropical climate facilitate ozone production all year [59] and contribute to the formation of secondary particulate matter. A review of several MMC short-term pilot studies showed that the existing heavy-duty diesel fleet emits high amounts of UFPM [65]. In addition, measurements of UFPM emissions from light gasoline vehicles at smoke checking workshops have also shown that old vehicles are high $PM_{0.1}$ emitters [65].

In this study, children and adult cohorts included residents in MMC, while subjects from small control cities represented the typical provincial areas where air pollution emissions are minimal. MMC northern industrialized and southern residential zones were represented in our samples. Southern MMC children are exposed to significant concentrations of ozone, secondary tracers (NO_3^-) and particles with lipopolysaccharides (PM-LPS), while northern children are exposed to higher concentrations of volatile organic compounds (VOCs) and $PM_{2.5}$ and its constituents: organic and elemental carbon, including polycyclic aromatic hydrocarbons, secondary inorganic aerosols (SO_4^{2-}, NO_3^-, NH_4^+) and metals (zinc, copper, lead, titanium, manganese, chromium and vanadium) [55,56,62,64]. Across MMC, residents are exposed to volatile organic compounds (VOCs) and polycyclic aromatic hydrocarbons (PAHs) complex mixtures containing over 100 compounds associated with fine particle-bound PAHs [58,64]. These PAHs are abundant in indoor and outdoor air and busy roadways and are associated with frying oils and snacks and a wide range of occupational exposures [64]. MMC residents are also exposed on daily bases to high outdoor concentrations of Hg in $PM_{2.5}$ [62].

2.2. CSF and Brain Samples

This prospective study was approved by the review boards and ethics committees at the Universidad del Valle de Mexico, on the 18 November 2020, and the University of Montana, IRB-206R-09, on the 8 December 2016, and IRB 185-20, on the 23 November 2020.

Normal CSF samples were selected from two cohorts admitted for investigation of neurological involvement in the context of a hematological, neoplastic or infectious brain processes: (i) children admitted to the hospital from a clean air city or MMC, with a work-up diagnosis of acute lymphoblastic leukemia (ALL) entering a clinical protocol that included a spinal tap, and (ii) young and older adults admitted to the hospital for a work-up that required a spinal tap with varied diagnoses, including potential neoplastic and infectious CNS involvement. The cohort of young and older adults also included permanent residents in clean environments and lifetime residents in highly polluted MMC. The normal CSF samples studied were destined to be destroyed after the diagnosis of normal CSF in the laboratory. We also examined 19 CSF ALS cases from Dartmouth-Hitchcock Medical Center Cerebral Spinal Fluid Bank for research IRB #29104 and 5 Mexican ALS cases under the Universidad del Valle de Mexico 18 November 2020 IRB.

The autopsy cases with cerebello-medullary cisternal tap included 15 MMC subjects and 5 low pollution control cases; all had complete forensic autopsies, including full neuropathological examination. These autopsies were performed between 2004 and 2008 under a Consejo de la Judicatura del Distrito Federal permit (14571/2003).

2.2.1. CSF Spinal Taps

Spinal tap was performed on the left lateral decubitus from the intervertebral spaces L3-S1 using a standard 22 spinal needle. Spinal taps were performed between 8 and 10 am. CSF was collected dripping in free air in 1 mL aliquot into Nalge Nunc polypropylene CryoTubes. Lumbar puncture samples were collected during non-traumatic, non-complicated procedures. CSF samples were examined immediately to determine haematological, oncological or infectious involvement and then stored at -80 °C and kept frozen until the current analysis. CSF pleocytosis was defined as CSF white blood cell (WBC) counts of ≥ 7 cells per mm^3. All CSF samples in this study were read as normal. We performed the hTDP43 total ELISA (Cat. No. 847-0108000107, Roboscreen GmbH, Leipzig, Germany) according to the instructions for use. This ELISA uses two monoclonal antibodies directed at amino acids 79–91 and 259–271.

2.2.2. Pediatric Cohort for the Measurement of TDP-43 in CSF

This work includes CSF data from a pediatric cohort: 92 children from MMC (33F/59M, mean age = 10.27 years, SD = 4.73) and 26 low pollution control children (11F/15M, mean age = 11.5 years, SD = 4.4). The selected children had no previous oncologic and/or hematologic CNS or systemic treatments and their CSF samples were read as normal, with CNS involvement being ruled out at the time of their hospitalization. Children's clinical inclusion criteria were negative known smoking history and environmental tobacco exposure, lifelong residency in MMC or the control city, residency within a radius of 2.5 miles of one of the representative city monitoring stations, full-term birth and unremarkable clinical histories prior to their admission to the hospital. We specifically excluded children with a history of active participation in team sports with high incidences of head trauma, including soccer. Mothers had unremarkable, full-term pregnancies with uncomplicated vaginal deliveries and took no illicit drugs, including alcohol and tobacco. These children had a history of breast feeding for a minimum of 6 months and were introduced to solid foods after the age of 4 months. Participants were from middle class families, living in single-family homes with no indoor pets, used LP gas for cooking and kitchens were separated from the living and sleeping areas. Low and high pollution-exposed children were matched by age, gender and socioeconomic status.

2.2.3. Adult Cohort for the Measurement of TDP-43 in CSF

We had 19 ALS cases (9F/10M, average age 52.4 ± 14.1 y), of which 14 were from NH and 5 from MMC; 43 normal MMC CSF samples (27M/16F, average age 43.2 ± 15.9 y); and 14 samples from residents in low pollution cities (9M/5F average age 33.1 ± 12.0 y).

2.2.4. Children and Adult Forensic Autopsies for the Measurement of Cisternal CSF TDP-43 and Complete Brain Examination Including Immunohistochemistry for TDP-43

This work included forensic cases from MMC and low pollution controls. A total of 20 subjects (1F, 19M) (mean age 42.3 years, $SD = 17.9$, age range 16 to 83 y) were examined: 15 MMC male residents, average age 41.13 ± 18.9 y, and 5 controls (1F/4M, 46 ± 16 y). The inclusion criteria for this cohort included lifelong residency in MMC or the control cities and a cause of death—i.e., accidents, homicides and suicides—that did not involve the brain directly. Immunohistochemistry was performed using the TDP-43 mab2G10 (847-0102007401, Cat. No. Roboscreen GmbH, Leipzig, Germany, 1:1000). This antibody is a recombinant human TDP-43 directed to the amino acids MTEDELREFFSQYGDVM of the TDP43 protein and able to identify prominent physiological nuclear immunostaining and neuronal pathological cytoplasmic immunoreactivity in neurons and glial cells in TDP-43 proteinopathy cases.

2.2.5. Data Analysis

We first calculated summary statistics of the TDP-43 concentrations, age and gender for the following cohorts: control children, MMC children, ALS patients, MMC adults and control adults. We then compared the means of TDP-43 concentration between the ALS cohort and controls and between the ALS and the MMC group. We performed two-sample t-tests for this purpose. Next, we investigated the role of age, gender and residency on TDP-43 concentrations in all subjects. For this purpose, we considered linear regression analysis. Since the TDP-43 values varied widely, an appropriate mathematical transformation was necessary so that linear regression analysis could be applied and interpreted reasonably. Logarithm transformation was a natural choice. We performed linear regression of the logarithm of TDP-43 concentration for age, gender and residency. Thereafter, we performed linear regression analysis of the logarithm of TDP-43 concentrations for age and gender. The statistical analyses were performed using the statistical software R.

3. Results

3.1. CSF TDP-43

CSF samples were colorless, with normal opening pressure. Table 1 shows the mean ± SD and 25th, median and 75th percentile results for ALS cases, MMC and lower pollution control children and adult samples.

Table 1. CSF TDP-43 ELISA results in pg/mL for control and MMC children, ALS patients and adult MMC and low pollution controls. In each cell, the first row shows the mean ± SD and the second row the 25th percentile, median and 75th percentile.

CSF Samples	Age and Gender	TDP-43 pg/mL
Control children n: 26	11.5 ± 4.4 y (8.25, 12.50, 15.00) y 11F/15M	102 ± 59 (58.14, 88.65, 129.77)
MMC children n: 92	10.27 ± 4.7 y (7.00, 11.00, 15.00) y 33F/59M	239 ± 152 (130.28, 229.39, 299.47)
ALS patients n: 19	52.4 ± 14.1 y (56.50, 61.00, 64.00) y 9F/10M	902 ± 269 (683.30, 906.07, 1085.79)
MMC adults n: 43	43.2 ± 15.9 y (28.50, 45.00, 54.00) y 16F/27M	373 ± 358 (159.86, 275.10, 473.55)
Control adults n: 14	33.14 ± 12.0 y (27.50, 32.00, 33.75) y 5F/9M	108 ± 67 (56.49, 81.75, 150.75)

Mean CSF TDP-43 concentration was significantly higher in ALS versus MMC and non-MMC controls ($p < 0.0001$). The logarithm of TDP-43 increased significantly with age ($p < 0.0001$) and it was higher for MMC residents ($p < 0.0001$). Excluding ALS cases, a log-transformed linear regression of TDP-43 concentration relative to age and residency showed that CSF TDP-43 increases significantly with age ($p = 0.0032$) (Figure 3).

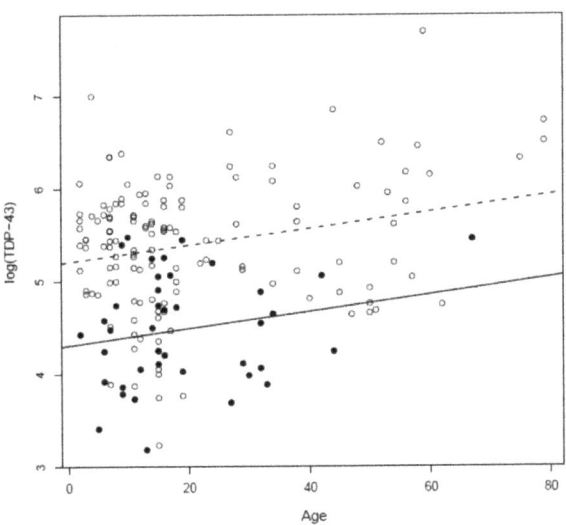

Figure 3. Linear regression of logarithm of TDP-43 CSF concentrations for age and residency (controls and MMC residents). Logarithm of TDP-43 increased significantly with age ($p = 0.0032$). Black circles represent controls and open circles MMC residents.

3.2. Cisternal CSF TDP-43 and Brain Pathology

The average age of the MMC adult cases was 41.1 ± 18.9 years and that of the controls was 46 ± 16 y. A 16-year-old MMC boy was also studied. Table 2 shows the neuropathological markers in each case and the concentrations of cisternal CSF TDP-43.

There was a significant difference between the CSF TDP-43 concentrations in controls without brain pathology versus the six MMC cases showing TDP-43 brain pathology: controls—265.2 ± 132 vs. MMC—572.5 ± 228.5 pg/mL. The mean MMC TDP-43 cisternal concentration was 350.8 ± 247 pg/mL.

Table 2. Autopsy cases with cisternal CSF TDP-43 and complete neuropathological examination using H&E, PHF-tau8 phosphorylated at Ser199-202-Thr205 and α-synuclein phosphorylated at Ser-129, LB509 and TDP-43 mab2G10.

ID	Age	Gender	APOE	AD pτ *	AD Aβ **	SN pτ §	SN αS §§	TDP-43 Brain ‡	TDP-43 Cisternal pg/mL
1	16	1	0	2	2	1	0	1	1013
2	21	1	0	5	3	0	0	0	392
3	24	1	0	2	2	1	1	1	375
4	25	1	0	1	2	0	0	1	565
5	27	1	0	2	2	1	1	0	218
6	37	0	0	5	4	1	1	0	42
7	38	1	0	4	3	1	0	0	306
8	39	1	0	3	2	1	1	0	167
9	40	1	0	4	3	1	1	1	562
10	42	1	0	3	2	1	0	1	496
11	47	1	0	3	2	0	0	0	194
12	48	1	0	4	3	1	1	0	293
13	55	1	0	5	3	0	1	0	150
14	75	0	0	4	3	1	1	1	424
15	83	0	0	4	3	1	0	0	66
1 CTL	29	0	0	0	0	0	0	0	364
2 CTL	34	1	0	0	0	0	0	0	191
3CTL	43	1	0	0	0	0	0	0	435
4 CTL	56	1	0	0	0	0	0	0	226
5 CTL	68	1	0	0	0	0	0	0	110

* AD staging—pτ stage: 0 = absent; 1 = pre-tangle stages a–c; 2 = pre-tangle stages 1a and 1b; 3 = NFT stages I and II; 4 = NFT stages III and IV; 5 = NFT stages V and VI. ** AD staging—Aβ phase: 0 = absent; 1 = basal temporal neocortex; 2 = all cerebral cortex; 3 = subcortical portions—forebrain; 4 = mesencephalic components; 5 = reticular formation and cerebellum. § Substantia nigrae pτ was evaluated as pre-tangles, positive neurites and tangles using the PHF-tau8 phosphorylated at Ser199-202-Thr205 (Innogenetics, Belgium, AT-8 1:1000). §§ Substantia nigrae α-S was evaluated as neuronal immunoreactive (IR) aggregates in the somato-dendritic compartment, cytoplasmic inclusions, core-halo Lewy bodies and dystrophic neurites (Lewy neurites) using α-synuclein phosphorylated at Ser-129, LB509 (In Vitrogen, Carlsbad, CA 1:1000). ‡ Brain TDP-43 was evaluated as dash-like IR particles in the vicinity of the cell nucleus, with or without complete loss of nuclear TDP-43 expression and somatic skein inclusions and glial pathology using mab2G10 (Roboscreen GmbH, Leipzig, Germany 1:1000).

Remarkably, concentrations of TDP-43 in cisternal CSF with an average of 572 ± 208 pg/mL forecasted cortical and subcortical TDP-43 pathology, while averages of 232 ± 130 pg/mL were associated with negative TDP-43 brain pathology in MMC residents and controls.

Table 3 shows the TDP-43 immunoreactivity in the 6 MMC cases with TDP-43-related brain pathology and targeted anatomical locations. A total of 25 cortical and subcortical regions were immunoassayed with a TDP-43 antibody and/or counter-stained with hematoxylin. Regions were evaluated for: (1) complete loss of nuclear TDP-43 expression; (2) dash immunoreactive (IR) particles in the vicinity of neuronal nuclei; (3) skein-like tangles in neurons; (4) glial pathology, including oligodendroglia coil tangles. We sectioned the entire brainstem up to cervical levels C1–C2 and included the olfactory bulb; frontal, temporal and parietal cortices; hippocampus, caudate and putamen; substantia nigrae; locus coeruleus; cranial nerve nuclei; trigeminal ganglia; and cervical sections C1 and C2 in our immunohistochemistry studies.

Table 3. Neuropathology findings in the six MMC males with cisternal CSF TDP-43 data and TDP-43 neuropathology. Numbers represent: (1) complete loss of nuclear TDP-43 expression; (2) dash-like immunoreactive (IR) particles in the vicinity of neuronal nuclei; (3) skein-like tangles in neurons; (4) glial pathology, including oligodendroglia coil tangles. * Cranial nerve nuclei.

Anatomical Areas	16 1013 pg/mL	24 375 pg/mL	25 565 pg/mL	40 562 pg/mL	42 496 pg/mL	75 424 pg/mL
Frontal motor	1	1	1	1	1, 2	1, 2
Frontal non-motor	1	1	1	1	1	1
Parietal	1	0	0	1	1	1
Temporal	1	1	0	1	1, 2	1
Hippocampus	1	1	1, 2, 4	1, 2	1, 2	1, 2, 4
Caudate	1	0	1	0	0	0
Putamen	0	0	1	0	0	1
Globus pallidus	0	0	1	0	1	0
XII *	1, 2	1, 2	1	1	1, 2	1
X *	1	1, 2	1	1	1	1
IX *	0	0	1	1	0	0
VIII *	1	1	1	0	0	1
VII *	1	0	1, 2	1, 2	1	1
VI *	0	1	1	0	0	0
V *	1, 2	1	1, 2	1	1	1
IV *	1	1	1	0	1	1
III *	1	1	1, 2	1	1	1
II *	0	0	0	0	0	0
I *	1	1	1, 2, 3, 4	1	1, 2	1
Substantia nigrae pc	1, 2	1, 2	1	1, 2	1, 2	0
Locus coeruleus	1, 2	1	1	1, 2	1, 2	1, 2
Pons neurons	1, 2, 4	1, 2, 4	1, 2	1, 2	1, 2	1, 2
Mesencephalic reticular formation	1, 2	1	1, 2	1, 2	1, 2	1
Area postrema	1	1	1, 2	1, 2	1	1
Trigeminal ganglia	0	1	1	1, 2	1, 2	1, 2
Inferior olivary complex	1	1	1	1	1	1
Cervical, anterior horn	1	1, 2	1, 2	1	1	1

Representative immunohistochemistry photographs are shown in Figures 4–6. Positive TDP-43 pathology in the six MMC autopsy cases was characterized by complete loss of nuclear TDP-43 expression and/or dash-like IR in the vicinity of neuronal nuclei (Figure 4). We documented olfactory bulb granule cell short tangles in young adults (Figure 4A).

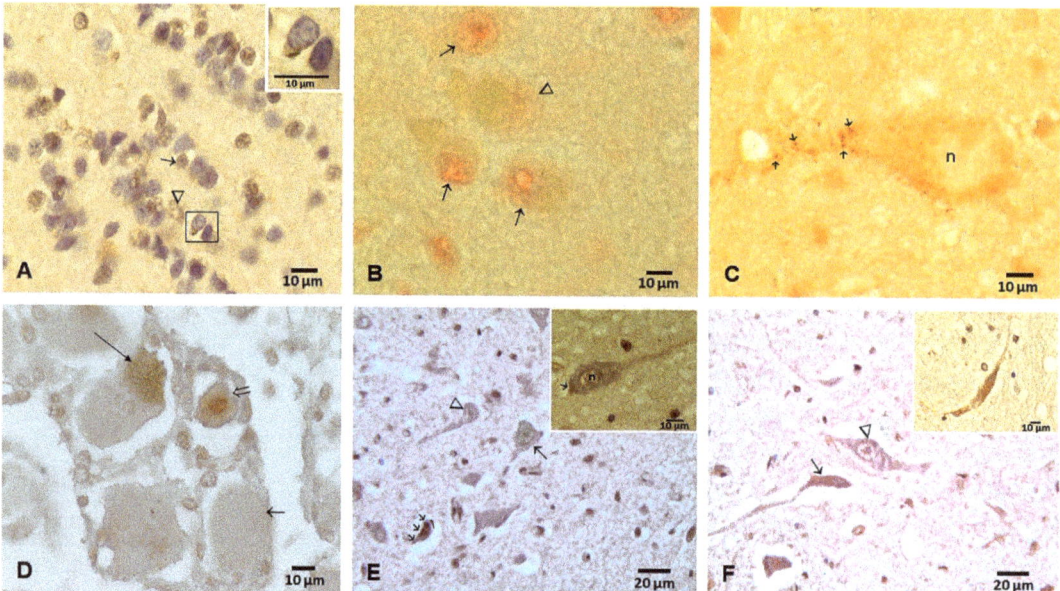

Figure 4. Olfactory bulb, trigeminal ganglia and brainstem motor nuclei immunohistochemistry for TDP-43 in young Metropolitan Mexico City residents. (**A**) Olfactory bulb granule cells in a 25 y old male showing complete loss of nuclear TDP-43 IR (arrowhead) alternating with nuclear TDP-43 (short arrow), the presence of short tangles and loss of nuclear expression (square and insert, the arrow points to a short TDP-43 positive tangle in a granule neuron). TDP-43 and DAB (brown staining). (**B**) Oculomotor nucleus (III cranial nerve) in the 16 y old showing a neuron (arrowhead) with complete loss of nuclear IR surrounded by three neurons with strongly stained red nuclei (short arrows). (**C**) 40 y old male trigeminal spinal neurons with negative nuclei and cytoplasmic dash-like IR, mostly in the axonal region (short arrows). (**D**) 45 y old male trigeminal ganglia neurons with negative nuclei and cytoplasmic positivity (long arrow), alternating with negative nuclear IR (short arrow) and strong nuclear TDP-43 IR (arrowhead). (**E**) 16 y male vagal neurons with negative nuclei (arrowhead), neurons with weak nuclear IR (long arrow) and neurons with intense cytoplasmic inclusions (three short arrows). DAB, brown product. Insert: Vagal neuron with a negative nucleus (n) and positive cytoplasmic IR (short arrow). (**F**) 16 y old male hypoglossal neurons with negative IR nuclei (arrowhead) alongside a neuron with intense cytoplasmic IR (arrow). Insert. hypoglossal neuron with intense IR granular material. DAB, brown product.

The pathology was mostly seen in brainstem levels, including the medulla and pons, substantia nigrae and locus coeruleus, and in relation to the mesencephalic reticular formation, ventral tegmental area-parabrachial pigmented nucleus complex and caudal-rostral linear nucleus of the raphe (Figure 5).

The cortical and hippocampal pathology was characterized by loss of nuclear TDP-43 expression and/or dash-like IR cytoplasmic neurons. The 24 and 25 y old subjects showed negative IR nuclei in frontal and temporal neurons, cytoplasmic IR and oligodendroglia tangles (Figure 6A,B), while the 16 y old boy exhibited cervical motor neurons with IR negativity and cytoplasmic IR (Figure 6F).

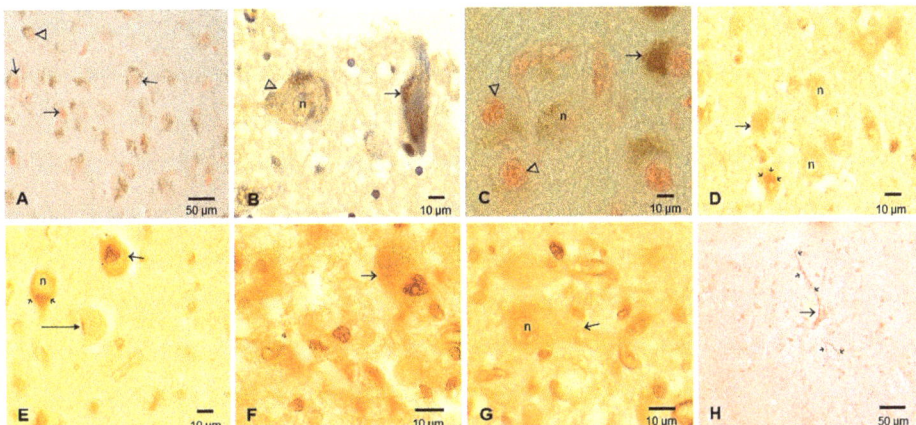

Figure 5. TDP-43 immunohistochemistry in locus coeruleus (LC), substantia nigrae (SN), pons and medulla. (**A**) Locus coeruleus in a 24 y old showing the spectrum of TDP-43 nuclear pathology from positive nuclear staining (short arrows) to negative nuclear IR (arrowhead). (**B**) Sixteen y old male with LC neurons showing negative nuclei and scanty dash-like IR (arrowhead), along with negative nuclear IR and prominent granular cytoplasmic IR (arrow). DAB, brown product. (**C**) 42 y old male SN neuron with IR negative nucleus (n) contrasting with IR-positive nuclei (arrowheads) with a few melanin granules and a neuron with abundant neuromelanin and IR-positive nucleus (arrow). Red product. (**D**) Cluster of pontine neurons in a 42 y old with IR-negative nuclei (n), fine granular cytoplasmic IR (arrow) and paranuclear strong IR (three arrows). DAB, brown product. (**E**) 42 y old male inferior olivary complex with unremarkable neurons (short arrow), nuclear IR negativity (n) and strong granular paranuclear IR (two short arrows). One neuron with a short tangle and a negative IR nucleus (long horizontal arrow) is also identified. (**F**) Seventy-five y old male area postrema with large neuron with strong nuclear IR (arrow). (**G**) Same subject as F with area postrema showing a large neuron (arrow) with nuclear (n) IR negativity. (**H**) Forty y old male medullary reticular neuron (long arrow) with nuclear IR negativity and extensive granular IR along axonal and dendritic tree (short arrows).

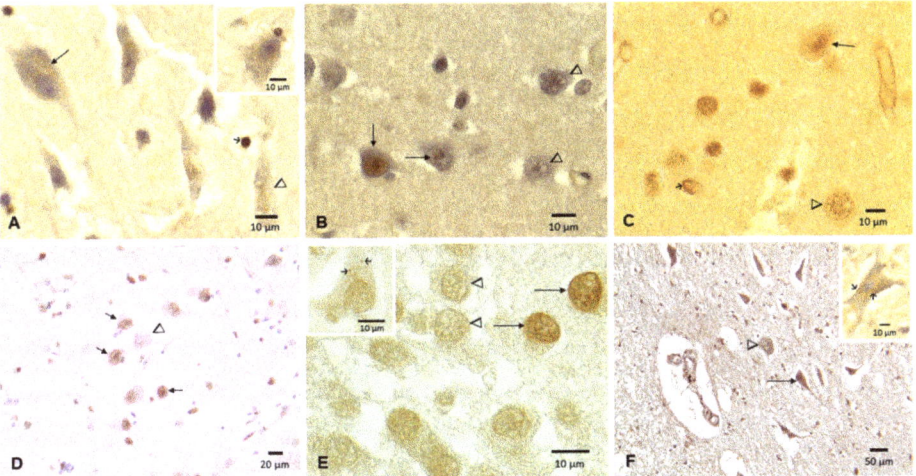

Figure 6. TDP-43 Immunohistochemistry in frontal and temporal cortex, hippocampus and cervical motor neurons. (**A**) Twenty-four y old male showing a frontal pyramidal neuron with negative nuclear

IR and dash-like cytoplasmic positive IR (long arrow), a pyramidal neuron with cytoplasmic IR and negative IR nucleus (arrowhead) and a glial cell with strong nuclear IR (short arrow). Insert shows a coil tangle in an oligodendroglia cell close to a frontal motor neuron with negative IR nucleus and a cytoplasmic IR. DAB counterstained with hematoxylin. (**B**) Twenty-five y old male temporal cortex showing unremarkable neurons with strong nuclear IR (long vertical arrow) contrasting with nuclear negative IR (arrowheads) and one neuron with negative nuclear IR and a small cluster of IR positive granules (horizontal arrow). (**C**) Forty-two y old male temporal cortex with normal neurons with strong nuclear IR (long arrow), neuronal negative nuclear IR (arrowhead) and coil tangle in an oligodendroglia (short arrow). (**D**) Seventy-five y old hippocampus CA2 neurons with nuclear IR (short arrows) and negative nuclear IR (arrowhead). (**E**) Same case as (**D**), dentate hippocampal gyrus neurons with strong nuclear IR (arrows) contrasting with nuclear negative IR (arrowheads). Insert is a hippocampal neuron in CA3 in the same subject showing a negative nuclear IR and a few positive cytoplasmic granules. (**F**) Sixteen y old male cervical (C2) anterior horn motor neuron with negative nuclei (arrowhead) and one neuron with cytoplasmic IR (long arrow). Insert: This cervical motor neuron in the same child exhibits a negative IR nucleus and a few positive IR cytoplasmic granules.

4. Discussion

Intracellular accumulation of abnormal misfolded proteins is the critical neuropathological feature of ALS, FTD, Alzheimer's and Parkinson's diseases and exposure to particulate matter air pollution has been described as a strong risk factor for Metropolitan Mexico City (MMC) young residents [1–4]. Mexican urbanites exposed to complex mixtures of air pollutants, including $PM_{2.5}$ above current EPA US standards and highly toxic UFPM have CSF TDP-43 concentrations exponentially increasing with age. TDP-43 is the target protein associated with ALS and fronto-temporal dementia (FTD) [39–44,66–68]. Remarkably, concentrations of TDP-43 in cisternal CSF with averages of 572 ± 208 pg/mL forecasted cortical and subcortical TDP-43 pathology, while averages of 232 ± 130 pg/mL were associated with no TDP-43 brain pathology in any of the study subjects. Our neuropathology findings in the six MMC individuals included loss of normal nuclear TDP-43 expression and development of cytoplasmic aggregations in non-motor and motor neuronal groups and involved the olfactory bulb, brainstem and cervical motor neurons. Our previously published MMC cases [2] with TDP-43 pathology involved non-motor nuclei, as described in the work by Pandya [67]. Pandya et al. investigated 79 ALS cases using a network diffusion model (NDM) to define whether a process of focal pathological "seeding", followed by structural network-based spread, recapitulated postmortem histopathological staging, and if there was any correlation with the pattern of expression of a panel of genes implicated in ALS across the healthy brain. Remarkably, the critical seed regions for spread within the model were the thalamus, insula, pallidum, putamen and caudate [67]. This information is very relevant to our Mexico City studies, since we have a significant overlap of abnormal neural proteins [1,2], and non-primary motor regions are among the earliest sites of cerebral TDP-43 pathology. Moreover, the involvement of the frontal and temporal cortex and cerebellum in frontotemporal lobe dementia FTLD-TDP patients should be noted, as described in the work of Hasan et al. [68]. Equally relevant to our previous MRI and magnetic NPs quantification in MMC residents' cerebellum [2,47,69], Hasan et al. identified strong cerebellar involvement [68], which most certainly can be used as early evidence of neurodegeneration in MMC residents [2,4,46,69].

The global connectome architecture of FTD subjects is a relevant issue in early TDP-43 pathology, as it allowed researchers such as Shafiei et al. [70] to identify regional early atrophy; i.e., insula—which was identified as the predominant group epicenter of brain atrophy using data-driven and simulation-based methods—with secondary regions in frontal ventromedial and antero-medial temporal areas [70]. These critical observations [70] associating atrophy patterns in sporadic and genetic bvFTD with global connectome architecture and local transcriptomic vulnerability provide an explanation as to how quadruple pathology could account for overlapping clinical pictures [2,4,45,46,71]. Scarioni and colleagues [72] were able to dissect 20 standard neuropathology regions associated with FTLD-TDP, FTLD-tau and FTLD-fused-in-sarcoma (FTLD-FUS) and stained them for phosphorylated TDP-43, phosphorylated tau, FUS, amyloid-beta and alpha-synuclein. Their results showed TDP-43 pathology in the hippocampal granular layer correlates with hallucinations, CA1 with mania, CA3 with depression and parahippocampal tau with delusions. In the brainstem, the presence of alpha-synuclein co-pathology in the substantia nigra (SN) correlated with disinhibition, tau pathology in the SN with depression and tau pathology in the locus coeruleus with both depression and perseverative/compulsive behavior. The results of Scarioni et al. [72] strongly support that a subcortical TDP-43 burden contributes to configuring the clinical phenotype of FTLD. Recent important publications have described end-stage FTLD with tau or TDP-43 pathology [73,74], emphasizing laminar distributions of lower laminar tau, higher TDP pathology and Fe-rich cortical inflammation in tau vs. TDP cases. We were unable to corroborate such distributions in our cases. Our MMC cases demonstrated significant concentrations of highly reactive, magnetic Fe nanoparticles distributed throughout cortical, olfactory, brainstem and cerebellum regions [2,24,25,46].

Our TDP-43 CSF findings and the previously documented quadruple brain pathology [1–4] are in keeping with the presence of several abnormal CSF proteins in the seemingly CNS-uncompromised MMC versus low pollution control children [30–34] with low amyloid-β1-42 and BDNF [32,33] and elevated MIF, IL6, IL1ra, IL2 and PrP(C) levels [30].

The abnormal CSF proteins found in MMC children and young adults are very concerning because they are involved in several pathophysiological mechanisms of early neural damage with eventual impacts on cognitive, neurological and psychiatric outcomes [71,75,76].

At the core of our results, we report accumulation of TDP-43 starting at an early age in individuals highly exposed to complex environmental emissions, including UFPM [1–4]. The TDP-43 pathology observed in young MMC children [2] and the correlation between cisternal TDP-43 levels and the distribution of pathology in children and young adults cannot be dismissed.

Non-fibrillary TDP-43 accumulates in the rough endoplasmic reticulum (RER), as described by Kon and colleagues [77], and the ER is one of the targets of UFPM/NPs in MMC young residents [1,2,24]. To this end, the work of Scarioni and colleagues is key [72]. Their robust data established associations between clinical symptoms and TDP-43 pathology. Strikingly, MMC residents have cellular, subcellular and immunoreactive pathology in precisely the same regions [2,46,69]. Moreover, Andrew and colleagues [78] identified contaminants found to have a strong association with ALS risk in the US, including airborne lead (false discovery rate (FDR) = 0.00077), primarily produced by small aircraft, and polychlorinated biphenyls (PCBs), such as heptachlorobiphenyl (FDR = 3.60E-05) emitted by power plants burning biomass and industrial boilers. This analysis supports neurotoxic airborne metals and PCBs as risk factors for ALS.

Neuropathological information in conjunction with the social brain hypothesis [79] and the application of targeted cognitive behavioral function tests [80] for highly exposed cohorts is a path we could explore, knowing social and criminal transgressions are recorded in bvFTD patients [81]. Mendez discussed precisely this impairment in an innate sense of morality and the predominantly right-hemisphere pathology in frontal (ventromedial, orbitofrontal, inferolateral frontal), anterior temporal (amygdala, temporal pole), limbic (anterior cingulate, amygdala) and insular regions in bvFTD patients [81]. MMC subjects show involvement of these key areas, as explored by brain MRI [69], and social violence in MMC is significant [82]. According to a 2020 report by the Mexico City-based Citizen Council for Public Safety and Criminal Justice, seven out of the ten "most violent" cities in the world were located in Mexico [83]. For the country as a whole, 2019 and 2020 were the most violent on record, with more than 34,000 intentional homicides each year, and the Mexico state—a very polluted particulate matter region—has the highest incidence of violence [83].

The involvement of TDP-43 in the complex reticular formation in MMC residents must be pursued further, given the complexity of the brainstem reticular nuclei and their connections with supra- and infra-cortical structures involving major integration and relay centers coordinating survival functions and key connections between the cerebral cortex, the cerebellum and the spinal cord [84–96]. We are particularly concerned about the associations between reticular brainstem-impaired connectivity and isolated sleep behavior disorder (iRBD) [88], one of the earliest manifestations of α synucleinopathies, which is present in MMC young adults [46], as well as the higher risk of falls [90,94] in young MMC adults [69,97].

Research regarding TDP-43, including novel nuclear pore articles, muscle TDP-43 involvement and the anatomical targets [39–45,98–111], must be revisited in the context of potential early involvement in pollution-exposed populations. For example, it could be particularly intriguing to look for nuclear NPs in motor neurons of highly exposed city dwellers [107] and hypothalamic TDP-43 lesions [111].

There is an urgent need for noninvasive, reliable fluid biomarkers to diagnose early TDP-43 pathology to improve the differential diagnosis with overlapping neurodegenerative diseases that undoubtedly exhibit an extreme variability in clinical phenotypes, as described by Virgilio et al., for tau [112]. Since TDP-43 pathology increases linearly with age in older adults with and without dementia [113], the issue of prevention at early ages is certainly crucial. Identifying the individuals at highest risk of MMC TDP-43 pathology is one of our goals, and to the exploration of cognitive behavioral function tests we could add lipid metabolic traits and body complexions causally associated with the risk of FTD, as in the work of Esteban-García et al. [114]. Increased trunk-predicted mass and fat-free mass, as well as higher circulating triglyceride levels, impact differentially on the risk of FTD and ALS [114].

The work of researchers exploring correlations between fluid biomarkers is highly relevant [115–122]. In particular, our interest is focused on plasma biomarkers to help distinguish between MCI + AD and controls and between FTD and progressive supranuclear palsy (PSP); i.e., P-tau181 [122]—the positive correlation between CSF and plasma values for NfL ($p < 0.0001$), with NfL values higher for all phenotypes of symptomatic FTD-ALS spectrum (FAS) patients compared to primary psychiatric disorders (PPD) [121].

Since, our MMC cases have AD hallmarks, and given that cognition, gait and balance; auditory-evoked brainstem potentials; and brain MRI changes are striking in the young MMC residents [1,2,16,46,69,97,123–125]—we are obligated to include AD biomarkers [118,126,127]. Since CSF samples continue to be the gold standard of neurodegenerative biomarkers, exploration of normal CSF samples in the hospital setting will continue to be an excellent source of samples. Thus, multi-marker synaptic proteins [128], CSF phosphorylated-tau levels (associated with cerebral tau burden in FTLD) and TDP-43 may help to define, in autopsy materials, the burden of TDP-43 pathology and identify risk factors [129,130]. Forensic autopsy-confirmed neurodegenerative biomarkers and neuropathology hallmarks are crucial to define the pathology burden in a population at large.

There were advantages and limitations to this study. A major advantage was the multidisciplinary collaborators and the efforts made to exchange viewpoints regarding the importance of early clinical detection of young individuals at risk, key in understanding the impact of our findings in future multidisciplinary studies. The current particle number concentration (PNC) in MMC is crucial environmental information for the responsible authorities. Residents continue to be exposed to an average of 44,000 particles per cm^{-3} [63], with all the health-associated risks. There is a need to define the presence of the major ALS mutations, including the C9orf72 expansion mutations, SOD1 and TARDBP gene mutations, in MMC residents, and this study further highlights the need to consider early TDP-43 pathological changes as an opportunity to explore pathomechanistic avenues where we could intervene to halt neurodegenerative processes.

5. Concluding Remarks

1. Particulate matter exposures—specifically, UFPM/NP sustained exposures from utero—are likely key in aberrant neural protein pathology. The CSF TDP-43 results identify logarithmic increases related to age across young megacity urbanites, crucial information in view of the 18% TDP-43 pathology reported in 202 forensic MMC autopsies aged 27.29 ± 11.8 y and the overlap of aberrant hyperphosphorylated tau, beta amyloid, α synuclein and TDP-43. These data are striking in view of the work of Karanth et al. [71] and Carlos et al. [113]. Karanth and coworkers pointed out that quadruple misfolded proteins, including tau neurofibrillary tangles, amyloid-β [Aβ], α-synuclein and TDP-43, in the same brain are relatively common in aging. Moreover, dementia frequency was highest among those with quadruple misfolded proteins [71]. Carlos et al. [113] made a calculation of the frequency and distribution of TDP-43 pathology in 1072 cases, average age 87 years, with AD and TDP-43 pathology and antemortem cognitive studies, including 58% with dementia, 15% with mild cognitive impairment and 27% who were cognitively intact. Carlos and colleagues showed a linear increase in TDP-43 pathology with age: 30% of subjects aged 70 had TDP-43 pathology, 42% by age 80 y and 49% by age 90. Strikingly, these cases were white residents in a low-polluted area, reflecting that elderly TDP-43 increases linearly, notwithstanding the low cumulative exposures to environmental air pollutants, in sharp contrast with our logarithmic increases in pediatric and young adults with high UFPM/NP exposures already exhibiting quadruple misfolded protein pathology.

2. We identified a significant relationship between cisternal CSF TDP-43, an average of 572 ± 208 pg/mL, and TDP-43 brain pathology. This is particularly serious for highly exposed children, as with the 16 y old boy (1013 pg/mL) who had extensive nonmotor and motor TDP43 pathology. As toxicologists working with forensic colleagues, we suggest that forensic cases are very helpful to explore the extent of brain pathology in a population at large, and taking a cisternal sample is simple and quick.

3. Defining early markers of the quadruple aberrant neurodegenerative diseases, including TDP-43 pathology, ought to be the core of our future efforts. MMC residents are showing early clinical symptomatology—including gait and balance alterations, cognitive deficits and MRI volumetric cortical and subcortical abnormalities, all of which may help identify young subjects at higher risk.

4. Exposed children and young adults in highly polluted areas need early neuroprotection and multidisciplinary prevention efforts. Control of combustion and friction UFPM sources and engineered NPs (food products, cosmetics, toothpaste, sun protectors, surface disinfectants, paints, e-waste) is becoming increasingly important and urgent to diminish the human and economic costs of a global neurodegenerative epidemic.

5. UFPM/NP exposure should be included in any assessment of the neurodegenerative risk profile of exposed individuals. No matter the portal of entry, chronic delivery of exogenous particles to the brain induces oxidative stress and neuroinflammation.

6. We have described the overlap of multiple neurodegenerative pathologies; the presence of anthropogenic UFPM in fetal brains; and the early development of AD, PD and TDP-43 pathology, along with their progression and their neuropsychiatric consequences: this body of knowledge resulting from multidisciplinary studies cannot be disregarded by those concerned with public health.

7. We urgently need to practice preventive medicine and develop tools to identify children at risk in order to implement neuroprotective strategies. As neurotoxicologists, we ought to define the mechanistic pathways involving complex NPs containing metalloids, metals, organic compounds, plastics, etc., that can cause extensive brain pathology. As physicians, our focus should be protecting the brains of our future citizens and our younger generations, identifying neurotoxic emission sources and being active players in multidisciplinary teams to prevent, ameliorate or halt neurodegenerative diseases.

Author Contributions: L.C.-G. and R.D.-C.: Conceptualization, Data curation, Formal analysis, Methodology, Investigation, Original draft preparation, Writing—reviewing and editing, Visualization, Supervision. P.S.M.: Formal analysis, Visualization, Investigation, Statistics, Writing—reviewing and editing. R.T.-J.: Air pollution analysis, Data curation, Formal analysis, Writing—reviewing and editing. A.G.-M.: Data curation, Imaging. E.W.S., I.L., K.W., C.-K.C. and E.G.-R.: Data curation, Investigation, Writing—reviewing and editing, Visualization. All authors have read and agreed to the published version of the manuscript.

Funding: This research received no external funding.

Institutional Review Board Statement: The study was conducted in accordance with the Declaration of Helsinki and approved by the review boards and ethics committees at the Universidad del Valle de Mexico, 18 November 2020, and the University of Montana, IRB-206R-09 and IRB 185-20.

Informed Consent Statement: Informed consent was obtained from all subjects involved in the study.

Data Availability Statement: All data necessary to understand and assess the conclusions of this study are available in the main text.

Conflicts of Interest: The authors declare no conflict of interest.

References

1. Calderón-Garcidueñas, L.; Gónzalez-Maciel, A.; Reynoso-Robles, R.; Delgado-Chávez, R.; Mukherjee, P.S.; Kulesza, R.J.; Torres-Jardón, R.; Ávila-Ramírez, J.; Villarreal-Ríos, R. Hallmarks of Alzheimer disease are evolving relentlessly in Metropolitan Mexico City infants, children and young adults. APOE4 carriers have higher suicide risk and higher odds of reaching NFT stage V at ≤40 years of age. *Environ. Res.* **2018**, *164*, 475–487. [CrossRef] [PubMed]
2. Calderón-Garcidueñas, L.; González-Maciel, A.; Reynoso-Robles, R.; Hammond, J.; Kulesza, R.; Lachmann, I.; Torres-Jardón, R.; Mukherjee, P.S.; Maher, B.A. Quadruple abnormal protein aggregates in brainstem pathology and exogenous metal-rich magnetic nanoparticles (and engineered Tirich nanorods). The substantia nigrae is a very early target in young urbanites and the gastrointestinal tract a key brainstem portal. *Environ. Res.* **2020**, *191*, 110139. [CrossRef] [PubMed]
3. Calderón-Garcidueñas, L.; Pérez-Calatayud, A.; González-Maciel, A.; Reynoso-Robles, R.; Silva-Pereyra, H.G.; Ramos-Morales, A.; Torres-Jardón, R.; Soberanes-Cerino, C.D.J.; Carrillo-Esper, R.; Briones-Garduño, J.C.; et al. Environmental Nanoparticles Reach Human Fetal Brains. *Biomedicines* **2022**, *10*, 410. [CrossRef] [PubMed]
4. Calderón-Garcidueñas, L.; Ayala, A. Air Pollution, Ultrafine Particles, and Your Brain: Are Combustion Nanoparticle Emissions and Engineered Nanoparticles Causing Preventable Fatal Neurodegenerative Diseases and Common Neuropsychiatric Outcomes? *Environ. Sci. Technol.* **2022**, *56*, 6847–6856. [CrossRef]
5. Ehsanifar, M.; Yavari, Z.; Rafati, M. Exposure to urban air pollution particulate matter: Neurobehavioral alteration and hippocampal inflammation. *Environ. Sci. Pollut. Res.* **2022**, *29*, 50856–50866. [CrossRef]
6. Jung, C.R.; Lin, Y.T.; Hwang, B. Ozone, particulate matter, and newly diagnosed Alzheimer's disease: A population-based cohort study in Taiwan. *J. Alzheimers Dis.* **2015**, *44*, 573–584. [CrossRef]
7. Lee, P.-C.; Liu, L.-L.; Sun, Y.; Chen, Y.-A.; Liu, C.-C.; Li, C.-Y.; Yu, H.-L.; Ritz, B. Traffic-related air pollution increased the risk of Parkinson's disease in Taiwan: A nationwide study. *Environ. Int.* **2016**, *96*, 75–81. [CrossRef]
8. Chen, H.; Kwong, J.C.; Copes, R.; Tu, K.; Villeneuve, P.J.; van Donkelaar, A.; Hystad, P.; Martin, R.V.; Murray, B.J.; Jessiman, B.; et al. Living near major roads and the incidence of dementia, Parkinson's disease, and multiple sclerosis: A population-based cohort study. *Lancet* **2017**, *389*, 718–726. [CrossRef]
9. Shi, L.; Steenland, K.; Li, H.; Liu, P.; Zhang, Y.; Lyles, R.H.; Requia, W.J.; Ilango, S.D.; Chang, H.H.; Wingo, T.; et al. A national cohort study (2000–2018) of long-term air pollution exposure and incident dementia in older adults in the United States. *Nat. Commun.* **2021**, *12*, 6754. [CrossRef]
10. Mortamais, M.; Gutierrez, L.-A.; de Hoogh, K.; Chen, J.; Vienneau, D.; Carrière, I.; Letellier, N.; Helmer, C.; Gabelle, A.; Mura, T.; et al. Long-term exposure to ambient air pollution and risk of dementia: Results of the prospective Three-City Study. *Environ. Int.* **2021**, *148*, 106376. [CrossRef]
11. Russ, T.C.; Cherrie, M.P.; Dibben, C.; Tomlinson, S.; Reis, S.; Dragosits, U.; Vieno, M.; Beck, R.; Carnell, E.; Shortt, N.K.; et al. Life Course Air Pollution Exposure and Cognitive Decline: Modelled Historical Air Pollution Data and the Lothian Birth Cohort 1936. *J. Alzheimer's Dis.* **2021**, *79*, 1063–1074. [CrossRef] [PubMed]
12. Gładka, A.; Rymaszewska, J.; Zatoński, T. Impact of air pollution on depression and suicide. *Int. J. Occup. Med. Environ. Health* **2018**, *31*, 711–721. [CrossRef] [PubMed]
13. Petkus, A.J.; Resnick, S.M.; Wang, X.; Beavers, D.P.; Espeland, M.A.; Gatz, M.; Gruenewald, T.; Millstein, J.; Chui, H.C.; Kaufman, J.D.; et al. Ambient air pollution exposure and increasing depressive symptoms in older women: The mediating role of the prefrontal cortex and insula. *Sci. Total Environ.* **2022**, *823*, 153642. [CrossRef]
14. Nguyen, A.-M.; Malig, B.J.; Basu, R. The association between ozone and fine particles and mental health-related emergency department visits in California, 2005–2013. *PLoS ONE* **2021**, *16*, e0249675. [CrossRef] [PubMed]

15. Hautekiet, P.; Saenen, N.D.; Demarest, S.; Keune, H.; Pelgrims, I.; Van der Heyden, J.; De Clercq, E.M.; Nawrot, T.S. Air pollution in association with mental and self-rated health and the mediating effect of physical activity. *Environ. Health* **2022**, *21*, 29. [CrossRef]
16. Calderón-Garcidueñas, L.; Mora-Tiscareño, A.; Ontiveros, E.; Gómez-Garza, G.; Barragán-Mejía, G.; Broadway, J. Air pollution, cognitive deficits and brain abnormalities: A pilot study with children and dogs. *Brain Cogn.* **2008**, *68*, 117–127. [CrossRef]
17. Porta, D.; Narduzzi, S.; Badaloni, C.; Bucci, S.; Cesaroni, G.; Colelli, V.; Davoli, M.; Sunyer, J.; Zirro, E.; Schwartz, J.; et al. Air pollution and cognitive development at age seven in a prospective Italian birth cohort. *Epidemiology* **2015**, *27*, 228–236. [CrossRef] [PubMed]
18. Kicinski, M.; Vermeir, G.; Van Larebeke, N.; Hond, E.D.; Schoeters, G.; Bruckers, L.; Sioen, I.; Bijnens, E.; Roels, H.A.; Baeyens, W.; et al. Neurobehavioral performance in adolescents is inversely associated with traffic exposure. *Environ. Int.* **2014**, *75*, 136–143. [CrossRef]
19. Beckwith, T.; Cecil, K.; Altaye, M.; Severs, R.; Wolfe, C.; Percy, Z.; Maloney, T.; Yolton, K.; Lemasters, G.; Brunst, K.; et al. Reduced gray matter volume and cortical thickness associated with traffic-related air pollution in a longitudinally studied pediatric cohort. *PLoS ONE* **2020**, *15*, e0228092. [CrossRef]
20. Carter, S.A.; Rahman, M.; Lin, J.C.; Shu, Y.-H.; Chow, T.; Yu, X.; Martinez, M.P.; Eckel, S.P.; Chen, J.-C.; Chen, Z.; et al. In utero exposure to near-roadway air pollution and autism spectrum disorder in children. *Environ. Int.* **2021**, *158*, 106898. [CrossRef]
21. Gartland, N.; Aljofi, H.E.; Dienes, K.; Munford, L.A.; Theakston, A.L.; van Tongeren, M. The Effects of Traffic Air Pollution in and around Schools on Executive Function and Academic Performance in Children: A Rapid Review. *Int. J. Environ. Res. Public Health* **2022**, *19*, 749. [CrossRef] [PubMed]
22. Maitre, L.; Julvez, J.; López-Vicente, M.; Warembourg, C.; Tamayo-Uria, I.; Philippat, C.; Gützkow, K.B.; Guxens, M.; Andrusaityte, S.; Basagaña, X.; et al. Early-life environmental exposure determinants of child behavior in Europe: A longitudinal, population-based study. *Environ. Int.* **2021**, *153*, 106523. [CrossRef] [PubMed]
23. Ritz, B.; Yan, Q.; He, D.; Wu, J.; Walker, D.I.; Uppal, K.; Jones, D.P.; Heck, J.E. Child serum metabolome and traffic-related air pollution exposure in pregnancy. *Environ. Res.* **2021**, *203*, 111907. [CrossRef] [PubMed]
24. Stone, V.; Miller, M.R.; Clift, M.J.D.; Elder, A.; Mills, N.L.; Møller, P.; Schins, R.P.F.; Vogel, U.; Kreyling, W.G.; Jensen, K.A.; et al. Nanomaterials versus ambient ultrafine particles: An op-portunity to exchange toxicology knowledge. *Environ. Health Perspect.* **2017**, *125*, 106002. [CrossRef] [PubMed]
25. Maher, B.A.; Ahmed, I.A.M.; Karloukovski, V.; MacLaren, D.A.; Foulds, P.G.; Allsop, D.; Mann, D.M.A.; Torres-Jardón, R.; Calderon-Garciduenas, L. Magnetite pollution nanoparticles in the human brain. *Proc. Natl. Acad. Sci. USA* **2016**, *113*, 10797–10801. [CrossRef]
26. Ayala, A. Ultrafine Particles and Air Pollution Policy. In *Ambient Combustion Ultrafine Particles and Health*; Brugge, D., Fuller, C.H., Eds.; Nova Science Publishers: Hauppauge, NY, USA, 2021; ISBN 978-1-53618-831-8.
27. Javdani, N.; Rahpeyma, S.S.; Ghasemi, Y.; Raheb, J. Effect of superparamagnetic nanoparticles coated with various electric charges on α-synuclein and β-amyloid proteins fibrillation process. *Int. J. Nanomed.* **2019**, *14*, 799–808. [CrossRef]
28. Mohammadi, S.; Nikkhah, M. TiO$_2$ Nanoparticles as Potential Promoting Agents of Fibrillation of α-Synuclein, a Parkinson's Disease-Related Protein. *Iran. J. Biotechnol.* **2017**, *15*, 87–94. [CrossRef]
29. Yarjanli, Z.; Ghaedi, K.; Esmaeili, A.; Rahgozar, S.; Zarrabi, A. Iron oxide nanoparticles may damage to the neural tissue through iron accumulation, oxidative stress, and protein aggregation. *BMC Neurosci.* **2017**, *18*, 51. [CrossRef]
30. Calderón-Garcidueñas, L.; Cross, J.V.; Franco-Lira, M.; Aragón-Flores, M.; Kavanaugh, M.; Torres-Jardón, R.; Chao, C.K.; Thompson, C.; Chang, J.; Zhu, H.; et al. Brain immune interactions and air pollution: Macrophage inhibitory factor (MIF), prion cellular protein (PrPc), interleukin-6 (IL6), interleukin 1 receptor antagonist (IL-1Ra), and interleukin-2 (IL-2) in cerebrospinal fluid and MIF in serum differentiate urban children exposed to severe vs. low air pollution. *Front Neurosci.* **2013**, *7*, 183–194. [CrossRef]
31. Calderón-Garcidueñas, L.; Chao, C.; Thompson, C.; Rodríguez-Díaz, J.; Franco-Lira, M.; Mukherjee, P.S.; Perry, G. CSF biomarkers: Low amyloid β $_{1-42}$ and BDNF and High IFNγ differentiate children exposed to Mexico City High air pollution v controls. Alzheimer's disease uncertainties. *Alzheimer's Dis. Parkinsonism* **2015**, *5*, 2.
32. Calderón-Garcidueñas, L.; Avila-Ramírez, J.; González-Heredia, T.; Acuña-Ayala, H.; Chao, C.-K.; Thompson, C.; Ruiz-Ramos, R.; Cortés-González, V.; Martínez-Martínez, L.; García-Pérez, M.A.; et al. Cerebrospinal Fluid Biomarkers in Highly Exposed PM2.5 Urbanites: The Risk of Alzheimer's and Parkinson's Diseases in Young Mexico City Residents. *J. Alzheimer's Dis.* **2016**, *54*, 597–613. [CrossRef] [PubMed]
33. Calderón-Garcidueñas, L.; Mukherjee, P.S.; Waniek, K.; Holzer, M.; Chao, C.-K.; Thompson, C.; Ruiz-Ramos, R.; Franco-Lira, M.; Reynoso-Robles, R.; Gónzalez-Maciel, A.; et al. Non-Phosphorylated Tau in Cerebrospinal Fluid is a Marker of Alzheimer's Disease Continuum in Young Urbanites Exposed to Air Pollution. *J. Alzheimer's Dis.* **2018**, *66*, 1437–1451. [CrossRef] [PubMed]
34. Calderón-Garcidueñas, L.; Vojdani, A.; Blaurock-Busch, E.; Busch, Y.; Friedle, A.; Franco-Lira, M.; Sarathi-Mukherjee, P.; Martínez-Aguirre, X.; Park, S.; Torres-Jardón, R.; et al. Air pollution and children: Neural and tight junction antibodies and combustion metals, the role of barrier breakdown and brain immunity in neurodegeneration. *J. Alzheimer. Dis.* **2015**, *43*, 1039–1058. [CrossRef] [PubMed]

35. Calderón-Garcidueñas, L.; Serrano-Sierra, A.; Torres-Jardón, R.; Zhu, H.; Yuan, Y.; Smith, D.; Delgado-Chávez, R.; Cross, J.V.; Medina-Cortina, H.; Kavanaugh, M.; et al. The impact of environmental metals in young urbanites' brains. *Exp. Toxicol. Pathol.* **2013**, *65*, 503–511. [CrossRef] [PubMed]
36. Reiber, H. Non-linear ventriculo–Lumbar protein gradients validate the diffusion-flow model for the blood-CSF barrier. *Clin. Chim. Acta* **2020**, *513*, 64–67. [CrossRef]
37. Reiber, H. Blood-cerebrospinal fluid (CSF) barrier dysfunction means reduced CSF flow not barrier leakage-conclusions from CSF protein data. *Arq. De Neuro-Psiquiatr.* **2021**, *79*, 56–67. [CrossRef]
38. Peyron, P.-A.; Hirtz, C.; Baccino, E.; Ginestet, N.; Tiers, L.; Martinez, A.Y.; Lehmann, S.; Delaby, C. Tau protein in cerebrospinal fluid: A novel biomarker of the time of death? *Int. J. Legal. Med.* **2021**, *135*, 2081–2089. [CrossRef]
39. Brettschneider, J.; Del Tredici, K.; Toledo, J.B.; Robinson, J.L.; Irwin, D.J.; Grossman, M.; Suh, E.R.; Van Deerlin, V.M.; Wood, E.M.; Baek, Y.; et al. Stages of pTDP-43 pathology in amyotrophic lateral sclerosis. *Ann. Neurol.* **2013**, *74*, 20–38. [CrossRef]
40. Braak, H.; Del Tredici, K. Anterior Cingulate Cortex TDP-43 Pathology in Sporadic Amyotrophic Lateral Sclerosis. *J. Neuropathol. Exp. Neurol.* **2017**, *77*, 74–83. [CrossRef]
41. James, B.D.; Wilson, R.S.; Boyle, P.A.; Trojanowski, J.Q.; Bennett, D.A.; Schneider, J.A. TDP-43 stage, mixed pathol-ogies, and clinical Alzheimer's-type dementia. *Brain* **2016**, *139*, 2983–2993. [CrossRef]
42. Nelson, P.T.; Dickson, D.W.; Trojanowski, J.Q.; Jack, C.R.; Boyle, P.A.; Arfanakis, K.; Rademakers, R.; Alafuzoff, I.; Attems, J.; Brayne, C.; et al. Limbic-predominant age-related TDP-43 encephalopathy (LATE): Consensus working group report. *Brain* **2019**, *142*, 1503–1527. [CrossRef] [PubMed]
43. Jamshidi, P.; Kim, G.; Shahidehpour, R.K.; Bolbolan, K.; Gefen, T.; Bigio, E.H.; Mesulam, M.-M.; Geula, C. Distribution of TDP-43 Pathology in Hippocampal Synaptic Relays Suggests Transsynaptic Propagation in Frontotemporal Lobar Degeneration. *J. Neuropathol. Exp. Neurol.* **2020**, *79*, 585–591. [CrossRef] [PubMed]
44. Geula, C.; Keszycki, R.; Jamshidi, P.; Kawles, A.; Minogue, G.; Flanagan, M.E.; Zaccard, C.R.; Mesulam, M.M.; Gefen, T. Propagation of TDP-43 proteinopathy in neurodegenerative disorders. *Neural Regen. Res.* **2022**, *17*, 1498. [CrossRef] [PubMed]
45. Calderón-Garcidueñas, L.; Rajkumar, R.P.; Stommel, E.W.; Kulesza, R.; Mansour, Y.; Rico-Villanueva, A.; Flores-Vázquez, J.O.; Brito-Aguilar, R.; Ramírez-Sánchez, S.; García-Alonso, G.; et al. Brain-stem Quadruple Aberrant Hyperphosphorylated Tau, Beta-Amyloid, Alpha-Synuclein and TDP-43 Pathology, Stress and Sleep Behavior Disorders. *Int. J. Environ. Res. Public Health* **2021**, *18*, 6689. [CrossRef] [PubMed]
46. Calderón-Garcidueñas, L.; González-Maciel, A.; Reynoso-Robles, R.; Silva-Pereyra, H.G.; Torres-Jardón, R.; Brito-Aguilar, R.; Ayala, A.; Stommel, E.W.; Delgado-Chávez, R. Environmentally Toxic Solid Nanoparticles in Noradrenergic and Dopaminergic Nuclei and Cerebellum of Metropolitan Mexico City Children and Young Adults with Neural Quadruple Misfolded Protein Pathologies and High Exposures to Nano Particulate Matter. *Toxics* **2022**, *10*, 164. [CrossRef]
47. Garcia-Gomar, M.G.; Videnovic, A.; Singh, K.; Stauder, M.; Lewis, L.D.; Wald, L.L.; Rosen, B.R.; Bianciardi, M. Disruption of Brain-stem Structural Connectivity in REM Sleep Behavior Disorder Using 7 Tesla Magnetic Resonance Imaging. *Mov. Disord.* **2022**, *37*, 847–853. [CrossRef]
48. Singh, K.; Cauzzo, S.; García-Gomar, M.G.; Stauder, M.; Vanello, N.; Passino, C.; Bianciardi, M. Functional connectome of arousal and motor brainstem nuclei in living humans by 7 Tesla resting-state fMRI. *NeuroImage* **2022**, *249*, 118865. [CrossRef]
49. Llibre-Guerra, J.J.; Behrens, M.I.; Hosogi, M.L.; Montero, L.; Torralva, T.; Custodio, N.; Longoria-Ibarrola, E.M.; Giraldo-Chica, M.; Aguillón, D.; Hardi, A.; et al. Frontotemporal Dementias in Latin America: History, Epidemiology, Genetics, and Clinical Research. *Front. Neurol.* **2021**, *12*, 710332. [CrossRef]
50. Cervantes-Aragón, I.; Ramírez-García, S.A.; Baltazar-Rodríguez, L.M.; García-Cruz, D.; Castañeda-Cisneros, G. Genetic approach in amyotrophic lateral sclerosis. *Gac. Med. Mex.* **2020**, *155*, 475–482. [CrossRef]
51. Bos, M.V.D.; Geevasinga, N.; Higashihara, M.; Menon, P.; Vucic, S. Pathophysiology and Diagnosis of ALS: Insights from Advances in Neurophysiological Techniques. *Int. J. Mol. Sci.* **2019**, *20*, 2818. [CrossRef]
52. Barker, M.S.; Gottesman, R.T.; Manoochehri, M.; Chapman, S.; Appleby, B.S.; Brushaber, D.; Devick, K.L.; Dickerson, B.C.; Domoto-Reilly, K.; Fields, J.A.; et al. Proposed research criteria for prodromal behavioural variant frontotemporal dementia. *Brain* **2022**, *145*, 1079–1097. [CrossRef] [PubMed]
53. Caudillo, L.; Salcedo, D.; Peralta, O.; Castro, T.; Alvarez-Ospina, H. Nanoparticle size distributions in Mexico city. *Atmos. Pollut. Res.* **2019**, *11*, 78–84. [CrossRef]
54. Velasco, E.; Retama, A.; Segovia, E.; Ramos, R. Particle exposure and inhaled dose while commuting by public transport in Mexico City. *Atmos. Environ.* **2019**, *219*, 117044. [CrossRef]
55. Mugica-Álvarez, V.; Figueroa-Lara, J.; Romero-Romo, M.; Sepúlveda-Sánchez, J.; López-Moreno, T. Concentrations and properties of airborne particles in the Mexico City subway system. *Atmos. Environ.* **2012**, *49*, 284–293. [CrossRef]
56. Hernández-López, A.E.; Miranda Martín del Campo, J.; Mugica Álvarez, V.; Valle-Hernández, B.L.; Mejía-Ponce, L.V.; Pineda-Santamaría, J.C.; Reynoso-Cru, S.; Mendoza-Flores1, J.A.; Rozanes-Valenz, D. A study of PM2.5 elemental composition in southwest Mexico City and development of receptor models with positive matrix factorization. *Rev. Int. Contam. Ambie.* **2021**, *37*, 67–88. [CrossRef]
57. Molina, L.T.; Velasco, E.; Retama, A.; Zavala, M. Experience from Integrated Air Quality Management in the Mexico City Metropolitan Area and Singapore. *Atmosphere* **2019**, *10*, 512. [CrossRef]

58. Zavala, M.; Brune, W.H.; Velasco, E.; Retama, A.; Cruz-Alavez, L.A.; Molina, L.T. Changes in ozone production and VOC reactivity in the atmosphere of the Mexico City Metropolitan Area. *Atmos. Environ.* **2020**, *238*, 117747. [CrossRef]
59. Velasco, E.; Retama, A. Ozone's threat hits back Mexico City. *Sustain. Cities Soc.* **2017**, *31*, 260–263. [CrossRef]
60. Dunn, M.J.; Jiménez, J.-L.; Baumgardner, D.; Castro, T.; McMurry, P.H.; Smith, J.N. Measurements of Mexico City nanoparticle size distributions: Observations of new particle formation and growth. *Geophys. Res. Lett.* **2004**, *31*. [CrossRef]
61. Kleinman, L.I.; Springston, S.R.; Wang, J.; Daum, P.H.; Lee, Y.N.; Nunnermacker, L.J.; Senum, G.I.; Weinstein-Lloyd, J.; Alexander, M.L.; Hubbe, J.; et al. The time evolution of aerosol size distribution over the Mexico City plateau. *Atmos. Chem. Phys.* **2009**, *9*, 4261–4278. [CrossRef]
62. Morton-Bermea, O.; Garza-Galindo, R.; Hernández-Álvarez, E.; Ordoñez-Godínez, S.L.; Amador-Muñoz, O.; Beramendi-Orosco, L.; Miranda, J.; Rosas-Pérez, I. Atmospheric PM2.5 Mercury in the Metropolitan Area of Mexico City. *Bull. Environ. Contam. Toxicol.* **2018**, *100*, 588–592. [CrossRef] [PubMed]
63. Kumar, P.; Morawska, L.; Birmili, W.; Paasonen, P.; Hu, M.; Kulmala, M.; Harrison, R.M.; Norford, L.; Britter, R. Ultrafine particles in cities. *Environ. Int.* **2014**, *66*, 1–10. [CrossRef] [PubMed]
64. Mugica, V.; Hernández, S.; Torres, M.; García, R. Seasonal Variation of Polycyclic Aromatic Hydrocarbon Exposure Levels in Mexico City. *J. Air Waste Manag. Assoc.* **2010**, *60*, 548–555. [CrossRef] [PubMed]
65. Cárdenas, B.; Alberto, A.; Benitez, S.; González, E.H.; Jaimes, M.; Retama, A. Ultrafine Particles in Mexico City Metropolitan Area: A review. In Proceedings of the 7th International Symposium on Ultrafine Particles, Air Quality and Climate, Brüssel, Belgien, 15–16 May 2019.
66. Steinacker, P.; Hendrich, C.; Sperfeld, A.D.; Jesse, S.; von Arnim, C.A.F.; Lehnert, S.; Pabst, A.; Uttner, I.; Tumani, H.; Lee, V.M.-Y.; et al. TDP-43 in Cerebrospinal Fluid of Patients With Frontotemporal Lobar Degeneration and Amyotrophic Lateral Sclerosis. *Arch. Neurol.* **2008**, *65*, 1481–1487. [CrossRef] [PubMed]
67. Pandya, S.; Maia, P.D.; Freeze, B.; Menke, R.A.L.; Talbot, K.; Turner, M.R.; Raj, A. Modeling seeding and neuroanatomic spread of pathology in amyotrophic lateral sclerosis. *NeuroImage* **2022**, *251*, 118968. [CrossRef]
68. Hasan, R.; Humphrey, J.; Bettencourt, C.; Newcombe, J.; NYGC ALS Consortium; Lashley, T.; Fratta, P.; Raj, T. Transcriptomic analysis of frontotemporal lobar degeneration with TDP-43 pathology reveals cellular alterations across multiple brain regions. *Acta Neuropathol.* **2022**, *143*, 383–401. [CrossRef] [PubMed]
69. Calderón-Garcidueñas, L.; Hernández-Luna, J.; Mukherjee, P.S.; Styner, M.; Chávez-Franco, D.A.; Luévano-Castro, S.C.; Crespo-Cortés, C.N.; Stommel, E.W.; Torres-Jardón, R. Hemispheric Cortical, Cerebellar and Caudate Atrophy Associated to Cognitive Impairment in Metropolitan Mexico City Young Adults Exposed to Fine Particulate Matter Air Pollution. *Toxics* **2022**, *10*, 156. [CrossRef]
70. Shafiei, G.; Bazinet, V.; Dadar, M.; Manera, A.L.; Collins, D.L.; Dagher, A.; Borroni, B.; Sanchez-Valle, R.; Moreno, F.; Laforce, R.; et al. Network structure and transcriptomic vulnerability shape atrophy in frontotemporal dementia. *Brain* **2022**, awac069. [CrossRef]
71. Karanth, S.; Nelson, P.T.; Katsumata, Y.; Kryscio, R.J.; Schmitt, F.A.; Fardo, D.W.; Cykowski, M.D.; Jicha, G.A.; Van Eldik, L.J.; Abner, E.L. Prevalence and Clinical Phenotype of Quadruple Misfolded Proteins in Older Adults. *JAMA Neurol.* **2020**, *77*, 1299–1307. [CrossRef]
72. Scarioni, M.; Gami-Patel, P.; Peeters, C.F.W.; de Koning, F.; Seelaar, H.; Mol, M.O.; van Swieten, J.C.; Rozemuller, A.J.M.; Hoozemans, J.J.M.; Pijnenburg, Y.A.L.; et al. Psychiatric symptoms of frontotemporal dementia and subcortical (co-)pathology burden: New insights. *Brain* **2022**, awac043. [CrossRef]
73. Ohm, D.T.; Cousins, K.A.Q.; Xie, S.X.; Peterson, C.; McMillan, C.T.; Massimo, L.; Raskovsky, K.; Wolk, D.A.; Van Deerlin, V.M.; Elman, L.; et al. Signature laminar distributions of pathology in frontotemporal lobar degeneration. *Acta Neuropathol.* **2022**, *143*, 363–382. [CrossRef] [PubMed]
74. Tisdall, M.D.; Ohm, D.T.; Lobrovich, R.; Das, S.R.; Mizsei, G.; Prabhakaran, K.; Ittyerah, R.; Lim, S.; McMillan, C.T.; Wolk, D.A.; et al. Ex vivo MRI and histopathology detect novel iron-rich cortical inflammation in frontotemporal lobar degeneration with tau versus TDP-43 pathology. *NeuroImage: Clin.* **2021**, *33*, 102913. [CrossRef] [PubMed]
75. Bayram, E.; Shan, G.; Cummings, J.L. Associations between Comorbid TDP-43, Lewy Body Pathology, and Neuropsychiatric Symptoms in Alzheimer's Disease. *J. Alzheimers Dis.* **2019**, *69*, 953–961. [CrossRef] [PubMed]
76. Sennik, S.; Schweizer, T.A.; Fischer, C.E.; Munoz, D.G. Risk Factors and Pathological Substrates Associated with Agitation/Aggression in Alzheimer's Disease: A Preliminary Study using NACC Data. *J. Alzheimers Dis.* **2017**, *55*, 1519–1528. [CrossRef] [PubMed]
77. Kon, T.; Mori, F.; Tanji, K.; Miki, Y.; Nishijima, H.; Nakamura, T.; Kinoshita, I.; Suzuki, C.; Kurotaki, H.; Tomiyama, M.; et al. Accumulation of Nonfibrillar TDP-43 in the Rough En-doplasmic Reticulum Is the Early-Stage Pathology in Amyotrophic Lateral Sclerosis. *J. Neuropathol. Exp. Neurol.* **2022**, *81*, 271–281. [CrossRef]
78. Andrew, A.; Zhou, J.; Gui, J.; Harrison, A.; Shi, X.; Li, M.; Guetti, B.; Nathan, R.; Tischbein, M.; Pioro, E.; et al. Airborne lead and polychlorinated biphenyls (PCBs) are associated with amyotrophic lateral sclerosis (ALS) risk in the U.S. *Sci. Total Environ.* **2022**, *819*, 153096. [CrossRef] [PubMed]
79. Vandenbulcke, M.; Van de Vliet, L.; Sun, J.; Huang, Y.-A.; Bossche, M.J.A.V.D.; Sunaert, S.; Peeters, R.; Zhu, Q.; Vanduffel, W.; de Gelder, B.; et al. A paleo-neurologic investigation of the social brain hypothesis in frontotemporal dementia. *Cereb. Cortex* **2022**, bhac089. [CrossRef]

80. Lulé, D.; Michels, S.; Finsel, J.; Braak, H.; Del Tredici, K.; Strobel, J.; Beer, A.J.; Uttner, I.; Müller, H.-P.; Kassubek, J.; et al. Clinicoanatomical substrates of selfish behaviour in amyotrophic lateral sclerosis—An observational cohort study. *Cortex* 2021, *146*, 261–270. [CrossRef]
81. Mendez, M.F. Behavioral Variant Frontotemporal Dementia and Social and Criminal Transgressions. *J. Neuropsychiatry Clin. Neurosci.* 2022, 21080224. [CrossRef]
82. Fondevila, G.; Meneses-Reyes, R. Lethal Violence, Childhood, and Gender in Mexico City. *Int. Crim. Justice Rev.* 2017, *29*, 33–47. [CrossRef]
83. Violencia en México. Available online: http://www.seguridadjusticiaypaz.org.mx/ (accessed on 10 May 2022).
84. Mangold, S.A.; Das, J.M. Neuroanatomy, Reticular Formation. In *StatPearls [Internet]*; StatPearls Publishing: Treasure Island, FL, USA, 2022.
85. Cauzzo, S.; Singh, K.; Stauder, M.; García-Gomar, M.G.; Vanello, N.; Passino, C.; Staab, J.; Indovina, I.; Bianciardi, M. Functional connectome of brainstem nuclei involved in autonomic, limbic, pain and sensory processing in living humans from 7 Tesla resting state fMRI. *NeuroImage* 2022, *250*, 118925. [CrossRef] [PubMed]
86. Wang, N.; Perkins, E.; Zhou, L.; Warren, S.; May, P.J. Reticular Formation Connections Underlying Horizontal Gaze: The Central Mesencephalic Reticular Formation (cMRF) as a Conduit for the Collicular Saccade Signal. *Front. Neuroanat.* 2017, *11*, 36. [CrossRef] [PubMed]
87. Leisman, G.; Melillo, R. Front and center: Maturational dysregulation of frontal lobe functional neuroanatomic connections in attention deficit hyperactivity disorder. *Front. Neuroanat.* 2022, *16*, 936025. [CrossRef] [PubMed]
88. Brown, R.E.; Spratt, T.J.; Kaplan, G.B. Translational approaches to influence sleep and arousal. *Brain Res. Bull.* 2022, *185*, 140–161. [CrossRef]
89. Liu, S.; Ye, M.; Pao, G.M.; Song, S.M.; Jhang, J.; Jiang, H.; Kim, J.-H.; Kang, S.J.; Kim, D.-I.; Han, S. Divergent brainstem opioidergic pathways that coordinate breathing with pain and emotions. *Neuron* 2021, *110*, 857–873.e9. [CrossRef]
90. Bourilhon, J.; Mullie, Y.; Olivier, C.; Cherif, S.; Belaid, H.; Grabli, D.; Czernecki, V.; Karachi, C.; Welter, M.L. Stimulation of the pe-dunculopontine and cuneiform nuclei for freezing of gait and falls in Parkinson disease: Cross-over single-blinded study and long-term follow-up. *Parkinsonism Relat Disord* 2022, *96*, 13–17. [CrossRef]
91. Burdge, J.; Jhumka, Z.A.; Bravo, I.M.; Abdus-Saboor, I. Taking a deep breath: How a brainstem pathway integrates pain and breathing. *Neuron* 2022, *110*, 739–741. [CrossRef]
92. Özkan, M.; Köse, B.; Algın, O.; Oğuz, S.; Erden, M.E.; Çavdar, S. Non-motor connections of the pedunculopontine nucleus of the rat and human brain. *Neurosci. Lett.* 2021, *767*, 136308. [CrossRef]
93. Robinson, D.A. Neurophysiology of the saccadic system: The reticular formation. *Prog. Brain Res.* 2022, *267*, 355–378. [CrossRef]
94. He, S.; Deli, A.; Fischer, P.; Wiest, C.; Huang, Y.; Martin, S.; Khawaldeh, S.; Aziz, T.Z.; Green, A.L.; Brown, P.; et al. Gait-Phase Modulates Alpha and Beta Oscillations in the Pedunculopontine Nucleus. *J. Neurosci.* 2021, *41*, 8390–8402. [CrossRef]
95. Singh, K.; Garcia-Gomar, M.G.; Bianciardi, M. Probabilistic Atlas of the Mesencephalic Reticular Formation, Isthmic Reticular Formation, Microcellular Tegmental Nucleus, Ventral Tegmental Area Nucleus Complex, and Caudal-Rostral Linear Raphe Nucleus Complex in Living Humans from 7 Tesla Magnetic Resonance Imaging. *Brain Connect* 2021, *11*, 613–623. [PubMed]
96. Coulombe, V.; Saikali, S.; Goetz, L.; Takech, M.A.; Philippe, E.; Parent, A.; Parent, M. A Topographic Atlas of the Human Brainstem in the Ponto-Mesencephalic Junction Plane. *Front. Neuroanat.* 2021, *15*, 627656. [CrossRef]
97. Calderón-Garcidueñas, L.; Torres-Solorio, A.K.; Kulesza, R.J.; Torres-Jardón, R.; González-González, L.O.; García-Arreola, B.; Chávez-Franco, D.A.; Luévano-Castro, S.C.; Hernández-Castillo, A.; Carlos-Hernández, E.; et al. Gait and balance disturbances are common in young urbanites and associated with cognitive impairment. Air pollution and the historical development of Alzheimer's disease in the young. *Environ. Res.* 2020, *191*, 110087. [CrossRef] [PubMed]
98. Braak, H.; Ludoph, A.; Thal, D.R.; Del Tredeci, K. Amyotrophic lateral sclerosis: Dash-like accumulation of phosphorylated TDP-43 in somatodendritic and axonal compartments of somatomotor neurons of the lower brainstem and spinal cord. *Acta Neuropathol.* 2010, *120*, 67–74. [CrossRef] [PubMed]
99. Thal, D.R.; Del Tredici, K.; Ludolph, A.C.; Hoozemans, J.; Rozemuller, A.J.; Braak, H.; Knippschild, U. Stages of granulovacuolar degeneration: Their relation to Alzheimer's disease and chronic stress response. *Acta Neuropathol.* 2011, *122*, 577–589. [CrossRef]
100. Brettschneider, J.; Arai, K.; Del Tredici, K.; Toledo, J.B.; Robinson, J.L.; Lee, E.B.; Kuwabara, S.; Shibuya, K.; Irwin, D.J.; Fang, L.; et al. TDP-43 pathology and neuronal loss in amyotrophic lateral sclerosis spinal cord. *Acta Neuropathol.* 2014, *128*, 423–437. [CrossRef]
101. Eisen, A.; Braak, H.; Del Tredici, K.; Lemon, R.; Ludolph, A.C.; Kiernan, M.C. Cortical influences drive amyotrophic lateral sclerosis. *J. Neurol. Neurosurg. Psychiatry* 2017, *88*, 917–924. [CrossRef]
102. Del Tredici, K.; Braal, H. Neuropathology and neuroanatomy of TDP-43 amyotrophic lateral sclerosis. *Curr. Opin. Neurol.* 2022, *35*, 660–671. [CrossRef]
103. Šušnjar, U.; Škrabar, N.; Brown, A.-L.; Abbassi, Y.; Phatnani, H.; Fratta, P.; Kwan, J.; Sareen, D.; Broach, J.R.; Simmons, Z.; et al. Cell environment shapes TDP-43 function with implications in neuronal and muscle disease. *Commun. Biol.* 2022, *5*, 314. [CrossRef]
104. Koper, M.J.; Tomé, S.O.; Gawor, K.; Belet, A.; Van Schoor, E.; Schaeverbeke, J.; Vandenberghe, R.; Vandenbulcke, M.; Ghebremedhin, E.; Otto, M.; et al. LATE-NC aggravates GVD-mediated necroptosis in Alzheimer's disease. *Acta Neuropathol. Commun.* 2022, *10*, 128. [CrossRef]

105. Kawles, A.; Nishihira, Y.; Feldman, A.; Gill, N.; Minogue, G.; Keszycki, R.; Coventry, C.; Spencer, C.; Lilek, J.; Ajroud, K.; et al. Cortical and subcortical pathological burden and neuronal loss in an autopsy series of FTLD-TDP-type C. *Brain* **2021**, *145*, 1069–1078. [CrossRef] [PubMed]
106. Sainouchi, M.; Tada, M.; Fitrah, Y.A.; Hara, N.; Tanaka, K.; Idezuka, J.; Aida, I.; Nakajima, T.; Miyashita, A.; Akazawa, K.; et al. Brain TDP-43 pathology in corticobasal degeneration: Topographical correlation with neuronal loss. *Neuropathol. Appl. Neurobiol.* **2021**, *48*, e12786. [CrossRef]
107. Aizawa, H.; Teramoto, S.; Hideyama, T.; Kato, H.; Terashi, H.; Suzuki, Y.; Kimura, T.; Kwak, S. Nuclear pore destruction and loss of nuclear TDP-43 in FUS mutation-related amyotrophic lateral sclerosis motor neurons. *J. Neurol. Sci.* **2022**, *436*, 120187. [CrossRef]
108. Keating, S.S.; Gil, R.S.; Swanson, M.E.; Scotter, E.L.; Walker, A.K. TDP-43 pathology: From noxious assembly to therapeutic removal. *Prog. Neurobiol.* **2022**, *211*, 102229. [CrossRef] [PubMed]
109. Altman, T.; Ionescu, A.; Ibraheem, A.; Priesmann, D.; Gradus-Pery, T.; Farberov, L.; Alexandra, G.; Shelestovich, N.; Dafinca, R.; Shomron, N.; et al. Axonal TDP-43 condensates drive neuromuscular junction disruption through inhibition of local synthesis of nuclear encoded mitochondrial proteins. *Nat. Commun.* **2021**, *12*, 6914. [CrossRef] [PubMed]
110. Homma, H.; Tanaka, H.; Jin, M.; Jin, X.; Huang, Y.; Yoshioka, Y.; Bertens, C.J.; Tsumaki, K.; Kondo, K.; Shiwaku, H.; et al. DNA damage in embryonic neural stem cell determines FTLDs' fate via early-stage neuronal necrosis. *Life Sci. Alliance* **2021**, *4*, e202101022. [CrossRef] [PubMed]
111. Ahmed, R.M.; Halliday, G.; Hodges, J.R. Hypothalamic symptoms of frontotemporal dementia disorders. *Handb. Clin. Neurol.* **2021**, *182*, 269–280. [CrossRef] [PubMed]
112. Virgilio, E.; De Marchi, F.; Contaldi, E.; Dianzani, U.; Cantello, R.; Mazzini, L.; Comi, C. The Role of Tau beyond Alzheimer's Disease: A Narrative Review. *Biomedicines* **2022**, *10*, 760. [CrossRef]
113. Carlos, A.F.; Tosakulwong, N.; Weigand, S.D.; Boeve, B.F.; Knopman, D.S.; Petersen, R.C.; Nguyen, A.; Reichard, R.R.; Murray, M.E.; Dickson, D.W.; et al. Frequency and distribution of TAR DNA-binding protein 43 (TDP-43) pathology increase linearly with age in a large cohort of older adults with and without dementia. *Acta Neuropathol.* **2022**, *144*, 159–160. [CrossRef]
114. Esteban-García, N.; Fernández-Beltrán, L.C.; Godoy-Corchuelo, J.M.; Ayala, J.L.; Matias-Guiu, J.A.; Corrochano, S. Body Complexion and Circulating Lipids in the Risk of TDP-43 Related Disorders. *Front. Aging Neurosci.* **2022**, *14*, 838141. [CrossRef]
115. Zetterberg, H. Biofluid-based biomarkers for Alzheimer's disease-related pathologies: An update and synthesis of the literature. *Alzheimers Dement* **2022**, *18*, 1687–1693. [CrossRef] [PubMed]
116. Körtvelyessy, P.; Heinze, H.J.; Prudlo, J.; Bittner, D. CSF Biomarkers of Neurodegeneration in Progressive Non-fluent Aphasia and Other Forms of Frontotemporal Dementia: Clues for Pathomechanisms? *Front. Neurol.* **2018**, *9*, 504. [CrossRef] [PubMed]
117. Del Campo, M.; Galimberti, D.; Elias, N.; Boonkamp, L.; Pijnenburg, Y.A.; van Swieten, J.C.; Watts, K.; Paciotti, S.; Beccari, T.; Hu, W.; et al. Novel CSF biomarkers to discriminate FTLD and its pathological subtypes. *Ann. Clin. Transl. Neurol.* **2018**, *5*, 1163–1175. [CrossRef] [PubMed]
118. Molinuevo, J.L.; Ayton, S.; Batrla, R.; Bednar, M.M.; Bittner, T.; Cummings, J.; Fagan, A.M.; Hampel, H.; Mielke, M.M.; Mikulskis, A.; et al. Current state of Alzheimer's fluid biomarkers. *Acta Neuropathol.* **2018**, *136*, 821–853. [CrossRef] [PubMed]
119. Foiani, M.S.; Cicognola, C.; Ermann, N.; Woollacott, I.O.C.; Heller, C.; Heslegrave, A.J.; Keshavan, A.; Paterson, R.W.; Ye, K.; Kornhuber, J.; et al. Searching for novel cerebrospinal fluid biomarkers of tau pathology in frontotemporal dementia: An elusive quest. *J. Neurol. Neurosurg. Psychiatry* **2019**, *90*, 740–746. [CrossRef] [PubMed]
120. Khosla, R.; Rain, M.; Sharma, S.; Anand, A. Amyotrophic Lateral Sclerosis (ALS) prediction model derived from plasma and CSF biomarkers. *PLoS ONE* **2021**, *16*, e0247025. [CrossRef] [PubMed]
121. Escal, J.; Fourier, A.; Formaglio, M.; Zimmer, L.; Bernard, E.; Mollion, H.; Bost, M.; Herrmann, M.; Ollagnon-Roman, E.; Quadrio, I.; et al. Comparative diagnosis interest of NfL and pNfH in CSF and plasma in a context of FTD–ALS spectrum. *J. Neurol.* **2021**, *269*, 1522–1529. [CrossRef]
122. Chouliaras, L.; Thomas, A.; Malpetti, M.; Donaghy, P.; Kane, J.; Mak, E.; Savulich, G.; Prats-Sedano, M.A.; Heslegrave, A.J.; Zetterberg, H.; et al. Differential levels of plasma biomarkers of neurodegeneration in Lewy body dementia, Alzheimer's disease, frontotemporal dementia and progressive supranuclear palsy. *J. Neurol. Neurosurg. Psychiatry* **2022**, *93*, 651–658. [CrossRef]
123. Calderón-Garcidueñas, L.; Mukherjee, P.S.; Kulesza, R.J.; Torres-Jardón, R.; Hernández-Luna, J.; Ávila-Cervantes, R.; Macías-Escobedo, E.; González-González, O.; González-Maciel, A.; García-Hernández, K.; et al. Mild Cognitive Impairment and Dementia Involving Multiple Cognitive Domains in Mexican Urbanites. *J. Alzheimers Dis.* **2019**, *68*, 1113–1123. [CrossRef]
124. Calderón-Garcidueñas, L.; Chávez-Franco, D.A.; Luévano-Castro, S.C.; Macías-Escobedo, E.; Hernández-Castillo, A.; Carlos-Hernández, E.; Franco-Ortíz, A.; Castro-Romero, S.P.; Cortés-Flores, M.; Crespo-Cortés, C.N.; et al. Metals, Nanoparticles, Particulate Matter, and Cognitive Decline. *Front. Neurol.* **2022**, *12*, 794071. [CrossRef]
125. Calderón-Garcidueñas, L.; González-González, L.O.; Kulesza, R.J.; Fech, T.M.; Pérez-Guillé, G.; Luna, M.A.J.-B.; Soriano-Rosales, R.E.; Solorio, E.; Miramontes-Higuera, J.D.J.; Chew, A.G.-M.; et al. Exposures to fine particulate matter (PM2.5) and ozone above USA standards are associated with auditory brainstem dysmorphology and abnormal auditory brainstem evoked potentials in healthy young dogs. *Environ. Res.* **2017**, *158*, 324–332. [CrossRef] [PubMed]
126. Milà-Alomà, M.; Suárez-Calvet, M.; Molinuevo, J.L. Latest advances in cerebrospinal fluid and blood biomarkers of Alzheimer's disease. *Ther. Adv. Neurol. Disord.* **2019**, *12*, 1756286419888819. [CrossRef] [PubMed]

127. Smirnov, D.S.; Ashton, N.J.; Blennow, K.; Zetterberg, H.; Simrén, J.; Lantero-Rodriguez, J.; Karikari, T.K.; Hiniker, A.; Rissman, R.A.; Salmon, D.P.; et al. Plasma biomarkers for Alzheimer's Disease in relation to neuropathology and cognitive change. *Acta Neuropathol.* **2022**, *143*, 487–503. [CrossRef] [PubMed]
128. González, A.C.; Irwin, D.J.; Alcolea, D.; McMillan, C.T.; Chen-Plotkin, A.; Wolk, D.; Sirisi, S.; Dols-Icardo, O.; Querol-Vilaseca, M.; Illán-Gala, I.; et al. Multimarker synaptic protein cerebrospinal fluid panels reflect TDP-43 pathology and cognitive performance in a pathological cohort of frontotemporal lobar degeneration. *Mol. Neurodegener.* **2022**, *17*, 29. [CrossRef]
129. Irwin, D.J.; Lleó, A.; Xie, S.X.; McMillan, C.T.; Wolk, D.A.; Lee, E.B.; Van Deerlin, V.M.; Shaw, L.M.; Trojanowski, J.Q.; Grossman, M. Ante mortem cerebrospinal fluid tau levels correlate with postmortem tau pathology in frontotemporal lobar degeneration. *Ann. Neurol.* **2017**, *82*, 247–258. [CrossRef]
130. Re, D.B.; Yan, B.; Calderón-Garciduéñas, L.; Andrew, A.S.; Tischbein, M.; Stommel, E.W. A perspective on persistent toxicants in veterans and amyotrophic lateral sclerosis: Identifying exposures determining higher ALS risk. *J. Neurol.* **2022**, *269*, 2359–2377. [CrossRef]

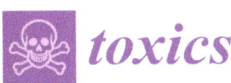

Article

Exposure to Volatile Organic Compounds in Paint Production Plants: Levels and Potential Human Health Risks

Safiye Ghobakhloo [1], Amir Hossein Khoshakhlagh [2,*], Simone Morais [3] and Ashraf Mazaheri Tehrani [1]

[1] Department of Environmental Health Engineering, School of Health, Kashan University of Medical Sciences, Kashan 8715988141, Iran
[2] Department of Occupational Health Engineering, School of Health, Kashan University of Medical Sciences, Kashan 8715988141, Iran
[3] REQUIMTE-LAQV, Instituto Superior de Engenharia do Porto, Instituto Politécnico do Porto, Rua Dr. António Bernardino de Almeida, 431, 4249-015 Porto, Portugal
* Correspondence: ah.khoshakhlagh@gmail.com

Abstract: A wide range of volatile organic solvents, including aliphatic and aromatic hydrocarbons, alcohols, and ketones, are used in the production of paints, and they comprise more than 30% of the ingredients of paints. The present study was designed to evaluate the occupational exposure to 15 volatile organic compounds (VOCs, including benzene, toluene, ethylbenzene, xylene, styrene, n-hexane, n-heptane, n-nonane, trichloroethylene, tetrachloroethylene, n-butyl acetate, n-octane, n-decane, dichlorofluoromethane, and acetone) in Iranian paint production factories and subsequently, the associated health risks. The samples were collected from the respiratory zone of workers using the NIOSH 1501 method, and their qualitative and quantitative characterization was performed using gas chromatography-mass spectrometry and gas chromatography-flame ionization detector, respectively. The individual concentrations of VOCs ranged from 23.76 ± 0.57 µg m^{-3} (acetone) to 92489.91 ± 0.65 µg m^{-3} (m,p-xylene). The predominant compounds were m,p-xylene (up to 92489.91 ± 0.65 µg m^{-3}), ethylbenzene (up to 91188.95 ± 0.34 µg m^{-3}), and toluene (up to 46088.84 ± 0.14 µg m^{-3}). The non-cancer risks of benzene, n-nonane, trichloroethylene, tetrachloroethylene, xylene, and ethylbenzene surpassed the reference value in most of the sectors. In addition, total lifetime risks of cancer were in the range of 1.8×10^{-5}–3.85×10^{-3}, suggesting that there was a risk of carcinogenesis in all studied sections, mainly due to ethylbenzene and benzene. Considering their high exposure concentrations and their associated non-carcinogenic and carcinogenic risks, biological monitoring of workers and the use of technical and modern engineering control measures are recommended.

Keywords: paint production plant; volatile organic compounds (VOCs); inhalation exposure; cancer risk; non-cancer risk

1. Introduction

Volatile organic compounds (VOCs) are a wide variety of chemical substances that are derived from natural processes and human activities [1]. In the occupational context, these compounds are widely used in industrial processes, such as rubber manufacturing, plastic manufacturing, paint production, and automobile manufacturing [2–4]. Benzene, toluene, ethylbenzene, and xylene, which are among the most common VOCs, are known to pose risks to human health [5,6]. In addition to hydrocarbons, halocarbons and oxygenated hydrocarbons, such as styrene (vinyl benzene), are also classified as harmful compounds to human health. Styrene is an economically industrial chemical that is utilized in the synthesis and manufacturing of polystyrene and hundreds of different copolymers, as well as in many other industrial resins. Short-term exposure to high concentrations of VOCs may irritate the eyes, nose, throat, and lungs, as well as damage the liver, kidneys, and central nervous system. Additionally, long-term exposure to low concentrations of pollutants can lead to asthma, reduced lung function, cardiovascular disease, and cancer [7]. The International Agency for Research on Cancer (IARC) and the United States Environmental Protection Agency (USEPA) have classified benzene as a known human carcinogen (Group A), ethylbenzene and styrene as possibly carcinogenic to humans (Group 2B), and tetrachloroethylene and trichloroethylene as probable carcinogens to humans (Group 2A) [8]. Many studies have shown that inhalation is the main route of exposure to VOCs [9,10], and that significant risks for workers of different industries (gas station workers, tire-manufacturing factories, and dyeing industrial complex, among others) may exist [6,11–13]. Considering the potential toxic effects of VOCs on people's health in work environments, monitoring these compounds and assessing their health risks is the first way to adopt control measures for occupational exposure and regulatory purposes at the national and international level [14]. There are different methods to determine exposure to chemicals in work environments, and the direct measurement of pollutant concentration in a person's respiratory area is considered the most reliable method. By combining data related to exposure and the dose-response of the chemicals, risks from exposure to chemicals can be calculated [15]. Hu et al. found that the lifetime cancer risks of benzene, tetrachloromethane, trichloromethane, and trichloroethylene in different functional zones (traffic, industrial, development, resident, and ground zone) of a typical developing city in China were above the acceptable risk level (1.0×10^{-6}) set by USEPA [16]. Shuai et al. reported that the prevalence of respiratory, allergic, and cardiovascular diseases near the dyeing industrial complex in South Korea was significantly higher than in the control area [12]. The results of Tunsaringkarn et al. showed that occupational exposure to BTEX increased the risk of cancer in gas station workers [6]. Hosseini et al. reported unacceptable occupational cancer risks due to benzene exposure in two tire-manufacturing factories [11]. Other similar studies indicated significant risks of VOC exposure in different occupational and non-occupational environments [17–20]. Because organic solvents are still one of the main constituents of paints, workers from the paint and painting industries are regularly and occupationally exposed to them [21]. Golbabai et al. showed that the carcinogenic risks for benzene and ethylbenzene and the non-cancer risks for benzene and xylene in the paint section of an automotive industry were higher than the recommended level [13]. On the other hand, the market has been moving towards industrial paint applications in industries such as construction, automotive, general, coils, wood, aerospace, fences, and packaging coatings, which leads to the growth of demand [22]. Considering that the workforce is considered the capital of every society, providing, maintaining, and improving their health is one of the most important goals of every society [23]. Thus, in this study, and due to the limited information on the subject, the USEPA model [24,25] was used to assess the health risks of VOC exposure (to 15 compounds, including benzene, toluene, ethylbenzene, m/p-xylene, styrene, n-hexane, n-heptane, n-nonane, trichloroethylene, tetrachloroethylene, n-butyl acetate, n-octane, n-decane, dichlorofluoromethane, and acetone) in paint factories of Iran during 2022.

2. Materials and Methods

2.1. Site Description

This cross-sectional study was conducted on workers (all male) from two paint plants in the Semnan province of Iran in 2022. The characterized production processes were those conventionally used in Iran and took place on two closed floors of the plant. The workers of the production line were classified according to job operations. These people worked in units called raw materials, mixing and dispersion, and filling lines. Workers in the raw materials line began the process by emptying the paint materials into tanks connected to buckets in the mixing and dispersing department by pipes. In the second part, colored liquors were mixed with porcelain clays. The paint then went to the filling line and was emptied into cans for sealing and shipping. The manufacturing process was maintained, and air from the respiratory zone of the workers was collected for 8 h during the working shift. A temperature of 80 °C produced significant paint fumes in the work area. The paint production unit of the studied industry had 8 sections, including 3 different paint production salons [Plastic Color production (PC), Cathodic Electrodeposition production (CED), and Original Equipment Manufacturer Color production (OEM)], 2 paint warehouses (dispatch and topcoat), a washing salon (washing PC salon), and 2 paint laboratories (lab OEM and PC lab).

2.2. Sampling Method

The NIOSH-1501 method was used to assess the occupational exposure. None of the workers used personal protective equipment (PPE), including facemasks and protective clothing. VOC samples were collected in each factory section using tubes containing solid adsorbents of activated carbon (SKC Inc., Pittsburgh, PA, USA) and an individual sampling pump, calibrated at a flow rate of 200 mL min^{-1} (SKC Inc., Pittsburgh, PA, USA). Sampler specifications included a glass tube with a length of 7 cm, an inner diameter of 6 mm OD, and an outer diameter of 4 mm ID and flamed sealed ends with plastic caps containing two sections of 20/40 mesh-activated (600 °C) coconut shell charcoal (front = 100 mg, back = 50 mg) separated by a 2 mm urethane foam plug. A total of 75 individual samples of air were collected during sampling, and the environmental factors, such as temperature, humidity, air pressure, airflow speed, and the condition of the existing ventilation system on the concentration of pollutants in the workplace air were recorded.

2.3. Sample Preparation and Analysis

After collection, the samples were transported to the laboratory. Both the front and back sections of the activated carbon tube were transferred to different 2 mL vials. Samples were extracted, with 1 mL carbon disulfide (99.5%) (Merck Inc., Darmstadt, Germany) as eluent under ultrasonic waves for at least 30 min to complete extraction. Qualitative information about the predominant VOCs was obtained by gas chromatography-mass spectrometry (6890N/5973; Agilent, Palo Alto, Santa Clara, CA, USA). Analysis was performed using gas chromatography (GC 7890 Agilent, Santa Clara, CA, USA) equipped with a flame ionization detector (FID) using a capillary column (length = 30 m, internal diameter = 0.25 mm). Helium gas was used as a carrier gas, with a flow rate of 2 mL min^{-1}. The injection volume was 1 µL, and a split ratio of 5/1 was applied. The initial temperature of the column was 50 °C, which increased to 100 °C after 5 min. The injector was set at a temperature of 250 °C. Standard solutions of benzene, ethylbenzene, xylene, toluene, styrene, n-hexane, n-heptane, n-nonane, trichloroethylene, tetrachloroethylene, n-butyl acetate, n-octane, n-decane, dichlorofluoromethane, and acetone (Merck Inc., Darmstadt, Germany) were used to obtain the calibration curves.

2.4. Quality Control (QC)/Quality Assurance (QA)

In this study, the concentration of BTEX compounds was read according to the ISO/IEC 17025 standard method using the carbon disulfide extraction method and a gas chromatograph (GC) coupled with an FID in the laboratory. In this method, the detection limits for VOCs were in the range of 0.04 and 30 µg m^{-3} (for a sample preconcentration of 1 m^3) [26]. Additionally, control samples and duplicate samples (obtained from all study sites) were used. The relative deviation of all VOCs in duplicate samples was less than 11%. Five blank samples were taken to check the presence of any possible contamination during the sampling, transportation, and storage of air samples. In this study, the total concentration of VOCs in each blank sample was found to be <0.5 ppbv. Spiked samples were used to assess the recovery rate and accuracy. Accuracy and precision were determined by analyzing 15 replicates of QC samples on three different days. The results showed that the analyte recovery percentage was >95% for most compounds.

2.5. Health Risk Assessment

The cancer risk assessment for benzene, ethylbenzene, styrene, trichloroethylene, and tetrachloroethylene and the non-carcinogenic health risk assessment for all VOCs were performed using the EPA method [24,25]. After determining the concentration of pollutants, the adjusted air exposure concentration (EC, mg m^{-3}) was calculated in order to represent the duration of exposure through Equation (1), based on USEPA recommendations [25].

$$EC \ (mg \ m^{-3}) = (C \times ET \times EF \times ED/AT) \qquad (1)$$

where C (mg m^{-3}) is the concentration of the considered compound in the collected personal air sample; ET (h day^{-1}) is the exposure time per day; EF (days year^{-1}) is the exposure frequency per year; ED (years) is the exposure duration; and AT (hours) is the average lifetime (Table 1).

The hazard quotient (HQ) index was calculated to estimate the potential risk posed by the non-carcinogenic effects of the chemical compounds (Equation (2)). The total hazard quotient (THQ) is the sum of the individual HQs.

$$Hazard \ Quotient \ (HQ) = EC \ (mg \ m^{-3})/RFC \ (mg \ m^{-3}) \qquad (2)$$

where RFC is the reference concentration for inhalation exposure (Table 2).

The chronic daily intake (CDI) was calculated by:

$$CDI \ (mg \ kg^{-1} \ day^{-1}) = (C \times IR \times EF \times ED/LT \times BW) \qquad (3)$$

where BW is the body weight (kg), IR is the inhalation rate (m^3 day^{-1}), and LT is the lifetime (day) (Table 1).

If the lifetime risk of cancer (LTCR; Equation (4)) was less than or equal to one in a million (1×10^{-6}), it had no significant effects on human health, so cancer risk was negligible. A LTCR more than 1×10^{-4} was established as "definite risk," between 1×10^{-4} and 1×10^{-6} as "probable risk," between 1×10^{-5} and 1×10^{-6} as "possible risk," and less than 1×10^{-6} as "negligible risk" for human health [27]. The cancer slop factor (CSF) for benzene, ethylbenzene, styrene, trichloroethylene, and tetrachloroethylene are shown in Table 2 [10].

$$LTCR = CDI \ (mg \ kg^{-1} \ day^{-1}) \times CSF \ [(mg \ kg^{-1} \ day^{-1})]^{-1} \qquad (4)$$

Table 1. Information for risk assessment.

Parameter	Values	Data Collection
Exposure time to VOCs (hours/days)—ET	8	Questionnaire
Exposure frequency (day/year)—EF	300	Questionnaire
Exposure duration (years)—ED	30	USEPA, 2002 [25]
Lifetime (day)—LT	25,600	USEPA, 2011 [28]
Inhalation rate (m^3 day^{-1})—IR	16	USEPA, 2011 [25]
Body weight (kg)—BW	72 ± 9.42	Questionnaire
Average lifetime (hours)—AT	33,650	USEPA, 2011 [28]

Table 2. Inhalation dose reference exposure (RFC) and cancer inhalation unit risk for the characterized VOCs.

Agent	RFC (mg m^{-3})	Cancer Slop Factor (mg kg^{-1} day^{-1})	USEPA/IARC Class	Reference
Benzene	0.03	0.029	A	IRIS [a]
Toluene	5	...		IRIS
Ethylbenzene	1	0.0087	2B	IRIS
m,p-Xylene	0.1	...		IRIS
Styrene	1	5.7×10^{-4}	2B	CEP [b]
n-Hexane	0.7	...		IRIS

Table 2. Cont.

Agent	RFC (mg m^{-3})	Cancer Slop Factor (mg kg^{-1} day^{-1})	USEPA/IARC Class	Reference
n-Heptane	0.4	...		IRIS
n-Nonane	0.02	...		IRIS
Trichloroethylene	0.002	1.1×10^{-2}	2A	IRIS
Tetrachloroethylene	0.04	2.07×10^{-2}	2A	IRIS
n-Butyl acetate	1.429	...		WHO [c]
n-Octane	1.111	...		MHLW [d]
n-Decane	0.836	...		Sagunski and Mangelsdorf [29]
Dichlorofluoromethane	0.330	...		IRIS
Acetone	56	...		OECD [e]

[a] IRIS: Integrated Risk Information System from USEPA. [b] CEP: Cumulative Exposure Project from USEPA. [c] WHO: World Health Organization. [d] MHLW: Ministry of Health, Labor, and Welfare. [e] OECD: Organization for Economic Co-operation and Development.

3. Statistical Analysis

The analysis results of VOCs were expressed as mean ± standard deviation using SPSS 22 (Chicago, IL, USA). One-way analysis of variance (ANOVA) was used to determine the difference between the average exposure to VOCs in different units. The relationship between the data was checked at a significance level of 0.05.

4. Result and Discussion

4.1. Levels of the VOCs in the Personal Air in the Paint Factories

Based on the results of the qualitative analysis of the gas chromatography-mass spectrometric detection, 15 compounds were identified and quantified by GC-FID (Table 3). The concentrations of VOCs ranged from 23.76 ± 0.57 (dispatch) to 92,489.91 ± 0.65 µg m^{-3} (production). The analysis of VOCs showed that the decreasing order of the total concentrations of VOCs detected was the washing salon-pc ≫ PC production > CED production, the three of them being identified as the most polluted areas. The most abundant compounds, in order, were xylene (5.95% to 69.03%) > toluene (2.98% to 50.26%) > ethylbenzene (5.94% to 43.14%) (Figure 1). The maximum values detected for xylene (92,489.91 ± 0.65 µg m^{-3} and 81,200.06 ± 0.45 µg m^{-3} in the PC production and washing salons, respectively) and ethylbenzene (91,188.95 µg m^{-3}, 21.07 ppm in the paint-washing PC salon) exceeded the occupational exposure limit of 20 ppm provided by the Environmental and Occupational Health Center of Iran (EOHCI). The results obtained in this study are in line with those reported for other countries. Mo et al. [10] conducted a study to assess the human health risk of VOCs in the paint and coatings industry in the Yangtze River Delta, China. They found that toluene, m/p-xylene, and ethylbenzene were the prevalent compounds in the container coating sector (22.01%, 23.11%, and 17.73%, respectively), ship coating sector (28.73%, 22.76%, and 25.78%, respectively), and furniture coating sector (13.40%, 27.5%, and 27.16%, respectively) [10]. Omidi et al. reported that benzene concentrations in the energy, biochemical, and benzol refining sectors from Iran were higher than the set national occupational exposure limit, opposite to the levels of toluene, ethylbenzene, and xylene in other studied sectors (muffle furnace, battery, and material recycling) [30]. Additionally, Dehghani et al. reported benzene concentrations up to 3.035 mg m^{-3} (equivalent to 0.95 ppm) in the paint cabin section, which surpassed the occupational exposure limit (0.5 ppm) provided by the Environment and Labor Health Center of the Ministry of Health [31].

Table 3. Mean concentrations of the VOCs detected in several sections of the characterized paint factories.

[a] VOCs	[b] TLV-TWA (ppm)	[c] OEM Production	[d] Production	[e] CED Production	Washing Salon-PC	[f] OEM Lab	[g] PC Lab	Dispatch	[h] CED Topcoat
Benzene [i] (LOD = 0.5)	0.5	63.89 ± 0.27 (0.09%)	447.25 ± 0.21 (0.33%)	479.20 ± 0.23 (0.52%)	1277.87 ± 0.32 (0.51%)	31.94 ± 0.08 (0.24%)	63.89 ± 0.65 (8.75%)	63.89 ± 0.17 (0.37%)	543.09 ± 0.73 (1.25%)
Toluene (LOD = 0.7)	20	2110.36 ± 0.53 (2.98%)	14,056.53 ± 0.56 (10.49%)	46,088.84 ± 0.14 (50.26%)	37,873.49 ± 0.13 (16.87%)	527.59 ± 0.34 (4.04%)	37.68 ± 0.43 (5.16%)	452.22 ± 0.56 (2.63%)	19,219.3 ± 0.41 (44.41%)
Ethylbenzene (LOD = 0.5)	20	30,526.58 ± 0.18 (43.14%)	22,232.73 ± 0.32 (16.59%)	8337.27 ± 0.57 (9.09%)	91,188.95 ± 0.34 (39.95%)	2127.74 ± 0.45 (16.31%)	43.42 ± 0.75 (5.94%)	5992.41 ± 0.17 (34.85%)	4081.79 ± 0.37 (9.43%)
m,p-Xylene (LOD = 0.7)	20	37,473.61 ± 0.38 (52.95%)	92,489.91 ± 0.65 (69.03%)	35,997.24 ± 0.45 (39.260%)	81,200.06 ± 0.45 (39.95%)	8814.76 ± 0.76 (67.57%)	43.42 ± 0.33 (5.95%)	5688.34 ± 0.63 (33.09%)	18,411.1 ± 0.18 (42.55%)
Styrene (LOD = 0.4)	10	42.59 ± 0.42 (0.06%)	42.59 ± 0.12 (0.03%)	42.59 ± 0.24 (0.05%)	85.19 ± 0.26 (0.03%)	38.33 ± 0.18 (0.29%)	42.59 ± 0.34 (5.84%)	38.33 ± 0.69 (0.22%)	85.19 ± 0.58 (0.22%)
n-Hexane (LOD = 0.4)	50	35.24 ± 0.17 (0.05%)	35.24 ± 0.68 (0.03%)	70.49 ± 0.27 (0.08%)	105.74 ± 0.18 (0.04%)	35.24 ± 0.38 (0.27%)	35.24 ± 0.19 (4.83%)	35.24 ± 0.13 (0.21%)	105.74 ± 0.65 (0.24%)
n-Heptane (LOD = 0.06)	400	40.98 ± 0.14 (0.06%)	40.98 ± 0.23 (0.03%)	40.98 ± 0.18 (0.04%)	81.97 ± 0.61 (0.03%)	40.98 ± 0.37 (0.31%)	40.98 ± 0.23 (5.61%)	36.88 ± 0.25 (0.21%)	81.97 ± 0.23 (0.19%)
n-Nonane (LOD = 0.04)	200	52.43 ± 0.23 (0.07%)	52.43 ± 0.13 (0.04%)	52.43 ± 0.11 (0.06%)	104.86 ± 0.76 (0.04%)	314.6 ± 0.78 (2.41%)	52.43 ± 0.12 (7.18%)	41.94 ± 0.27 (0.24%)	104.86 ± 0.28 (0.24%)
Trichloroethylene (LOD = 0.6)	10	53.73 ± 0.23 (0.08%)	53.73 ± 0.16 (0.04%)	53.73 ± 0.23 (0.06%)	53.73 ± 0.43 (0.04%)	53.73 ± 0.17 (0.21%)	53.73 ± 0.52 (7.36%)	53.73 ± 0.48 (0.31%)	107.47 ± 0.56 (0.25%)
Tetrachloroethylene (LOD = 2)	25	67.82 ± 0.47 (0.10%)	67.82 ± 0.73 (0.05%)	47.47 ± 0.24 (0.05%)	67.82 ± 0.23 (0.03%)	67.828 ± 0.27 (0.36%)	67.82 ± 0.33 (9.29%)	67.828 ± 0.27 (0.39%)	33.91 ± 0.15 (0.08%)
n-Butyl acetate (LOD = 0.9)	150	47.51 ± 0.29 (0.07%)	47.51 ± 0.39 (0.04%)	47.51 ± 0.19 (0.05%)	47.51 ± 0.21 (0.02%)	28.51 ± 0.21 (0.22%)	47.51 ± 0.19 (6.51%)	28.51 ± 0.2 (0.17%)	47.51 ± 0.24 (0.11%)
n-Octane (LOD = 0.3)	300	46.72 ± 0.76 (0.07%)	46.72 ± 0.21 (0.03%)	46.72 ± 0.28 (0.05%)	93.44 ± 0.81 (0.04%)	280.32 ± 0.38 (2.15)	46.72 ± 0.52 (6.40%)	37.38 ± 0.84 (0.22%)	93.44 ± 0.19 (0.22%)
n-Decane (LOD = 0.06)	45	58.20 ± 0.65 (0.08%)	58.20 ± 0.13 (0.04%)	58.20 ± 0.72 (0.06%)	116.39 ± 0.33 (0.05%)	40.74 ± 0.73 (0.31%)	58.20 ± 0.84 (7.97%)	400.29 ± 0.12 (0.24%)	116.39 ± 0.14 (0.27%)
Dichlorofluoromethane (LOD = 30)	1000	97.65 ± 0.82 (0.14%)	97.65 ± 0.95 (0.07%)	97.65 ± 0.27 (0.11%)	146.48 ± 0.38 (0.06%)	48.83 ± 0.17 (0.37%)	48.83 ± 0.79 (6.69%)	4589.66 ± 0.29 (26.70%)	146.48 ± 0.48 (0.34%)
Acetone (LOD = 20)	500	47.52 ± 0.21 (0.07%)	4205.29 ± 0.64 (3.14%)	237.59 ± 0.84 (0.26%)	5702.09 ± 0.46 (2.31%)	641.48 ± 0.33 (4.92%)	47.52 ± 0.25 (6.51%)	23.76 ± 0.57 (0.14%)	95.03 ± 0.52 (0.22%)

[a] VOCs: volatile organic compounds. [b] TLV-TWA (ppm): threshold limit value–Time-Weighted Average. [c] OEM production: original equipment manufacturer color production. [d] PC production: plastic color production. [e] CED production: cathodic electro deposition production. [f] OEM lab: original equipment manufacturer color laboratory. [g] PC lab: plastic color laboratory. [h] CED topcoat: cathodic electro deposition topcoat. [i] Limit of detection ($\mu g\ m^{-3}$).

4.2. Health Risk Assessment

The data of EC, HQ, and CDI of the characterized VOCs in different parts of the factory are displayed in Table 4 and Figure 2 [32].

HQ ≤ 1 indicates that adverse health effects are unlikely to occur, whereas HQ > 1 means that there may be risks to sensitive individuals as a result of exposure. Sectors with relatively high non-cancer risk values and their exposed workers were identified. The non-cancer risk values of benzene, n-nonane, trichloroethylene, and tetrachloroethylene in all parts of the factory exceeded the safe level of one. Additionally, the non-cancer risk values of xylene, ethylbenzene, and toluene surpassed the reference value in most of the sectors, with the PC lab being the common safer site (HQ < 1). The non-cancer risks were higher in washing salon-PC, followed by production salon-PC, OEM salon, CED production, CED topcoat, OEM lab, dispatch, and PC lab. On the contrary, all the other compounds, i.e., styrene, dichlorofluoromethane, acetone, n-Hexane, n-heptane, n-octane, n-decane, and n-butylacetate within several sectors exhibited acceptable non-carcinogenic risks (HQ < 1). However, exposure to multiple hazardous pollutants may promote combined and/or synergistic effects. Possible associations were suggested between exposure to chlorinated solvents (such as tetrachloroethane, trichloroethylene, and tetrachloroethylene), benzene, lead, and asbestos and the risk of breast cancer in women (exposed workers) [33].

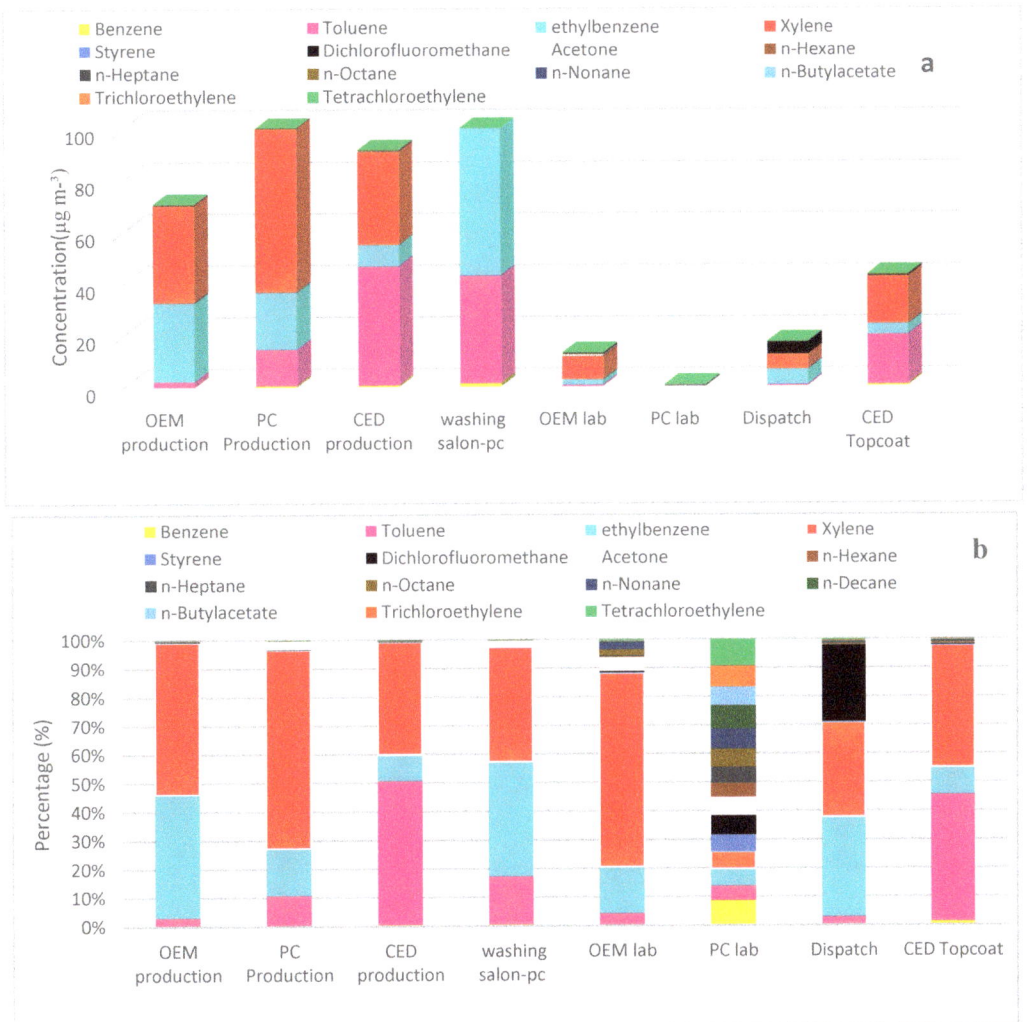

Figure 1. Comparison of (**a**) concentrations and (**b**) percentages of the characterized VOCs in different sectors of the paint factories.

Table 4. The exposure concentrations, hazard quotients (HQ), and chronic daily intakes of VOCs through inhalation in the characterized production zones.

Pollutant	OEM Salon	Production Salon-PC	CED Production	Washing Salon-PC	OEM Lab	PC Lab	Dispatch	CED Topcoat
			Exposure concentration (mg m^{-3})					
Benzene	0.137	0.957	1.025	2.734	0.068	0.137	0.137	1.162
Toluene	4.515	30.076	98.615	89.100	1.129	0.081	0.968	41.123
Ethylbenzene	65.317	47.571	17.839	210.910	4.553	0.093	12.822	8.734
Xylene	80.181	197.898	77.022	210.906	18.861	0.093	12.171	39.394
Styrene	0.091	0.091	0.091	0.182	0.082	0.091	0.082	0.182
Dichlorofluoromethane	0.209	0.209	0.209	0.313	0.104	0.104	9.820	0.313

Table 4. Cont.

Pollutant	OEM Salon	Production Salon-PC	CED Production	Washing Salon-PC	OEM Lab	PC Lab	Dispatch	CED Topcoat
Acetone	0.102	8.998	0.508	12.201	1.373	0.102	0.051	0.203
n-Hexane	0.075	0.075	0.151	0.226	0.075	0.075	0.075	0.226
n-Heptane	0.088	0.088	0.088	0.175	0.088	0.088	0.079	0.175
n-Octane	0.100	0.100	0.100	0.200	0.600	0.100	0.080	0.200
n-Nonane	0.112	0.112	0.112	0.224	0.673	0.112	0.090	0.224
n-Decane	0.125	0.125	0.125	0.249	0.087	0.125	0.087	0.249
n-Butylacetate	0.102	0.102	0.102	0.102	0.061	0.102	0.061	0.102
Trichloroethylene	0.115	0.115	0.115	0.230	0.057	0.115	0.115	0.230
Tetrachloroethylene	0.145	0.145	0.102	0.145	0.102	0.145	0.145	0.073
Hazard quotient								
Benzene	4.56	31.90	34.18	91.14	2.28	4.56	4.56	38.73
Toluene	0.90	6.02	19.72	17.82	0.23	0.02	0.19	8.22
Ethylbenzene	65.32	47.57	17.84	210.91	4.55	0.09	12.82	8.73
Xylene	801.81	1978.98	770.22	2109.06	188.61	0.93	121.71	393.94
Styrene	0.09	0.09	0.09	0.18	0.08	0.09	0.08	0.18
Dichlorofluoromethane	0.63	0.63	0.63	0.95	0.32	0.32	29.76	0.95
Acetone	0.00	0.16	0.01	0.22	0.02	0.00	0.00	0.00
n-Hexane	0.11	0.11	0.22	0.32	0.11	0.11	0.11	0.32
n-Heptane	0.22	0.22	0.22	0.44	0.22	0.22	0.20	0.44
n-Octane	0.12	0.12	0.12	0.24	0.72	0.12	0.10	0.24
n-Nonane	5.61	5.61	5.61	11.22	33.66	5.61	4.49	11.22
n-Decane	0.15	0.15	0.15	0.30	0.10	0.15	0.10	0.30
n-Butylacetate	0.07	0.07	0.07	0.07	0.04	0.07	0.04	0.07
Trichloroethylene	57.49	57.49	57.49	114.98	28.75	57.49	57.49	114.98
Tetrachloroethylene	3.63	3.63	2.54	3.63	2.54	3.63	3.63	1.81
Chronic daily intake ($\mu g\ kg^{-1}\ day^{-1}$)								
Benzene	0.001	0.010	0.010	0.027	0.001	0.001	0.001	0.012
Toluene	0.045	0.301	0.988	0.892	0.011	0.001	0.010	0.412
Ethylbenzene	0.654	0.476	0.179	2.112	0.046	0.001	0.128	0.087
Xylene	0.803	1.982	0.771	2.112	0.189	0.001	0.122	0.395
Styrene	0.001	0.001	0.001	0.002	0.001	0.001	0.001	0.002
Dichlorofluoromethane	0.002	0.002	0.002	0.003	0.001	0.001	0.098	0.003
Acetone	0.001	0.090	0.005	0.122	0.014	0.001	0.001	0.002
n-Hexane	0.001	0.001	0.002	0.002	0.001	0.001	0.001	0.002
n-Heptane	0.001	0.001	0.001	0.002	0.001	0.001	0.001	0.002
n-Octane	0.001	0.001	0.001	0.002	0.006	0.001	0.001	0.002
n-Nonane	0.001	0.001	0.001	0.002	0.007	0.001	0.001	0.002
n-Decane	0.001	0.001	0.001	0.002	0.001	0.001	0.001	0.002
n-Butylacetate	0.001	0.001	0.001	0.001	0.001	0.001	0.001	0.001
Trichloroethylene	0.001	0.001	0.001	0.002	0.001	0.001	0.001	0.002
Tetrachloroethylene	0.001	0.001	0.001	0.001	0.001	0.001	0.001	0.001

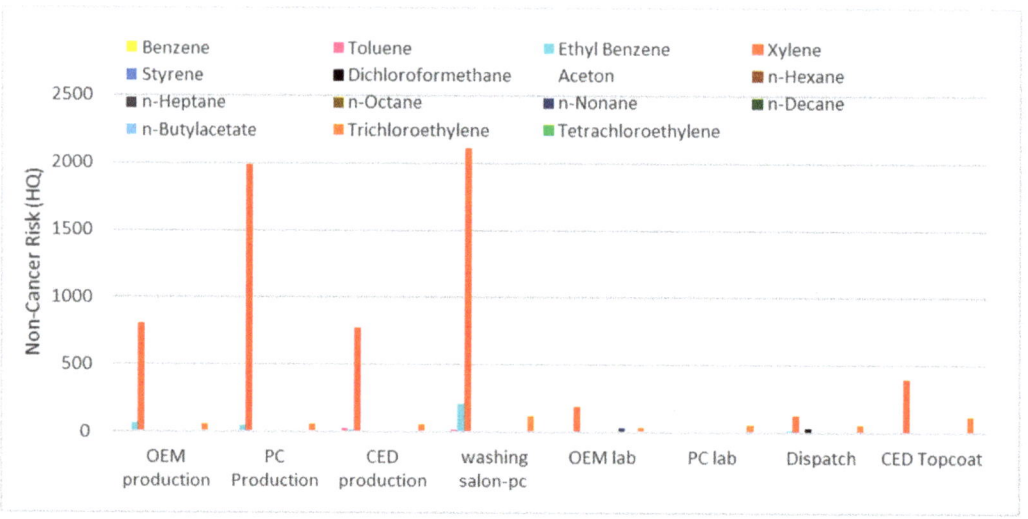

Figure 2. Comparison of non-cancer risk in different sectors of the factories.

Table 5 presents the total and individual carcinogenic risks of the VOCs in the selected paint factories. USEPA considers the acceptable risk level to be in the range of 1×10^{-6} to 1×10^{-4}. For carcinogens, USEPA considers excess cancer risks that are below 1 chance in 1,000,000 (1×10^{-6}) to be so small as to be negligible. However, for a residual cancer risk of less than 10^{-4}, it is recommended to ensure that there is no cumulative cancer risk of potentially carcinogenic compounds. According to the results of Table 5, total LTCR values were in the range of 1.8×10^{-5}–3.85×10^{-3}, suggesting that there was a risk of carcinogenesis in all studied sections. The cancer risk of ethylbenzene was higher than 1×10^{-4} in all sectors of the factories except in PC lab, while the cancer risks of tetrachloroethane and trichloroethylene were lower than 1×10^{-5} in all sectors of the factories. The cancer risk of styrene was higher than 1×10^{-6} only in the CED topcoat sector. The exposure to benzene presented cancer risks in the range of 1.99×10^{-5} to 7.94×10^{-4}. Thus, ethylbenzene was the predominant contributor to the determined increased risk of cancer. The washing salon-PC, CED production, dispatch, OEM production salon, PC production salon, CED topcoat, and OEM lab were the most polluted environments, with the highest risk of cancer being for ethylbenzene (5.28×10^{-2}, 4.47×10^{-3}, 3.21×10^{3}, 1.64×10^{-3}, 1.19×10^{-3}, 2.19×10^{-4}, and 1.14×10^{-4}, respectively). This means that workers in these sectors may suffer from a cancer risk 45–530 times higher than 1 additional case per 10,000 employees exposed (1×10^{-4}), i.e., the upper limit of acceptable cancer risk (1×10^{-4}) established by USEPA recommendations. These findings emphasize the role of ethylbenzene compounds in the occupational exposure in the paint industry in Iran. One of the reasons for the high level of ethylbenzene in this section is the presence of ethylbenzene impurity in the solvents and the excessive use of thinner in cleaning surfaces, despite the elimination/reduction in many raw materials. These data are consistent with the results reported by Golbabaei et al. [13]. It was also found that ethylbenzene in spray paints (9.71×10^{-4}), wooden furniture manufacturing (1.75×10^{-5}), municipal solid waste (1.71×10^{-6}), electronic waste dismantling processes (6.2×10^{-3}), the rubber footwear industry ($>1 \times 10^{-4}$), and the oil refinery (6.09×10^{-3}) originates high cancer risks [10]. In addition, considering the other determined VOCs, the only exceedance was detected for the LTCR of benzene in washing salon-PC (1.64×10^{-4}), which was in agreement with the reported information from Zhang et al. and Chen et al., who found average LTCR values of 3.4×10^{-4} and 4.1×10^{-5}, respectively, in the ambient air of Beijing, China and the petrochemical industrial complexes [34,35]. Benzene contributes significantly to the risk of cancer in petrochemical industries, rubber shoes, asphalt paving, and coking wastewater treatment industries [36,37], supporting its selection in this study. Exposure to benzene may cause a potential risk of adverse health effects during a thirty-year exposure period. Lan et al. [38] conducted a study to assess the risk of benzene in three clothes-manufacturing factories in the same region near Tianjin. Despite benzene levels being lower than the permissible limits, the relative risk of leukemia for employees was reported to be 1.1 times higher than in the non-exposed group.

Table 5. Lifetime risk of cancer (LTCR) of the characterized VOCs.

ELCR	OEM Salon	Production Salon-PC	CED Production	Washing Salon-PC	OEM Lab	PC Lab	Dispatch	CED Topcoat
Benzene	3.97×10^{-5}	2.78×10^{-4}	2.98×10^{-4}	7.94×10^{-4}	1.99×10^{-5}	3.97×10^{-5}	3.97×10^{-5}	3.37×10^{-4}
Ethylbenzene	1.64×10^{-3}	1.19×10^{-3}	4.47×10^{-3}	5.28×10^{-2}	1.14×10^{-4}	2.33×10^{-6}	3.21×10^{-3}	2.19×10^{-4}
Trichloroethylene	1.27×10^{-5}	1.27×10^{-5}	1.27×10^{-5}	2.53×10^{-5}	6.33×10^{-6}	1.27×10^{-5}	1.27×10^{-5}	2.53×10^{-5}
Tetrachloroethylene	2.91×10^{-5}	2.91×10^{-5}	2.03×10^{-5}	2.91×10^{-5}	2.03×10^{-5}	2.91×10^{-5}	2.91×10^{-5}	1.45×10^{-5}
Styrene	5.2×10^{-7}	5.2×10^{-7}	5.2×10^{-7}	1.04×10^{-6}	4.68×10^{-7}	5.2×10^{-7}	4.68×10^{-7}	1.04×10^{-6}
Total LTCR	1.15×10^{-3}	8.93×10^{-4}	3.77×10^{-4}	3.85×10^{-3}	8.87×10^{-5}	1.8×10^{-5}	2.4×10^{-4}	2.28×10^{-4}

During working hours, workers are exposed to various hazards, including contact with chemicals, biological and physical factors, and unfavorable ergonomic conditions, which are responsible for a variety of health outcomes [39]. Firoozeh et al. [40] found that chronic occupational exposure to excess amounts of mixed organic solvents can cause decreased motivation and mental fatigue in exposed individuals. The results of a study at a petrochemical plant in China showed that xylene, benzene, and toluene are potentially involved in causing lung dysfunction. Physiologically based pharmacokinetic results showed that the metabolism of ethylbenzene was strongly reduced by simultaneous exposure to high concentrations of xylene, leading to non-linear behavior [41]. Additionally, in recent years, various studies have been conducted to assess the health risk of exposure to organic solvents in paint factories. A cross-sectional study involving 97 workers from a paint plant in Mexico showed a significant association between macrocytosis and exposure to high doses of BTX mixtures (OR: 3.6, 95% CI: 1.08 to 13.9, p = 0.02) [42]. Hassan et al. found that neuropsychological symptoms were 63.04% in paint manufacturing workers, while it was only 2.1% in the control group. Additionally, the risk of neurological symptoms was higher in the production group than in the packaging group (OR = 13.94) [43]. Ikegwuonu et al. [44] showed that the serum levels of aspartate transaminase, alkaline phosphatase, sodium, and chloride in workers working in paint plants were significantly higher than in workers working in non-paint factories. Exposure to VOCs and heavy metals in the paint plant makes workers prone to liver and kidney disorders [45].

5. Conclusions and Implications

This study collected VOC samples in the respiratory zone of workers in paint factories under normal occupational conditions. Xylene, toluene, and ethylbenzene were the most abundant compounds in the production processes, which was generally consistent with previous, related studies. A total of 15 VOCs were selected to evaluate their non-carcinogenic and carcinogenic risks to workers from different sectors in paint factories. The highest concentration of total VOCs was observed in the washing salon-PC sector. Non-carcinogenic risks promoted by exposure to benzene, n-nonane, trichloroethylene, tetrachloroethylene, xylene, and ethylbenzene were found almost in all of the sectors of the factories. For carcinogens, the LTCR values significantly exceeded the value of the negligible risks, which was 1.0×10^{-6}. Ethylbenzene and benzene were the most critical pollutants that contributed to the high risk of cancer in these factories. Considering the high exposure concentrations and the high non-carcinogenic and carcinogenic risks of these compounds, the use of PPE, biological monitoring of workers, and the use of technical and modern engineering control measures are highly recommended. Additionally, in order to reduce VOC emissions directly at the source, paints with low VOC content or without VOCs (new environmentally friendly paints) are urgently needed.

Author Contributions: Conceptualization, S.G. and A.H.K.; methodology, S.G. and A.H.K.; software, S.G.; validation, S.G., A.H.K. and S.M.; formal analysis, S.G.; investigation, S.G., A.H.K. and S.M.; resources, A.M.T.; data curation, S.G. and A.M.T.; writing—original draft preparation, S.G. and A.H.K.; writing—review and editing, S.G., A.H.K. and S.M.; visualization, S.G. and A.H.K.; supervision, A.H.K.; project administration, S.G.; funding acquisition, S.G. and A.M.T. All authors have read and agreed to the published version of the manuscript.

Funding: This research received no external funding.

Institutional Review Board Statement: Not applicable.

Informed Consent Statement: Informed consent was obtained from all subjects involved in the study (IR.KAUMS.MEDNT.REC.1401.191).

Data Availability Statement: Not applicable.

Acknowledgments: The study is supported by Kashan University of medical sciences. The authors would like to express their gratitude to all the employees and managers of the paint manufacturing plants for their cooperation.

Conflicts of Interest: The authors declare no conflict of interest.

References

1. Agenson, K.O.; Oh, J.-I.; Urase, T. Retention of a wide variety of organic pollutants by different nanofiltration/reverse osmosis membranes: Controlling parameters of process. *J. Membr. Sci.* **2003**, *225*, 91–103. [CrossRef]
2. Aghaei, H.; Kakooei, H.; Shahtaheri, S.J.; Omidi, F.; Arefian, S.; Azam, K. Evaluating Poly-Aromatic Hydrocarbons in respiratory zone of the asphalt workers in Tehran city. *Saf. Health Work* **2014**, *3*, 31–40.
3. Jones, D.; Brischke, C. *Performance of Bio-based Building Materials*; Cost European Corporation in Science and Technology, Woodhead Publishing: Sawston, UK, 2017; Volume 7.
4. Carbonell, J.C. *Pinturas y Barnices: Tecnología Básica*; Ediciones Díaz de Santos: Madrid, Spain, 2014; Volume 2.
5. Edokpolo, B.; Yu, Q.J.; Connell, D. Health Risk Assessment of Ambient Air Concentrations of Benzene, Toluene and Xylene (BTX) in Service Station Environments. *Int. J. Environ. Res. Public Health* **2014**, *11*, 6354–6374. [CrossRef] [PubMed]
6. Tunsaringkarn, T.; Siriwong, W.; Rungsiyothin, A.; Nopparatbundit, S. Occupational exposure of gasoline station workers to BTEX compounds in Bangkok, Thailand. *Int. J. Occup. Environ. Med.* **2012**, *3*, 117–125.
7. Lloyd-Smith, M. Underground Coal Gasification (UCG). National Toxics Network. November 2015. Available online: https://ntn.org.au/wp-content/uploads/2015/11/Nov-Underground-Coal-Gasification-Nov-2015f-1 (accessed on 9 December 2022).
8. Lyon, F. *IARC Monographs on the Evaluation of Carcinogenic Risks to Humans. Some Industrial Chemicals*; WHO: Geneva, Switzerland, 1994; Volume 60, pp. 389–433.
9. Fang, L.; Norris, C.; Johnson, K.; Cui, X.; Sun, J.; Teng, Y.; Tian, E.; Xu, W.; Li, Z.; Mo, J.; et al. Toxic volatile organic compounds in 20 homes in Shanghai: Concentrations, inhalation health risks, and the impacts of household air cleaning. *Build. Environ.* **2019**, *157*, 309–318. [CrossRef]
10. Mo, Z.; Lu, S.; Shao, M. Volatile organic compound (VOC) emissions and health risk assessment in paint and coatings industry in the Yangtze River Delta, China. *Environ. Pollut.* **2020**, *269*, 115740. [CrossRef]
11. Hosseini, S.; Rezazadeh-azari, M.A.; Taifeh-Rahimian, R.A.; Tavakkol, E. Occupational risk assessment of benzene in rubber tire manufacturing workers. *Int. J. Occup. Hyg.* **2014**, *6*, 220–226.
12. Shuai, J.; Kim, S.; Ryu, H.; Park, J.; Lee, C.K.; Kim, G.-B.; Ultra, V.U., Jr.; Yang, W. Health risk assessment of volatile organic compounds exposure near Daegu dyeing industrial complex in South Korea. *BMC Public Health* **2018**, *18*, 528. [CrossRef]
13. Golbabaie, F.; Eskandari, D.; Rezazade Azari, M.; Jahangiri, M.; Rahimi, M.; Shahtaheri, J. Health risk assessment of chemical pollutants in a petrochemical complex. *Iran Occup. Health* **2012**, *9*, 11–21.
14. Guo, H.; Lee, S.; Chan, L.; Li, W. Risk assessment of exposure to volatile organic compounds in different indoor environments. *Environ. Res.* **2004**, *94*, 57–66. [CrossRef]
15. Nieuwenhuijsen, M.; Paustenbach, D.; Duarte-Davidson, R. New developments in exposure assessment: The impact on the practice of health risk assessment and epidemiological studies. *Environ. Int.* **2006**, *32*, 996–1009. [CrossRef]
16. Hu, R.; Liu, G.; Zhang, H.; Xue, H.; Wang, X. Levels, characteristics and health risk assessment of VOCs in different functional zones of Hefei. *Ecotoxicol. Environ. Saf.* **2018**, *160*, 301–307. [CrossRef]
17. Jia, C.; Fu, X.; Chauhan, B.; Xue, Z.; Kedia, R.J.; Mishra, C.S. Exposure to volatile organic compounds (VOCs) at gas stations: A probabilistic analysis. *Air Qual. Atmos. Health* **2022**, *15*, 465–477. [CrossRef]
18. He, Z.; Li, G.; Chen, J.; Huang, Y.; An, T.; Zhang, C. Pollution characteristics and health risk assessment of volatile organic compounds emitted from different plastic solid waste recycling workshops. *Environ. Int.* **2015**, *77*, 85–94. [CrossRef]
19. Jo, W.-K.; Park, K.-H. Heterogeneous photocatalysis of aromatic and chlorinated volatile organic compounds (VOCs) for non-occupational indoor air application. *Chemosphere* **2004**, *57*, 555–565. [CrossRef]
20. Qi, Y.-J.; Ni, J.-W.; Zhao, D.-X.; Yang, Y.; Han, L.-Y.; Li, B.-W. Emission Characteristics and Risk Assessment of Volatile Organic Compounds from Typical Factories in Zhengzhou. *Huan Jing Ke Xue* **2020**, *41*, 3056–3065.
21. de Oliveira, H.M.; Dagostim, G.P.; da Silva Mota, A.; Tavares, P.; da Rosa, L.A.; de Andrade, V.M. Occupational risk assessment of paint industry workers. *Indian J. Occup. Environ. Med.* **2011**, *15*, 52.
22. Jiménez-López, A.M.; Hincapié-Llanos, G.A. Identification of factors affecting the reduction of VOC emissions in the paint industry: Systematic literature review-SLR. *Prog. Org. Coat.* **2022**, *170*, 106945. [CrossRef]
23. Olayemi, S.O. Human capital investment and industrial productivity in Nigeria. *Int. J. Humanit. Soc. Sci.* **2012**, *2*, 298–307.
24. Means, B. *Risk-Assessment Guidance for Superfund. Volume Human Health Evaluation Manual. Part A. Interim Report (Final)*; Office of Solid Waste and Emergency Response; Environmental Protection Agency: Washington, DC, USA, 1989.
25. United States Environmental Protection Agency (US EPA). *Exposure Factors Handbook, Edition (Final)*; Office of the Emergency and Remedial Response: Washington, DC, USA, 2011.
26. Ribani, M.; Bottoli, C.B.; Collins, C.H.; Jardim, I.C.; Melo, L.F. Validação em métodos cromatográficos e eletroforéticos. *Química Nova* **2004**, *27*, 771–780. [CrossRef]
27. Lamplugh, A.D. Volatile Organic Compounds: Exposure and Mitigation in Colorado Nail Salons. Ph.D. Thesis, University of Colorado at Boulder, Boulder, CO, USA, 2019.
28. United States Environmental Protection Agency (US EPA). *Supplemental Guidance for Developing Soil Screen-ing Levels for Superfund Sites*; Oficce of Emergency and Remedial Response: Washington, DC, USA, 2002.
29. Sagunski, H.; Mangelsdorf, I. Richtwerte für die Innenraumluft: Aromatenarme Kohlenwasserstoffgemische (C9–C14). *Bundesgesundheitsblatt Gesundh. Gesundh.* **2005**, *48*, 803–812. [CrossRef] [PubMed]

30. Omidi, F.; Fallahzadeh, R.A.; Dehghani, F.; Harati, B.; Barati, C.S.; Gharibi, V. Carcinogenic and non-carcinogenic risk assessment of exposure to volatile organic compounds (BTEX) using Monte-Carlo simulation technique in a steel industry. *Saf. Health Work* **2018**, *8*, 299–308.
31. Dehghani, F.; Golbabaei, F.; Abolfazl Zakerian, S.; Omidi, F.; Mansournia, M.A. Health risk assessment of exposure to volatile organic compounds (BTEX) in a painting unit of an automotive industry. *Saf. Health Work* **2018**, *8*, 55–64.
32. Tong, R.; Ma, X.; Zhang, Y.; Shao, G.; Shi, M. Source analysis and health risk-assessment of ambient volatile organic compounds in automobile manufacturing processes. *Hum. Ecol. Risk Assess. Int. J.* **2018**, *26*, 359–383. [CrossRef]
33. Chuang, Y.S.; Lee, C.Y.; Lin, P.C.; Pan, C.H.; Hsieh, H.M.; Wu, C.F.; Wu, M.T. Breast cancer incidence in a national cohort of female workers exposed to special health hazards in Taiwan: A retrospective case-cohort study of ~300,000 occupational records spanning 20 years. *Int. Arch. Occup. Environ. Health* **2022**, *95*, 1979–1993. [CrossRef] [PubMed]
34. Zhang, Y.; Mu, Y.; Liu, J.; Mellouki, A. Levels, sources and health risks of carbonyls and BTEX in the ambient air of Beijing, China. *J. Environ. Sci.* **2012**, *24*, 124–130. [CrossRef]
35. Chen, W.-H.; Chen, Z.-B.; Yuan, C.-S.; Hung, C.-H.; Ning, S.-K. Investigating the differences between receptor and dispersion modeling for concentration prediction and health risk assessment of volatile organic compounds from petrochemical industrial complexes. *J. Environ. Manag.* **2016**, *166*, 440–449. [CrossRef]
36. Cui, P.; Schito, G.; Cui, Q. VOC emissions from asphalt pavement and health risks to construction workers. *J. Clean. Prod.* **2020**, *244*, 118757. [CrossRef]
37. Mo, Z.; Shao, M.; Lu, S.; Qu, H.; Zhou, M.; Sun, J.; Gou, B. Process-specific emission characteristics of volatile organic compounds (VOCs) from petrochemical facilities in the Yangtze River Delta, China. *Sci. Total Environ.* **2015**, *533*, 422–431. [CrossRef]
38. Lan, Q.; Zhang, L.; Li, G.; Vermeulen, R.; Weinberg, R.S.; Dosemeci, M.; Rappaport, S.M.; Shen, M.; Alter, B.P.; Wu, Y.; et al. Hematotoxicity in Workers Exposed to Low Levels of Benzene. *Science* **2004**, *306*, 1774–1776. [CrossRef]
39. Aliyu, A.A.; Shehu, A.U. Occupational hazards and safety measures among stone quarry workers in northern Nigeria. *Niger. Med. Pract.* **2007**, *50*, 42–47. [CrossRef]
40. Firoozeh, M.; Kavousi, A.; Hasanzadeh, S. Evaluation of relationship between occupational exposure to organic solvent and fatigue workers at a paint factory in Saveh city. *Iran Occup. Health* **2017**, *14*, 82–92.
41. Liao, Q.; Zhang, Y.; Ma, R.; Zhang, Z.; Ji, P.; Xiao, M.; Du, R.; Liu, X.; Cui, Y.; Xing, X.; et al. Risk assessment and dose-effect of co-exposure to benzene, toluene, ethylbenzene, xylene, and styrene (BTEXS) on pulmonary function: A cross-sectional study. *Environ. Pollut.* **2022**, *310*, 119894. [CrossRef]
42. Haro-García, L.; Vélez-Zamora, N.; Aguilar-Madrid, G.; Guerrero-Rivera, S.; Sánchez-Escalante, V.; Muñoz, S.R.; Mezones-Holguín, E.; Juárez-Pérez, C. Blood disorders among workers exposed to a mixture of benzene-toluene-xylene (BTX) in a paint factory. *Rev. Peru. Med. Exp. Y Salud Publica* **2012**, *29*, 181–187. [CrossRef]
43. Hassan, A.A.E.H.; Elnagar, S.A.E.M.; El Tayeb, I.M.; Bolbol, S.A.E.H. Health Hazards of Solvents Exposure among Workers in Paint Industry. *Open J. Saf. Sci. Technol.* **2013**, *03*, 87–95. [CrossRef]
44. Ikegwuonu, I.C.; Obi-George, C.J.; Ikebudu, A.P.; Ikegwuonu, P.T.; Ogbodo, S.O.; Mba, C.B.; Arinze, I.E. Correlative study on the effect of toxic paint chemicals on the hepatorenal of paint factory workers in Enugu, Nigeria. *World J. Adv. Res. Rev.* **2022**, *15*, 432–439. [CrossRef]
45. Zhang, Y.; Wei, C.; Yan, B. Emission characteristics and associated health risk assessment of volatile organic compounds from a typical coking wastewater treatment plant. *Sci. Total Environ.* **2019**, *693*, 133417. [CrossRef]

Disclaimer/Publisher's Note: The statements, opinions and data contained in all publications are solely those of the individual author(s) and contributor(s) and not of MDPI and/or the editor(s). MDPI and/or the editor(s) disclaim responsibility for any injury to people or property resulting from any ideas, methods, instructions or products referred to in the content.

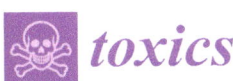

Article

Differential Expression of *AhR* in Peripheral Mononuclear Cells in Response to Exposure to Polycyclic Aromatic Hydrocarbons in Mexican Women

José Antonio Varela-Silva [1], Miguel Ernesto Martínez-Leija [1], Sandra Teresa Orta-García [2], Ivan Nelinho Pérez-Maldonado [2], Jesús Adrián López [3], Hiram Hernández-López [4], Roberto González-Amaro [5], Emma S. Calderón-Aranda [6], Diana Patricia Portales-Pérez [3] and Mariana Salgado-Bustamante [1,*]

1. Biochemistry Department, and Immunology, Department of Faculty of Medicine, UASLP, San Luis Potosí 78000, Mexico
2. Laboratory of Molecular Toxicology, Centro de Investigación Aplicada en, Ambiente y Salud (CIAAS), Coordinación para la Innovación y Aplicación de la, Ciencia y la Tecnología (CIACYT), UASLP, San Luis Potosí 78000, Mexico
3. Laboratorio de microRNAs y Cáncer, Unidad Académica de Ciencias Biológicas, Universidad Autónoma de Zacatecas, Zacatecas 98066, Mexico
4. Academic Unit of Chemistry Sciences, Universidad Autónoma de Zacatecas, Zacatecas 98606, Mexico
5. Laboratory of Immunology Cellular and molecular, Faculty of Chemistry, Universidad Autónoma de San Luis Potosí, San Luis Potosí 78000, Mexico
6. Toxicology Department, Centro de Investigación y Estudios Avanzados, IPN, México City 07360, Mexico
* Correspondence: mariana.salgado@uaslp.mx; Tel.: +52-444-826-2345 (ext. 6669)

Abstract: The exposure to air pollutants causes significant damage to health, and inefficient cooking and heating practices produce high levels of household air pollution, including a wide range of health-damaging pollutants such as fine particles, carbon monoxide and PAHs. The exposure to PAHs has been associated with the development of neoplastic processes, asthma, genotoxicity, altered neurodevelopment and inflammation. The effects on the induction of proinflammatory cytokines are attributed to the activation of *AhR*. However, the molecular mechanisms by which the PAHs produce proinflammatory effects are unknown. This study was performed on a group of 41 Mexican women from two rural communities who had stoves inside their houses, used wood as biomass fuel, and, thus, were vulnerable. According to the urinary 1-OHP concentration, the samples were stratified into two groups for determination of the levels of *TNF-α*, *AhR*, *CYP1B1*, miR-125b and miR-155 expression. Our results showed that the *CYP1B1*, *TNF-α*, miR-125b and miR-155 expression levels were not statistically different between women with the lowest and highest levels of 1-OHP. Interestingly, high levels of PAHs promoted augmented expression of AhR, which is a protein involved in the modulation of inflammatory pathways in vivo, suggesting that cell signaling of *AhR* may be implicated in several pathogenesis processes.

Keywords: pollutants; women exposure; microRNAs; PAHs

1. Introduction

Environmental pollutants are generated as a result of human activity; around 3 billion people still cook and heat their homes using solid fuels (i.e., wood, crop wastes, charcoal, coal and dung) in open fires and leaky stoves, and 4.3 million people a year die prematurely from illnesses attributable to household air pollution caused by the inefficient use of solid fuels [1,2]. Some compounds such as polycyclic aromatic hydrocarbons (PAHs) are generated by the incomplete combustion of organic matter and can travel together with coarse (10 PM), fine (2.5 PM) and ultrafine particles (0.1 PM) across long distances, being deposited and accumulating in various environmental matrices and entering into living organisms, bioaccumulating and becoming bioavailable to higher organisms such as

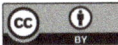

humans. Additionally, contact with PAHs causes a biomagnification as they enter the food chain [1–4].

Benzo [a] pyreno (BaP) is one of the PAHs most widely studied for its effects on health, including inflammatory diseases and cancer. The majority of its effects have been associated with the activation of AhR, which is a factor with bHLH domains (basic helix–loop–helix) [5]. AhR is a ligand-dependent transcription factor that is stripped from Hsp90, p23 and KAP2 proteins when activated and dimerizes with AhR nuclear translocator (ARNT)-recognizing DNA regulatory elements called XREs or DREs (xenobiotic response elements or dioxin response elements) of target genes, thereby increasing their transcription. The isoforms of Cytochromes p450 (CYP1A1, CYP1A2, CYP1B1) are targets of AhR that participate in PAH metabolism. CYP1A1 and CYP1B1 promote the transformation of B[a]P to B[a]P-7,8-oxide through a hydration reaction by the enzyme epoxide hydrolase B[a]P-7,8-oxide, and it is subsequently metabolized to B[a]P-trans-7,8-dihydrodiol (B [a] P-7,8-DHD). B [a] P-7,8-DHD is a substrate of CYPB in a second oxidation reaction generating the final carcinogenic metabolite [a] P-7,8-dihydroxy-9,10-epoxide (BPDE). BPDE joins the DNA chain, principally generating deoxyguanosine adducts [6,7].

Currently, most of the effects of BaP are attributed to the activation of AhR, which regulates the transcription of genes controlled by DRE sequences that have been found in promoter regions of different cytokines in murine models, including IL-2, IL-5, IL-10, TGF-$\beta 1$ and IFNγ [8]. However, it has been found that the expression of proinflammatory genes without DRE sequences in their promoters is upregulated with exposure to BaP, suggesting that there is another type of independent regulation of AhR through the regulation of protein and non-coding RNAs.

Epigenetic modification is one of the mechanisms by which gene expression is regulated, and it is characterized by the presence of changes in the composition and structure of chromatin, which can potentially be inherited [9]. Three of the most significant epigenetic modifications are DNA methylation, acetylation and expression of microRNA (miRNA). miRNAs are 18 to 22 nucleotides in length and regulate gene expression at the protein-translation and messenger RNA (mRNA)-level in P bodies by mRNA sequestration that results in a negative correlation between miRNA and mRNA. miRNA–mRNA interactions can explain the increase or decrease in protein levels [10]. Currently, in vitro models have demonstrated the involvement of microRNAs in the biological responses induced by toxic compounds such as BaP; therefore, altered expression of miRNAs is considered a biomarker [11]. In the present work, we analyzed the induction of the proinflammatory cytokine *TNF-α* attributed to the activation of *AhR* and *CYP1B1* as metabolic processors of PAH, and miR-125b and miR-155 expression related to these processes. We found that *AhR* expression is related to PAH exposure, which may be implicated in several pathogenesis processes.

2. Materials and Methods

2.1. Population

Forty-one samples were analyzed from healthy women with an age range of 18–45 years old, and all were residents of two rural communities (with little vehicular traffic) in the state of San Luis Potosi, Mexico (The Cañon, in the municipality of Xilitla, and Comoca Ahuacatitla, in the municipality of Axtla Terrazas). The women who participated in the study used wood as their only source of fuel for cooking, lived in traditional houses (usually wood) and usually spent most of the day inside their homes and an average of 6.5 h cooking. All the women who participated in the study had lived in their community since they were born. Therefore, their main source of exposure to PAHs was the combustion of biomass. After informed consent was obtained, a questionnaire was completed and urine samples were taken. The questionnaire included characteristics such as age, weight, height and exposure to snuff smoke. In addition, sociodemographic characteristics were described. The study was approved by the ethics committee of the Faculty of Medicine at the Autonomous University of San Luis Potosi.

2.2. Urine Collection

The first morning urine of each woman (at approximately 7:00 am) was collected. The urine was collected in airtight plastic bottles and stored in a freezer at −20 °C until analyzed. Before analysis, samples were thawed at room temperature, homogenized, and 10 ml of urine was transferred to a test tube (Corning®, New York, NY, USA).

2.3. Determination of Urinary 1-OHP

1-OHP (half-life ranged from 6 to 30 h) was taken as a representative biomarker of exposure to PAH mixtures [12,13]; it was taken into account that this compound is a pyrene metabolite, and, in turn, pyrene is often present in PAH mixtures. 1-OHP was quantified following the method described previously [13,14]. The analyses were performed using HPLC (HP1100, Agilent Technologies; Santa Clara, CA, USA) and a fluorescence detector (G1321A). A Zorbax SB-C18 pre-column (Agilent Technologies; Santa Clara, CA, USA) and a Zorbax Eclipse XDB-C18 column (Agilent Technologies; Santa Clara, CA, USA) were used. The analysis temperature was set at 40 °C, the flow was adjusted to 1 mL/min and the injection volume was 20 μL. 1-OHP was eluted with 88:12 methanol:water and 1% ascorbic acid. Data were collected and processed using HP ChemStation software (Dayton, OH). Urinary 1-OHP concentrations were adjusted to urinary creatinine, which was determined using the Jaffe colorimetric method [15]. Under our conditions, the detection and quantification limits were 1.0 nmol/L and 3.0 nmol/L, respectively. Quality control was certified using the standards IRIS Clin Cal Recipe (Munich, Germany) 50013, 8867 and 50014 (9.1, 15.6 and 32.5 nmol/L 1-OHP, respectively), and there was a recovery rate of 99%.

2.4. Peripheral Blood Mononuclear Cells (PBMCs) Isolation

Venous blood was collected by venipuncture from the antecubital area of the arm into tubes (Becton Dickinson Vacutainer®Mexico) containing EDTA. Peripheral blood mononuclear cells (PBMCs) were separated by density gradient centrifugation using Ficoll-Hypaque (Sigma-Aldrich by Merck, Darmstadt, Germany), and washed with phosphate-buffered saline (PBS) solution (Sigma-Aldrich by Merck, Darmstadt, Germany).

2.5. RNA Isolation and RT-qPCR

The PBMCs were collected and washed with PBS for total RNA and miRNA isolation using Trizol (Invitrogen by Thermo Fisher Scientific, Waltham, MA, USA) method; the concentration and quality was determined by spectrophotometric analysis in a Synergy HT Multi-Mode Microplate Reader, using Gen5™ Data Analysis Software (BioTek Instruments, Inc., a part of Agilent, Santa Clara, CA, USA), and the samples were stored at −80 °C until use. Complementary cDNA was synthesized with 1 μg total RNA using reverse transcriptase superscript II and reverse transcription reagents of Invitrogen (Thermo Fisher Scientific, Waltham, MA, USA) under the following conditions: 25 °C 10 min, 35 °C 90 min, 94 °C 5 min and 4 °C 5 min. The qPCR was performed by mixing 1 μL of cDNA (100 ng/μL), 0.1 μL sense and antisense primers (20 pM) (Invitrogen Thermo Fisher Scientific, Waltham, NA, USA) and 1X SYBR®Green PCR Master Mix (*Applied Biosystems* by Life Technologies Waltham, MA, USA) in a total volume of 10 μL. Primers were designed and checked for specificity by BLAST search, and the purity of the PCR products and specificity of the reaction were checked by agarose gel electrophoresis analysis. The expression of target genes was determined using the CFX96 BioRad thermocycler (Bio-Rad Laboratories Hercules, CA, USA). The cycling conditions were as follows: 10 min denaturing at 95 °C, followed by 40 cycles of denaturing at 95 °C for 15 s, 45 s primer annealing, and elongation at 60 °C for 18 s; specifically, the annealing temperatures were 67.5 °C for *TNFα* and *AhR* and 66.5 °C for *CYP1B1*. The melting curve was analyzed with CFX Manager™ software (Bio-Rad Laboratories Hercules, CA, USA). Transcript expressions were normalized to *18S* rRNA housekeeping gene and data were quantified by the method of $2^{-\Delta\Delta Ct}$. The primers used were as follows:

Genes	Forward sequence (5'-3')	Reverse sequence (5'-3')	Weight of the amplicon	Tm °C	Number of Cycles
18s	CGGCTACCACATCCAAGGAA	GCTGGAATTACCGCGGCT	189 pb	60	40
TNFα	CCCACGGCTCCACCCTCTCT	TCTGGGGGCCGATCACTCCA	215 pb	67.5	40
AhR	TCATTTGCTGGAGGTCACCC	GCCAAGGACTGTTGCTGTTG	254 pb	60	40
CyP1B1	TAGTGGTGCTGAATGGCGAG	CTCCGAGTAGTGGCCGAAAG	137 pb	66.5	40

2.6. miRNA Expression

For microRNA analysis, reverse transcription (RT) and real-time quantitative polymerase chain reaction (qRT-PCR) were performed using a TaqMan®MicroRNA Assay (Applied Biosystems by Life Technologies, Waltham, MA, USA; miR-155: 002623, miR125b:000449) according to the instructions supplied by the manufacturer. Small nuclear RNA U6 was used for normalization.

2.7. Statistical Analysis

Data are presented as mean ± SEM values. An unpaired t-test was performed to identify changes in the gene expression of AhR, CYP1A1, TNF-α, hsamiR-125 and hsamiR-155, and a Pearson coefficient test was applied to determine gene expression correlations. All statistical analysis was performed with the Graph Pad Prism version 8.0 for Windows (Prism Software, La Jolla, CA, USA, www.graphpad.com). A p value less than 0.05 was considered significant.

3. Results

3.1. 1-OHP Determination in Urine Samples

PAHs are generated during the incomplete combustion of organic matter. To determine the level of exposure to PAHs, we evaluated the concentration of urinary 1-OHP as a biomarker of exposure to the hydrocarbon mixture, as previously shown [16,17]. We assessed 41 urine samples of healthy women who had a traditional stove inside their house and used wood as a biomass fuel for cooking. Normalized data and non-normalized data with urine creatinine concentration (geometric mean ± SD 1.46 ± 2.11 µg/g creatinine; 1.09 ± 1.68 µg/L) and percentiles are shown in Table 1. Interestingly, in PC25, a value of 0.84 µg 1-OHP/g creatinine was found, despite limit values of 0.463 µg 1-OHP/g creatinine for occupationally unexposed non-smoking individuals and 1.46 µg 1-OHP/g creatinine for the occupationally unexposed smoking population having been previously established [13]. Considering that the women included in our study were occupationally unexposed but were in contact with a source of pollutants due to incomplete combustion, we stratified the population into two groups: group A, including individuals with less exposure to PAHs (levels below 1.46 µg 1-OHP/g creatinine), and group B, including individuals with greater exposure (levels above 1.46 µg 1-OHP/g creatinine) (Figure 1). The collected biochemical and anthropometric data from the studied population showed statistical difference solely for 1-OHP by the multiple t-tests, as seen in Table 2. Other features of the population, such as age, glucose level, cholesterol, height, weight, etc., were not statistically significant, reaffirming that 1-OHP could be used to stratify people exposed to PAHs.

Table 1. The 1-hydroxypyren urinary concentration of exposed women. The limit of detection (LOD) was 1 nmol/L (0.21825 µg/L).

Units	Mean	SD	PC25	PC50	PC75	PC95	Min	Max
µg/g creatinine	1.46	2.11	0.84	1.47	2.76	7.10	<LOD	10.87
µg/L of urine	1.09	1.68	0.61	0.96	2.10	6.08	<LOD	9.19

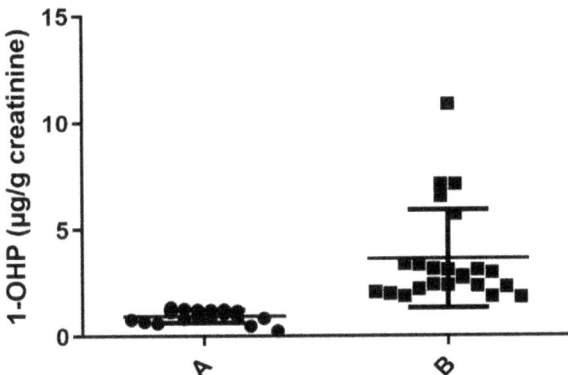

Figure 1. Determination of 1-OHP in μg/g creatinine in urine samples exposed to PAHs. Samples with urine concentration of 1-OHP ≤ 1.46 μg/g creatinine ($n = 18$) A. Samples with concentration of 1-OHP > 1.46 μg/g creatinine ($n = 23$), ($p = 0.0001$) B.

Table 2. Biochemical and anthropometric features analyzed by multiple t-tests of two-way ANOVA of urine samples exposed to PAHs.

	p Value	Mean of Group A	Mean of Group B
Age	0.109067	38.8261	46.3529
1-OHP	0.001267	0.848821	4.53468
Glucose	0.121731	92.8827	120.720
Total cholesterol	0.197449	165.233	181.997
HDL cholesterol	0.651043	46.2526	48.3669
LDL cholesterol	0.409356	94.2199	102.562
VLDL cholesterol	0.182865	25.3966	31.0680
Triglycerides	0.211349	126.983	153.343
Height	0.432416	1.46174	1.47686
Waist diameter	0.324131	85.4565	88.4571
Hip diameter	0.281592	97.9565	101.814
Weight	0.324085	55.5478	58.6314
BMI	0.508237	25.9577	26.7646

3.2. Determination and Correlation of AhR, CYP1B1 and TNF-α Expression by RT-qPCR

Once the 1-OHP concentration was determined and groups A and B were assigned as low and high 1-OHP concentration, respectively, we used the lower exposure group ("A") as a calibrator for the group with the highest exposure ("B"). We analyzed the expression levels of *TNF-α*, *AhR* and *CYP1B1* mRNAs in groups A and B. The difference in *AhR* expression between groups A and B was statistically significant, $p = 0.0412$; in group B, an increase was observed (Figure 2A). The expression of *CYP1B1* recorded similar expression in both groups, $p = 0.3570$ (Figure 2B), and *TNF-α* expression showed even more similarity between groups than *CYP1B1* (Figure 2C), $p = 0.2476$. Exposure to PAHs augmented *AhR* expression, suggesting a common gene regulation in response to contact with PAHs.

3.3. Evaluation of miR-125b and miR-155 Relative Expression in a Population Exposed to PAHs

It is well known that the regulation of gene expression is complex; currently, epigenetic regulators may explain part of the control. In this context, we evaluated the expression of miR-125b, an important master regulator of the methylation process, and miR-155, considered a pro-inflammatory regulator that is implicated in several pathologies. We did not find statistically significant differences in the expression of miR-125b and miR-155 between study groups (Figure 3A,B).

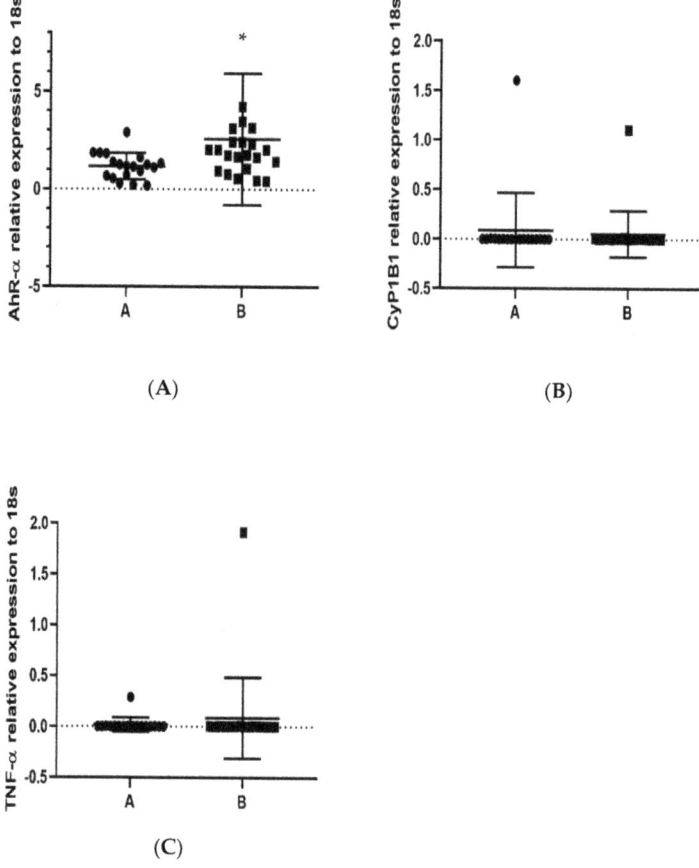

Figure 2. Determination by RT-qPCR of *AhR*, *CYP1B1* and *TNF-α* relative expression in PBMCs in population (groups A and B) exposed to PAHs: (**A**) *AhR*, * p = 0.0412; (**B**) *CYP1B1*, p = 0.3570; and (**C**) *TNF-α*, p = 0.2476. 18s RNA was used to normalize the expressed transcripts. * $p < 0.05$.

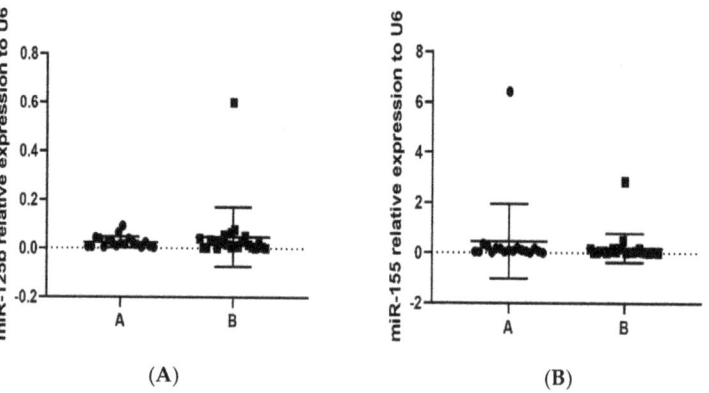

Figure 3. Determination by RT-qPCR of miR-125b and miR-155 relative expression in PBMCs in population (groups A and B) exposed to PAHs: (**A**) miR-125b, p = 0.2201; and (**B**) miR-155, p = 0.2227. Small nuclear RNA U6 was used for normalization.

4. Discussion

Women who use biomass as the main source of energy for cooking their food and heating their homes present different biomarkers of pollutants in their bodies such as 1-OHP. They are directly and chronically exposed to pollutants generated during their daily activities and spend a significant amount of time inside their kitchens every day. In this work, all of the samples tested presented values of 1-OHP higher than 0.463 µg/g creatinine, a limit value proposed for a non-occupationally exposed, non-smoking population [13]. We obtained levels almost three times higher (1.09 ± 1.68 µg/L) than Polanska et al., 2014, who reported 0.43 µg 1-OHP/g creatinine [18]. Furthermore, in 2016, Pruneda-Álvarez et al. reported a value of 0.92 ± 0.92 in a study performed in Mexican indigenous and rural communities [19]. Interestingly, in another study in the rural community El Leoncito, San Luis Potosí, the mean value of 1-OHP was 0.56 µg/L for 40 women who cooked on rustic stoves in their homes [20]; the value was similar to the 0.5 µg/L that was established in a German environmental survey for a general population without risk [21]. In both studies, Pruneda and Ruiz included indigenous Mexican women; however, the values were half of those found in the current study. The National Health and Nutrition Examination Survey IV (NHANES IV) reported a geometric mean of 0.074 µg/L for 1-OHP in people aged 20 years and older (n = 1301), a value ten times lower than our results; however, whether they are non-smokers and whether or not they are exposed to either source of PAHs were not specified [22]. Additionally, it should be considered that location, type of house, gender, age and genetic differences could all contribute to 1-OHP concentrations. Pruneda-Álvarez et al., 2012, showed that the levels of 1-OHP in indigenous women exposed either outdoors or indoors were 0.73 ± 0.45 µg/L and 4.81 ± 9.6 µg/L, respectively; the highest levels were in women who had a traditional stove inside their home and spent around 8 h cooking daily [23]. The exposure scenario is similar to our study; however, the mean for 1-OHP µg/L in the Pruneda-Álvarez 2012 report was significantly higher than what is reported here. Exposure to a mixture of PAHs could be an important human health risk factor, and this exposure has been associated with several adverse health effects [22]. The molecular mechanisms related to the health effects include DNA adducts, increased apoptosis, oxidative damage and pro-inflammatory responses [24–27]. In this regard, we evaluated mRNA levels of *TNF-α* as a pro-inflammatory biomarker in the women's samples and our results indicated slight upregulation of mRNA in the high-exposure group, suggesting a probable pro-inflammatory response to PAH exposure. In a recent study performed on 39 taxi drivers potentially exposed to emissions, a positive linear correlation between 1-OHP levels and pro-inflammatory cytokines (IL 1β (r = 0.37, p = 0.007), IL-6 (r = 0.32, p = 0.02) and TNFα (r = 0.33, p = 0.02)) was reported [28], suggesting a weak correlation between PAH exposure and TNFα mRNA and protein expression. The PAHs regulated gene expression at several levels, cell systems and cell-signaling pathways. It was shown that p,p'-Dichlorodiphenyldichloroethylene (DDE) and coplanar 3,3',4,4',5-pentachlorobiphenyl (PCBs) compounds were able to enhance *AhR* transcript expression [24,25]. Recently, enhanced AhR expression has been related to an inflammatory state as a consequence of 2,3,7,8-tetrachlorodibenzo-*p*-dioxin (TCDD), PCBs, DDE and metabolites exposure [6,26,29,30]. Here, we found an augmented expression of *AhR* in the high-exposure group, suggesting that PAHs promote responses through AhR activation. It has been shown that an increase in TNF-α expression contributes to keeping the activation of the AhR pathway and the chronic inflammatory state producing a positive feedback. AhR is a key regulatory element for some xenobiotic degradation enzymes, notably cytochromes P450 belonging to the CYP1 family. Cytochrome activation is induced by several ligands of AhR, such as TCDD or PAHs such as BaP, as potent inductors of CYP1B1 that could be considered as a biomarker for the activation of AhR [27]. AhR is mainly expressed in liver cells, but it is also present in different types of cells, such as blood cells [29–31], suggesting that it could be used as a biomarker for PAH exposure.

Recently, epigenetic mechanisms have emerged as an important response to pollutants. PAH exposure can alter epigenetic mechanisms, including miRNAs [32]. miR-125b is a methylation modulator upregulated in cell cultures exposed to BaP and having inflammatory regulation functions [10]. Overexpression of miR-125b induces the expression of TNF-α, IL-6 and IL-1β in plasma from rheumatoid arthritis patients, showing a strong positive correlation between miR-125b and TNF-α [33]. Here, we showed that *TNF-α* and miR-125b expression were not increased in women from the high PAH exposure group. The difference between the work of Zhang et al. and our results could be attributable to other mechanisms that modulate the expression of TNF-α, including other miRNAs or another epigenetic mechanism, lower sample numbers, a different population and environment, as well as feedback mechanisms activated during inflammatory chronic process. In addition, we analyzed the expression of miR-155, which is a multifunctional microRNA. Recent data indicated that miR-155 has different expression profiles and plays a crucial role in various physiological and pathological processes such as hematopoietic lineage differentiation, immunity, inflammation, cancer and cardiovascular diseases [34]. It has been reported that in human alveolar macrophages, co-culture with miR-155 inhibitors increases TNF-α expression [35], showing similarity to our work, despite the expression of *TNF-α* and miR-155 not being statistically significant.

AhR ligands such as PAHs induce biological effects, including the induction of cytochrome P450 (CYP1B1) and other AhR-regulated genes. Interestingly, it has been reported that other endogenous molecules such as TNF-α have a modulator effect in both cytochrome and AhR expression [26]. In previous studies, it has been shown that AhR ligands induce CYP1B production in cell cultures, and when TNF-α was added, the expression of CYP1B1 was induced. Interestingly, cells co-stimulated with both BaP and TNF-α showed synergized effect, significantly increasing CYP1B1 expression [36,37]. In our results, this association was not found. Interestingly, the *AhR* expression recorded in response to PAHs is similar in several works; therefore, *AhR* is an important biomarker for PAH exposure.

5. Conclusions

This study primarily describes women's exposure to PAHs in terms of urinary 1-OHP concentration, which was confirmed as a marker that can be used to classify PAH exposure. In fact, a stratification into two exposure groups has been proposed for the experimented levels of exposure, one at low levels of the 1-OHP indicator and one at high levels of 1-OHP. Even if these different levels were not explained by the type or intensity of the domestic source, the stratification was very useful to demonstrate that high levels of PAHs promote the expression of *AhR*, which is probably involved in pathway modulation in vivo, suggesting that cell signaling triggered by *AhR* may be implicated in several pathogenesis processes.

Author Contributions: Conceptualization, M.S.-B.; Methodology, J.A.V.-S., S.T.O.-G., J.A.L. and H.H.-L.; Formal analysis, J.A.V.-S., M.E.M.-L., S.T.O.-G., I.N.P.-M., J.A.L., H.H.-L., R.G.-A., E.S.C.-A., D.P.P.-P. and M.S.-B.; Investigation, J.A.V.-S., M.E.M.-L., J.A.L., E.S.C.-A., D.P.P.-P. and M.S.-B.; Data curation, I.N.P.-M., J.A.L., H.H.-L., R.G.-A., E.S.C.-A. and D.P.P.-P.; Writing—original draft, J.A.V.-S.; Supervision, I.N.P.-M., R.G.-A. and M.S.-B.; Funding acquisition, M.S.-B. All authors have read and agreed to the published version of the manuscript.

Funding: This research was funded by the Fondo Sectorial de Investigación en Salud y Seguridad Social SS/IMSS/ISSSTE-CONACYT-2010-01, grant number 141785 and Fortalecimiento de Infraestructura y Desarrollo de Capacidades Científicas, grant number 321616. The APC was funded by the Universidad Autónoma de Zacatecas.

Institutional Review Board Statement: The study was conducted in accordance with the Declaration of Helsinki and was approved by the ethics committee of the Faculty of Medicine at the Autonomous University of San Luis Potosi (protocol code 2014-004).

Informed Consent Statement: Informed consent was obtained from all subjects involved in the study.

Data Availability Statement: Data supporting the reported results may be requested from the corresponding author.

Conflicts of Interest: The authors declare no conflict of interest.

References

1. ADSTR. Toxicological Profile for Polycyclic Aromatic Hydrocarbons. U.S. Department of Health and Human Services Public Health Service. Agency for Toxic Substances and Disease Registry. 1995. Available online: https://www.atsdr.cdc.gov/toxprofiles/tp69.pdf (accessed on 11 November 2022).
2. U.S. EPA. *IRIS Toxicological Review of Benzo[A]Pyrene (Final Report)*; U.S. Environmental Protection Agency: Washington, DC, USA, 2017.
3. Dasari, S.; Ganjayi, M.S.; Yellanurkonda, P.; Basha, S.; Meriga, B. Role of glutathione S-transferases in detoxification of a polycyclic aromatic hydrocarbon, methylcholanthrene. *Chem. Biol. Interact.* **2018**, *294*, 81–90. [CrossRef]
4. Thuy, H.T.T.; Loan, T.T.C.; Phuong, T.H. The potential accumulation of polycyclic aromatic hydrocarbons in phytoplankton and bivalves in Can Gio coastal wetland, Vietnam. *Environ. Sci. Pollut. Res. Int.* **2018**, *25*, 17240–17249. [CrossRef] [PubMed]
5. Neavin, D.R.; Liu, D.; Ray, B.; Weinshilboum, R.M. The Role of the Aryl Hydrocarbon Receptor (AHR) in Immune and Inflammatory Diseases. *Int. J. Mol. Sci.* **2018**, *19*, 3851. [CrossRef] [PubMed]
6. Kobayashi, S.; Okamoto, H.; Iwamoto, T.; Toyama, Y.; Tomatsu, T.; Yamanaka, H.; Momohara, S. A role for the aryl hydrocarbon receptor and the dioxin TCDD in rheumatoid arthritis. *Rheumatology* **2008**, *47*, 1317–1322. [CrossRef] [PubMed]
7. Perumal Vijayaraman, K.; Muruganantham, S.; Subramanian, M.; Shunmugiah, K.P.; Kasi, P.D. Silymarin attenuates benzo(a)pyrene induced toxicity by mitigating ROS production, DNA damage and calcium mediated apoptosis in peripheral blood mononuclear cells (PBMC). *Ecotoxicol. Environ. Saf.* **2012**, *86*, 79–85. [CrossRef] [PubMed]
8. Tamaki, A.; Hayashi, H.; Nakajima, H.; Takii, T.; Katagiri, D.; Miyazawa, K.; Hirose, K.; Onozaki, K. Polycyclic aromatic hydrocarbon increases mRNA level for interleukin 1 beta in human fibroblast-like synoviocyte line via aryl hydrocarbon receptor. *Biol. Pharm. Bull.* **2004**, *27*, 407–410. [CrossRef]
9. Waddington, C.H. The epigenotype. 1942. *Int. J. Epidemiol.* **2012**, *41*, 10–13. [CrossRef]
10. Guo, H.; Ingolia, N.T.; Weissman, J.S.; Bartel, D.P. Mammalian microRNAs predominantly act to decrease target mRNA levels. *Nature* **2010**, *466*, 835–840. [CrossRef]
11. Lizarraga, D.; Gaj, S.; Brauers, K.J.; Timmermans, L.; Kleinjans, J.C.; van Delft, J.H. Benzo[a]pyrene-induced changes in microRNA-mRNA networks. *Chem. Res. Toxicol.* **2012**, *25*, 838–849. [CrossRef]
12. Jacob, J.; Seidel, A. Biomonitoring of polycyclic aromatic hydrocarbons in human urine. *J. Chromatogr. B Anal. Technol. Biomed. Life Sci.* **2002**, *778*, 31–47. [CrossRef]
13. Jongeneelen, F.J. Benchmark guideline for urinary 1-hydroxypyrene as biomarker of occupational exposure to polycyclic aromatic hydrocarbons. *Ann. Occup. Hyg.* **2001**, *45*, 3–13. [CrossRef] [PubMed]
14. Kuusimaki, L.; Peltonen, Y.; Mutanen, P.; Peltonen, K.; Savela, K. Urinary hydroxy-metabolites of naphthalene, phenanthrene and pyrene as markers of exposure to diesel exhaust. *Int. Arch. Occup. Environ. Health* **2004**, *77*, 23–30. [CrossRef] [PubMed]
15. Narayanan, S.; Appleton, H.D. Creatinine: A review. *Clin. Chem.* **1980**, *26*, 1119–1126. [CrossRef]
16. Perez-Maldonado, I.N.; Martinez-Salinas, R.I.; Pruneda Alvarez, L.G.; Perez-Vazquez, F.J. Urinary 1-hydroxypyrene concentration from Mexican children living in the southeastern region in Mexico. *Int. J. Environ. Health Res.* **2014**, *24*, 113–119. [CrossRef] [PubMed]
17. Perez-Maldonado, I.N.; Ochoa-Martinez, A.C.; Orta-Garcia, S.T.; Ruiz-Vera, T.; Varela-Silva, J.A. Concentrations of Environmental Chemicals in Urine and Blood Samples of Children from San Luis Potosi, Mexico. *Bull. Environ. Contam Toxicol.* **2017**, *99*, 258–263. [CrossRef]
18. Polanska, K.; Hanke, W.; Dettbarn, G.; Sobala, W.; Gromadzinska, J.; Magnus, P.; Seidel, A. The determination of polycyclic aromatic hydrocarbons in the urine of non-smoking Polish pregnant women. *Sci. Total Environ.* **2014**, *487*, 102–109. [CrossRef]
19. Pruneda-Alvarez, L.G.; Perez-Vazquez, F.J.; Ruiz-Vera, T.; Ochoa-Martinez, A.C.; Orta-Garcia, S.T.; Jimenez-Avalos, J.A.; Perez-Maldonado, I.N. Urinary 1-hydroxypyrene concentration as an exposure biomarker to polycyclic aromatic hydrocarbons (PAHs) in Mexican women from different hot spot scenarios and health risk assessment. *Environ. Sci. Pollut. Res. Int.* **2016**, *23*, 6816–6825. [CrossRef]
20. Ruiz-Vera, T.; Pruneda-Alvarez, L.G.; Ochoa-Martinez, A.C.; Ramirez-GarciaLuna, J.L.; Pierdant-Perez, M.; Gordillo-Moscoso, A.A.; Perez-Vazquez, F.J.; Perez-Maldonado, I.N. Assessment of vascular function in Mexican women exposed to polycyclic aromatic hydrocarbons from wood smoke. *Environ. Toxicol. Pharmacol.* **2015**, *40*, 423–429. [CrossRef]
21. Wilhelm, M.; Hardt, J.; Schulz, C.; Angerer, J.; Human Biomonitoring Commission of the German Federal Environment, A. New reference value and the background exposure for the PAH metabolites 1-hydroxypyrene and 1- and 2-naphthol in urine of the general population in Germany: Basis for validation of human biomonitoring data in environmental medicine. *Int. J. Hyg. Environ. Health* **2008**, *211*, 447–453. [CrossRef]
22. Kim, K.H.; Jahan, S.A.; Kabir, E.; Brown, R.J. A review of airborne polycyclic aromatic hydrocarbons (PAHs) and their human health effects. *Environ. Int.* **2013**, *60*, 71–80. [CrossRef]
23. Pruneda-Alvarez, L.G.; Perez-Vazquez, F.J.; Salgado-Bustamante, M.; Martinez-Salinas, R.I.; Pelallo-Martinez, N.A.; Perez-Maldonado, I.N. Exposure to indoor air pollutants (polycyclic aromatic hydrocarbons, toluene, benzene) in Mexican indigenous women. *Indoor Air* **2012**, *22*, 140–147. [CrossRef] [PubMed]

24. Alegria-Torres, J.A.; Diaz-Barriga, F.; Gandolfi, A.J.; Perez-Maldonado, I.N. Mechanisms of p,p'-DDE-induced apoptosis in human peripheral blood mononuclear cells. *Toxicol. In Vitro* **2009**, *23*, 1000–1006. [CrossRef] [PubMed]
25. Cardenas-Gonzalez, M.; Gaspar-Ramirez, O.; Perez-Vazquez, F.J.; Alegria-Torres, J.A.; Gonzalez-Amaro, R.; Perez-Maldonado, I.N. p,p'-DDE, a DDT metabolite, induces proinflammatory molecules in human peripheral blood mononuclear cells "in vitro". *Exp. Toxicol. Pathol.* **2013**, *65*, 661–665. [CrossRef] [PubMed]
26. Umannova, L.; Zatloukalova, J.; Machala, M.; Krcmar, P.; Majkova, Z.; Hennig, B.; Kozubik, A.; Vondracek, J. Tumor necrosis factor-alpha modulates effects of aryl hydrocarbon receptor ligands on cell proliferation and expression of cytochrome P450 enzymes in rat liver "stem-like" cells. *Toxicol. Sci.* **2007**, *99*, 79–89. [CrossRef]
27. Baird, W.M.; Hooven, L.A.; Mahadevan, B. Carcinogenic polycyclic aromatic hydrocarbon-DNA adducts and mechanism of action. *Environ. Mol. Mutagen.* **2005**, *45*, 106–114. [CrossRef]
28. Brucker, N.; Moro, A.M.; Charao, M.F.; Durgante, J.; Freitas, F.; Baierle, M.; Nascimento, S.; Gauer, B.; Bulcao, R.P.; Bubols, G.B.; et al. Biomarkers of occupational exposure to air pollution, inflammation and oxidative damage in taxi drivers. *Sci. Total Environ.* **2013**, *463–464*, 884–893. [CrossRef]
29. Vondracek, J.; Umannova, L.; Machala, M. Interactions of the aryl hydrocarbon receptor with inflammatory mediators: Beyond CYP1A regulation. *Curr. Drug Metab.* **2011**, *12*, 89–103. [CrossRef]
30. Vogel, C.F.; Khan, E.M.; Leung, P.S.; Gershwin, M.E.; Chang, W.L.; Wu, D.; Haarmann-Stemmann, T.; Hoffmann, A.; Denison, M.S. Cross-talk between aryl hydrocarbon receptor and the inflammatory response: A role for nuclear factor-kappaB. *J. Biol. Chem.* **2014**, *289*, 1866–1875. [CrossRef]
31. Prigent, L.; Robineau, M.; Jouneau, S.; Morzadec, C.; Louarn, L.; Vernhet, L.; Fardel, O.; Sparfel, L. The aryl hydrocarbon receptor is functionally upregulated early in the course of human T-cell activation. *Eur. J. Immunol.* **2014**, *44*, 1330–1340. [CrossRef]
32. Schembri, F.; Sridhar, S.; Perdomo, C.; Gustafson, A.M.; Zhang, X.; Ergun, A.; Lu, J.; Liu, G.; Zhang, X.; Bowers, J.; et al. MicroRNAs as modulators of smoking-induced gene expression changes in human airway epithelium. *Proc. Natl. Acad. Sci. USA* **2009**, *106*, 2319–2324. [CrossRef]
33. Zhang, B.; Wang, L.S.; Zhou, Y.H. Elevated microRNA-125b promotes inflammation in rheumatoid arthritis by activation of NF-kappaB pathway. *Biomed. Pharmacother.* **2017**, *93*, 1151–1157. [CrossRef] [PubMed]
34. Faraoni, I.; Antonetti, F.R.; Cardone, J.; Bonmassar, E. miR-155 gene: A typical multifunctional microRNA. *Biochim. Biophys. Acta* **2009**, *1792*, 497–505. [CrossRef] [PubMed]
35. Yang, Y.; Wu, B.Q.; Wang, Y.H.; Shi, Y.F.; Luo, J.M.; Ba, J.H.; Liu, H.; Zhang, T.T. Regulatory effects of miR-155 and miR-146a on repolarization and inflammatory cytokine secretion in human alveolar macrophages in vitro. *Immunopharmacol. Immunotoxicol.* **2016**, *38*, 502–509. [CrossRef] [PubMed]
36. Umannova, L.; Machala, M.; Topinka, J.; Novakova, Z.; Milcova, A.; Kozubik, A.; Vondracek, J. Tumor necrosis factor-alpha potentiates genotoxic effects of benzo[a]pyrene in rat liver epithelial cells through upregulation of cytochrome P450 1B1 expression. *Mutat. Res.* **2008**, *640*, 162–169. [CrossRef] [PubMed]
37. Umannova, L.; Machala, M.; Topinka, J.; Schmuczerova, J.; Krcmar, P.; Neca, J.; Sujanova, K.; Kozubik, A.; Vondracek, J. Benzo[a]pyrene and tumor necrosis factor-alpha coordinately increase genotoxic damage and the production of proinflammatory mediators in alveolar epithelial type II cells. *Toxicol. Lett.* **2011**, *206*, 121–129. [CrossRef] [PubMed]

Disclaimer/Publisher's Note: The statements, opinions and data contained in all publications are solely those of the individual author(s) and contributor(s) and not of MDPI and/or the editor(s). MDPI and/or the editor(s) disclaim responsibility for any injury to people or property resulting from any ideas, methods, instructions or products referred to in the content.

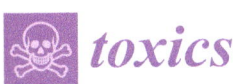

Article

Polycyclic Aromatic Hydrocarbons (PAHs) Exposure Triggers Inflammation and Endothelial Dysfunction in BALB/c Mice: A Pilot Study

Gabriel A. Rojas [1,2], Nicolás Saavedra [1], Kathleen Saavedra [1], Montserrat Hevia [1], Cristian Morales [1], Fernando Lanas [3] and Luis A. Salazar [1,*]

1. Center of Molecular Biology & Pharmacogenetics, Department of Basic Sciences, Scientific and Technological Bioresource Nucleus (BIOREN), Universidad de La Frontera, Temuco 4811230, Chile
2. Faculty of Health, School of Kinesiology, Universidad Santo Tomás, Valdivia 5090000, Chile
3. Department of Internal Medicine, Faculty of Medicine, Universidad de La Frontera, Temuco 4811230, Chile
* Correspondence: luis.salazar@ufrontera.cl

Abstract: The particulate matter present in air pollution is a complex mixture of solid and liquid particles that vary in size, origin, and composition, among which are polycyclic aromatic hydrocarbons (PAHs). Although exposure to PAHs has become an important risk factor for cardiovascular disease, the mechanisms by which these compounds contribute to increased cardiovascular risk have not been fully explored. The aim of the present study was to evaluate the effects of PAH exposure on systemic pro-inflammatory cytokines and markers of endothelial dysfunction. An intervention was designed using a murine model composed of twenty BALB/c male mice separated into controls and three groups exposed to a mixture of phenanthrene, fluoranthene, and pyrene using three different concentrations. The serum levels of the inflammatory cytokines and gene expression of adhesion molecules located on endothelial cells along with inflammatory markers related to PAH exposure in aortic tissue were determined. Furthermore, the expression of the ICAM-1 and VCAM-1 proteins was evaluated. The data showed significant differences in IL-6 and IFN-γ in the serum. In the gene expression, significant differences for ICAM-1, VCAM-1, and E-Selectin were observed. The results suggest that phenanthrene, fluoranthene, and pyrene, present in air pollution, stimulate the increase in serum inflammatory cytokines and the expression of markers of endothelial dysfunction in the murine model studied, both relevant characteristics associated with the onset of disease atherosclerosis and cardiovascular disease.

Keywords: air pollution; endothelium; inflammation; cardiovascular disease

1. Introduction

Air pollution is a serious global public health problem. According to the Ambient Air Quality Guide of the World Health Organization (WHO), 95% of the world population lives in areas exceeding the recommended values [1]. The most recent estimates revealed that 4.2 million deaths (7.6% of total global mortality and 700,000 more deaths in 2015 compared with 1990) are attributable to ambient particulate matter$_{2.5}$ (PM$_{2.5}$) [2]. PM is a widespread complex mixture of solid and liquid particles suspended in air that vary in size, shape, origin, and composition. PM is an air pollutant known as a human carcinogen (group I, IARC, 2013). The composition of PM can substantially vary between geographical regions, sources of emissions, and even weather or seasons [3]. Its chemical composition comprises inorganic ions (e.g., sulfates, nitrates, ammonium, and soluble metals), insoluble metals, elemental carbon, and organic compounds including PAHs, polychlorinated biphenyls, biological components (allergens), microbial agents, and water. The carbonaceous part of air pollution is regarded as more involved in adverse health effects, and some PAHs

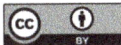

are considered as particularly important [4]. Thus, PM and PAH are among the most health-relevant air pollutants [5,6].

The three main ways in which air pollution causes damage to the cardiovascular system have been proposed: (a) secretion of pro-inflammatory mediators or oxidative stress in the circulatory system; (b) imbalance of the autonomic nervous system; and (c) direct penetration of particles or components in the circulatory system, which affect numerous tissues within the cardiovascular system [7]. Reports indicate that the smallest particles increase the risk of cardiovascular events, with $PM_{2.5}$ being specifically associated with an increased risk of myocardial infarction, stroke, arrhythmia, and exacerbation of heart failure symptoms in susceptible patients [8].

PM accumulation, especially redox active components (e.g., metals and PAHs), can cause oxidative stress and inflammation in lung tissue [9]. The inflammatory response to exposure to PM is characterized by the increased expression of pro-inflammatory cytokines such as tumor necrosis factor alpha (TNF-α) and interleukin-6 (IL-6), which are secreted by cells of the innate immune system [10]. In addition, the adaptive immune system releases interleukin-1β (IL-1β), interleukin-4 (IL-4), and IL-6 [11]. These cytokines are released into the circulatory system, increasing the liver production of C-reactive protein (CPR) and fibrinogen, IL-6, IL-1β, interferon-gamma (IFN-γ), interleukin-8 (IL-8), and TNF-α [8]. This increase in cytokines associated with exposure to PM has been described in various studies [12–15].

Pathological stimuli in the endothelium trigger a phenotype-modifying adaptive response, a process known as endothelial activation, characterized by increased expression of adhesion molecules Selectin-P (P-Selectin), Selectin-E (E-Selectin), intercellular adhesion molecule 1 (ICAM-1), and vascular cell adhesion molecule 1 (VCAM-1) [16,17]. This process compromises the barrier function of the endothelium, which promotes leukocyte diapedesis, increases vascular tone by decreasing nitric oxide production, and reduces resistance to thrombosis [18,19].

Among the toxic components found in $PM_{2.5}$ are PAHs, whose main emission sources are the domestic burning of coal and wood, power plants that burn fossil fuels and biomass, industrial processes, and vehicular traffic [20]. Concentrations of these compounds vary depending on multiple factors such as the season of the year, geographic location, and demographics, among others. Thus, for Temuco, Chile, it was determined that the dominant individual PAHs were phenanthrene (35–45%), fluoranthene (11–15%), and pyrene (9–12%), with the phenanthrene domain reflecting a typical characteristic of emissions from biomass combustion, especially burning wood for heating or cooking [21].

Most of these studies focused their interest on the PM relationship with cardiovascular disease development; however, the mechanisms by which PAH presents in PM contribute to the increased cardiovascular risk have not been explored in depth. Therefore, the objective was to evaluate the effects of PAH exposure on markers of inflammation and endothelial dysfunction in a murine model of BALB/c mice.

2. Materials and Methods

2.1. Animals

Twenty male BALB/c mice were randomly assigned to four equal groups of five animals each including a control group (C = no exposure) and three groups exposed to 10 µg, 30 µg, and 50 µg of a PAH mixture, composed of 55% phenanthrene (Sigma-Aldrich, St. Louis, MO, USA), 25% fluoranthene (Sigma-Aldrich, St. Louis, MO, USA), and 20% pyrene (Sigma-Aldrich, St. Louis, MO, USA), proportionally to the most representative distribution of the PAHs previously described [21]. Dimethylsulfoxide (DMSO, Sigma-Aldrich, St. Louis, MO, USA) was used as a solvent. The animals were kept in the Bioterio of the University of La Frontera, receiving a standard diet and ad libitum water.

2.2. Experimental Protocol

The animals received a 2-week acclimatization treatment according to the instillation protocol described above [22]. The intervention groups underwent nasal instillation of a volume of 10 µL using a micropipette. The intranasal instillation induced an apnea reflex followed by a deep inspiration. In addition, the control group was instilled with the vehicle solution (DMSO) using the same volume. The intervention protocol consisted of instillation for 5 days a week for 5 weeks. We recorded the weight of the animals once a week. To assess the animals' level of stress and spontaneous activity, the cylinder test was applied every two weeks, where the upright exploration attempts in a transparent cylinder were quantified [23]. Thus, low attempts or immobility indicated the level of activity of the animal. To assess the general condition of the animals, the Morton and Griffiths 'Animal Supervision Protocol' was applied once a week [24]. The Scientific Ethics Committee of the Universidad de La Frontera (No 105_18) approved the experimental protocol.

2.3. Sampling Extraction

Euthanasia was performed with a mixture of ketamine/xylazine using a lethal intraperitoneal dose of 200 mg/kg of ketamine-16 mg/kg of xylazine. Whole blood sampling was performed by cardiac puncture and centrifuged at 2000 rpm for 15 min. Once the serum was separated from the blood clot, the samples were stored at −80 °C for later analysis. The thoracic aorta was removed and stored at −80 °C in a sterile tube with 1 mL of RNAlaterTM stabilizer solution (Ambion Inc., Austin, TX, USA).

2.4. Cytokine Analysis

We analyzed the serum levels of IL-6, IL-10, IL-17A, INF-γ, and TNF-α with the 6-Plex Kit of the Bio-Plex Pro TM Mouse Cytokine Th17 Panel A (BioRad, Hercules, CA, USA) following the manufacturer's instructions, with the MAGPIX® system (Luminex, Austin, TX, USA). Twenty samples were tested in duplicate in a 96-well plate including an 8-point standard curve in duplicate and two wells as the negative control. Data collection was performed with xPONENT 4.2® software (Luminex, Austin, TX, USA). We adjusted the cytokine values according to the weight of each animal.

2.5. Gene Expression by RT-qPCR

Gene expression was analyzed by quantitative real-time polymerase chain reaction (RT-qPCR). Specific primers were used for ICAM-1, VCAM-1, E-Selectin, P-Selectin, platelet endothelial cell adhesion molecule (Pecam-1), endothelial nitric oxide synthase (eNOS), aryl hydrocarbon receptor (Ahr), Kelch-type ECH-associated protein 1 (Keap 1), transcription factor p65 (RelA), inhibitor of nuclear factor kappa-B kinase subunit beta (IKK-β), IL-6, and TNF-α, together with the reference genes for ribosomal protein L32 (RPL32) and beta2-microglobulin (B2M) (Table 1). Frozen aortic tissue samples were lysed using 2 mL prefilled tubes with ceramic beads (MP biomedical, Solon, OH, USA) in a benchtop BeadBugTM homogenizer (Benchmark Scientific, Sayreville, NJ, USA) for 60 s at 3500 rpm, adding 1 mL of TRIzol® reagent (Invitrogen, Waltham, MA, USA). Once the tissue was completely homogenized, the TRIzol® reagent protocol recommended by the manufacturer was followed to extract the total RNA, and subsequent evaluation by spectrophotometry (NanoQuant Infinite® 200 PRO, Tecan®, Männedorf, Switzerland) and fluorometry (Quantus™ Fluorometer, Promega, Madison, WI, USA) to determine the purity (260/280 nm ratio) and the amount of RNA extracted, respectively. A ratio between 1.8 and 2.0 was considered as acceptable. The total RNA samples were diluted to ensure a final concentration of 30 ng/µL. The synthesis of cDNA was carried out through reverse transcription using the High-Capacity cDNA Reverse Transcription Kit (Applied Biosystems, Foster City, CA, USA). A qPCR was performed to quantify the expression of each of the selected genes and housekeeping gene using the Fast SYBR® Green Master Mix Kit (Applied Biosystems, Foster City, CA, USA) following the manufacturer's protocols. For qPCR analysis, LinRegPCR® software was used, which established a linearity window and calculated the PCR efficiencies per sample. With the average PCR efficiency per sample, Ct value, and fluorescence threshold established, the initial concentration per sample expressed in arbitrary fluorescence units was calculated [25]. To analyze the specificity of the primers, the melting curve was evaluated.

Table 1. The primer sequences used for the PCR analysis.

Gene	Sequence Forward	Sequence Reverse
ICAM-1	TTCTCATGCCGCACAGAACT	TCCTGGCCTCGGAGACATTA
VCAM-1	CTGGGAAGCTGGAACGAAGT	GCCAAACACTTGACCGTGAC
E-Selectin	AGCCTGCCATGTGGTTGAAT	CTTTGCATGATGGCGTCTCG
P-Selectin	GAAGTGTGACGCTGTGCAAT	CAGCTGGAGTCGTAGGCAAA
PECAM-1	GGAAGTGTCCTCCCTTGAGC	GGAGCCTTCCGTTCTTAGGG
eNOS	GCTCCCAACTGGACCATCTC	TCTTGCACGTAGGTCTTGGG
Ahr	TAAAGTCCACCCCTGCTGAC	CATTCAGCGCCTGTAACAAGA
Keap1	GGCAGGACCAGTTGAACAGT	CATAGCCTCCGAGGACGTAG
RelA	CCTGGAGCAAGCCATTAGC	CGCACTGCATTCAAGTCATAG
IKK-β	GTGCCTGTGACAGCTTACCT	CTCCAGTCTAGAGTCGTGAAGC
IL-6	CCCCAATTTCCAATGCTCTCC	CGCACTAGGTTTGCCGAGTA
TNF-α	ATGGCCTCCCTCTCATCAGT	TTTGCTACGACGTGGGCTAC
RPL32	TAAGCGAAACTGGCGGAAAC	CATCAGGATCTGGCCCTTGA
B2M	ACTGACCGGCCTGTATGCTA	CAATGTGAGGCGGGTGGAA

ICAM-1—Intercellular adhesion molecule 1; VCAM-1—Vascular cell adhesion molecule 1; E-Selectin—Selectin, endothelial cell; P-Selectin—Selectin platelet; PECAM-1—Platelet/endothelial cell adhesion molecule 1; eNOS—Nitric oxide synthase endothelial cell; Ahr—Aryl-hydrocarbon receptor; Keap1—Kelch-like ECH-associated protein 1; RelA—Transcription factor p65; IKK-β—Inhibitor of nuclear factor kappa-B kinase subunit beta; IL-6—Interleukin 6; TNF-α—Tumor necrosis factor α; RPL32—Ribosomal protein L32; B2M—Beta-2 microglobulin.

2.6. Western Blotting

Protein levels of ICAM-1 and VCAM-1 were quantified using α/β-tubulin as a loading control. We performed total protein extraction from aortic tissue using the TRIzol® reagent protocol. Total proteins were quantified using the Pierce BCA Colorimetric Assay Kit (Thermo Scientific ™, Rockford, IL, USA) in a 96-well multiplate, in triplicate. The protein extract was diluted 3:1 in 4× Laemmli sample buffer (Bio-Rad, Hercules, CA, USA) before adding β-mercaptoethanol in a 1:9 ratio (Bio-Rad). The final protein concentration used for the immunodetection of each sample was 40 µg. The samples were denatured at 95 °C for 5 min, and then loaded onto a 4–20% Mini-PROTEAN® TGX ™ electrophoresis gel (Bio-Rad). Afterward, electrophoresis was applied at 100 V for 15 min and then 200 V for 30 min. To differentiate the molecular mass of the bands, the Precision Plus Protein ™ Kaleidoscope standard (Bio-Rad) with a volume of 10 µL was used. The proteins were then transferred to the PVDF immunoblot membrane (Bio-Rad) for 1.5 h at 350 mAmp. Once the transfer was complete, the membrane was stained with Ponceau Red Solution S (Biotium, Fremont, CA, USA) to verify the transfer. Subsequently, the membrane was blocked with 5% NFDM/TBS-Tween for 1 h and then incubated with the primary antibodies at 4 °C overnight according to the manufacturer's instructions. VCAM-1 (1:1000, 5% BSA, 1X TBS, 0.1% Tween®20; Cell Signaling 32653, Danvers, MA, USA), ICAM-1 (1:1000, 5% NFDM, 1X TBS, 0.1% Tween®20; Abcam, ab179707), and as the loading control α/β-tubulin (1:1000, 5% BSA, 1X TBS, 0.1% Tween®20; Cell Signaling 2148, Danvers, MA, USA). Subsequently, the membrane was washed with TBS-Tween and incubated with the HRP-conjugated secondary antibody (1:3000, 5% NFDM 1X TBS, 0.1% Tween®20, goat anti-rabbit IgG; Cell Signaling 7074, Danvers, MA, USA) for 1 h at room temperature. Antigen-antibody binding bands were detected using G: BOX Chemi XRQ (SYNGENE, Frederick, MD, USA) chemiluminescence equipment using the SuperSignal ™ West Femto Maximum Sensitivity Substrate Kit (Thermo Scientific ™, Rockford, IL, USA), following the manufacturer's recommendations. The densitometric analysis of the bands was performed using the ImageJ 1.51j8 open-source software (https://imagej.nih.gov/ij/index.html (accessed on 22 August 2022), National Institutes of Health, Bethesda, MD, USA)

2.7. Statistical Analysis

Data were analyzed using Prism 8.0.2 software (GraphPad, San Diego, CA, USA). The results are ex-pressed as the means ± standard error of the mean. To evaluate the distribution of the values obtained, the Shapiro–Wilk normality test was performed. For the comparison of the groups, Welch's ANOVA with the Dunnett's multiple comparisons test or its non-parametric simile Kruskal–Wallis and a multiple comparison analysis were used through Dunn's test. A two-way ANOVA was used for group comparison analyses with two variables. A p-value < 0.05 was established for statistical significance.

3. Results

3.1. Animals

The initial weight per group of animals did not show significant differences (p = 0.091). The mean weight was as follows: control = 24.20 ± 1.07 g; group 10 µg = 21.40 ± 0.40 g; group 30 µg = 21.80 ± 0.74 g; group 50 µg = 20.80 ± 0.37 g. The weekly weight of each animal was recorded, which did not show significant differences between the groups (p = 0.058). No differences were found in the spontaneous activity of the animals evaluated with the cylinder test (p = 0.919; Figure 1).

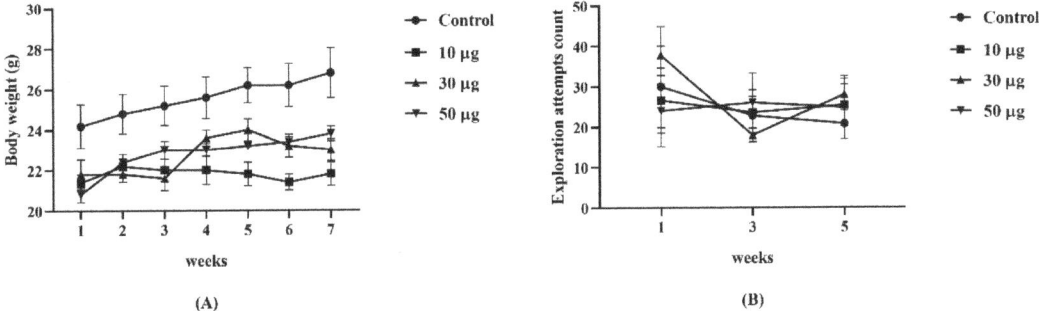

Figure 1. Monitoring of the general condition of the animals. (**A**) Evolution of weight per week by group (p = 0.058). (**B**) Comparison of the exploration attempts per group in the cylinder test (p = 0.919). Two-way ANOVA. (n = 5 per group).

3.2. Serum Cytokines

We observed significant differences between the intervention and the control groups for the IL-6 levels (p = 0.026) [Control v/s 10 µg, p = 0.025; Control v/s 30 µg, p = 0.024; Control v/s 50 µg, p = 0.256] and IFN-γ (p = 0.039) [Control v/s 10 µg, p = 0.039; Control v/s 30 µg, p = 0.050; Control v/s 50 µg, p = 0.195]. In contrast, TNF-α (p = 0.145), IL-10 (p = 0.576), and IL-17A (p = 0.296) did not show differences between the groups (Figure 2).

3.3. Gene Expression

We observed significant differences for the gene expression of ICAM-1 (p = 0.047) [Control v/s 10 µg, p = 0,944]; [Control v/s 30 µg, p = 0.655]; [Control v/s 50 µg, p = 0.041], VCAM-1 (p = 0.023) [Control v/s 10 µg, p = 0.981]; [Control v/s 30 µg, p = 0.910]; [Control v/s 50 µg, p = 0.023]; and E-Selectin (p = 0.048) [Control v/s 10 µg, p > 0.9999]; [Control v/s 30 µg, p > 0.999]; [Control v/s 50 µg, p = 0.033]. No differences were found for P-Selectin (p = 0.986), Pecam-1 (p = 0.705), and eNOS (p = 0.396) (Figure 3). Regarding markers related to PAH exposure and inflammatory indicators, no differences were identified in Ahr (p = 0.789); Keap1 (p = 0.507); RelA (p = 0.679); IKK-β (p = 0.450); IL-6 (p = 0.878); TNF-α (p = 0.760) (Figure 4).

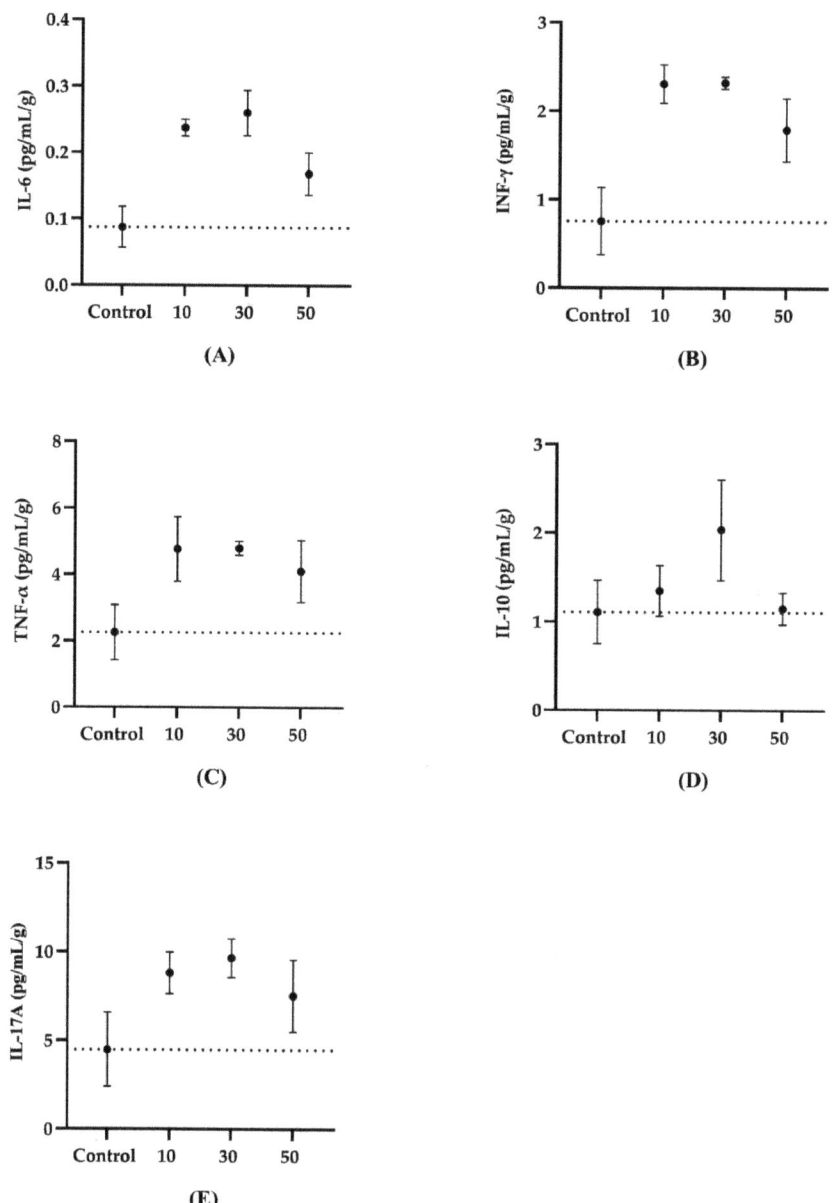

Figure 2. The quantification of weight-adjusted serum inflammatory cytokines in animals exposed to the PAHs and controls. (**A**) IL-6 ($p = 0.026$) [Control v/s 10 µg $p = 0.025$; Control v/s 30 µg $p = 0.024$; Control v/s 50 µg $p = 0.256$]. (**B**) IFN-γ ($p = 0.039$ [Control v/s 10 µg $p = 0.039$; Control v/s 30 µg $p = 0.050$; Control v/s 50 µg $p = 0.195$]). (**C**) TNF-α ($p = 0.145$). (**D**) IL-10 ($p = 0.576$). (**E**) IL-17A ($p = 0.296$). Data are presented as the mean ± SEM. The dashed line represents the mean value of the control group. Welch's ANOVA with Dunnett's multiple comparisons test (Control, $n = 4$; 10 µg, $n = 5$; 30 µg, $n = 4$; 50 µg, $n = 5$).

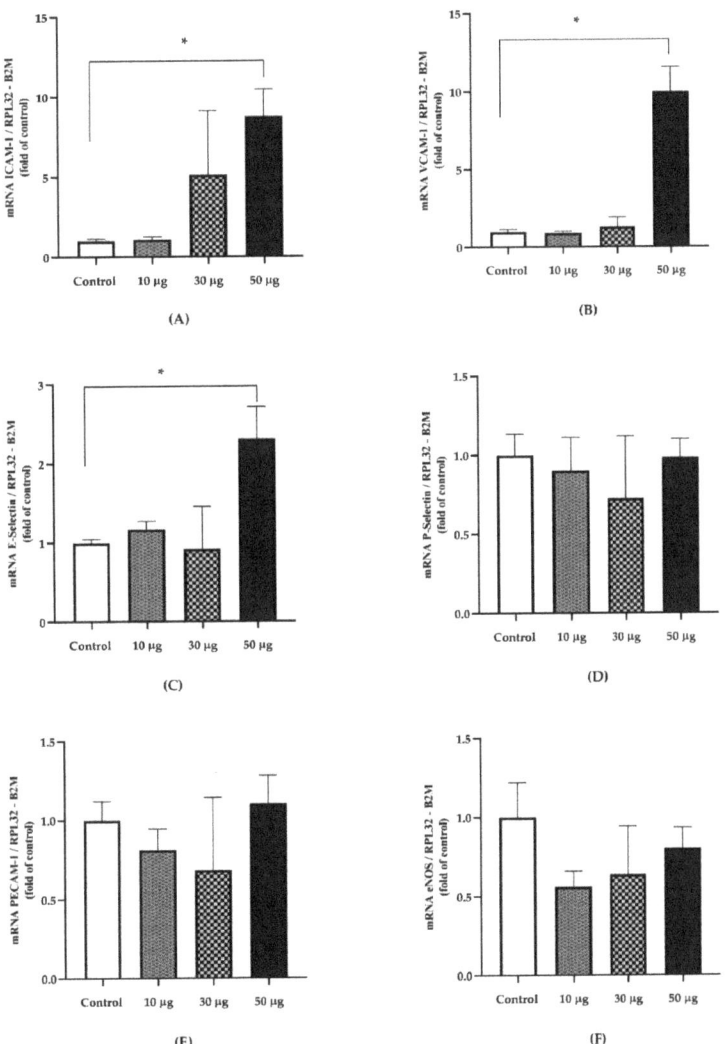

Figure 3. The relative gene expression of endothelial dysfunction markers in the aortic tissue of animals exposed to PAHs and controls. (**A**) ICAM-1 ($p = 0.047$) [†] [Control v/s 10 µg, $p = 0.944$]; [Control v/s 30 µg, $p = 0.655$]; [Control v/s 50 µg, $p = 0.041$]. (**B**) VCAM-1 ($p = 0.023$) [†] [Control v/s 10 µg, $p = 0.981$]; [Control v/s 30 µg, $p = 0.910$]; [Control v/s 50 µg, $p = 0.023$]. (**C**) E-Selectin ($p = 0.048$) [‡] [Control v/s 10 µg, $p > 0.9999$]; [Control v/s 30 µg, $p > 0.999$]; [Control v/s 50 µg, $p = 0.033$]. (**D**) P-Selectin ($p = 0.986$) [‡]. (**E**) Pecam-1 ($p = 0.705$) [‡]. (**F**) eNOS ($p = 0.396$) [†]. Relative quantification was calculated using the reference genes RPL32 and B2M. Data are presented as the means ± SEM. [†] Welch's ANOVA with Dunnett's multiple comparisons test. [‡] Kruskal–Wallis with Dunn's post hoc analysis (Control, $n = 4$; 10 µg, $n = 4$; 30 µg, $n = 4$; 50 µg, $n = 4$).* $p < 0.05$.

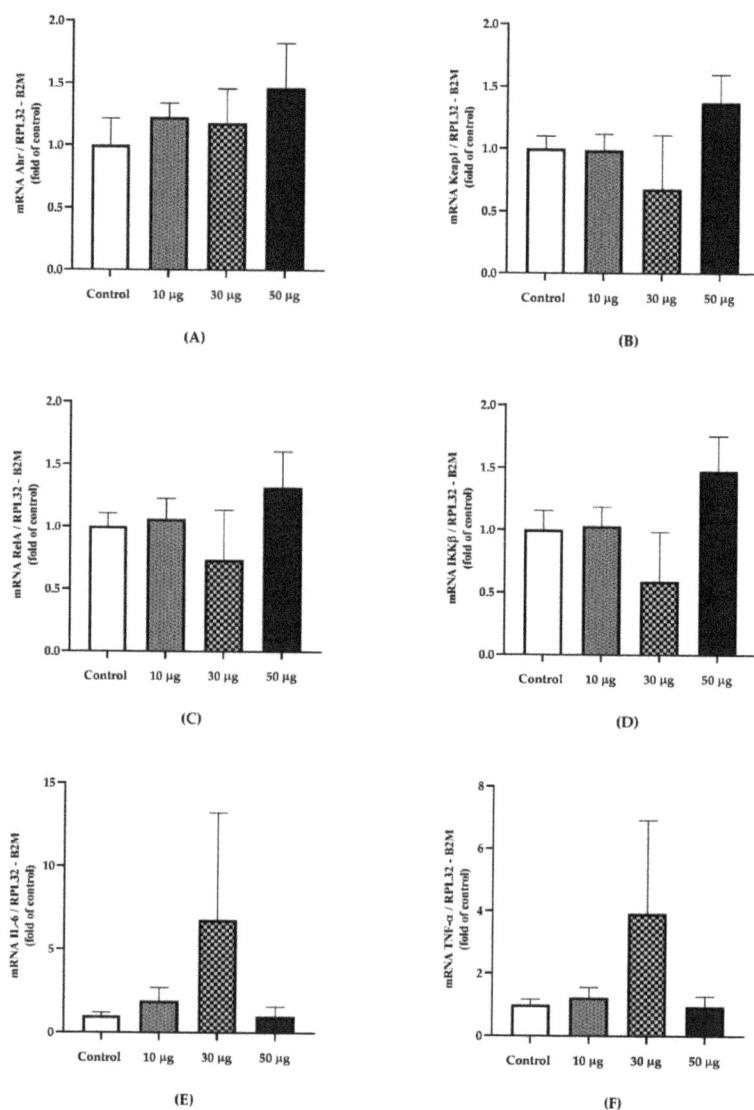

Figure 4. The relative gene expression of exposure-related PAHs and inflammatory markers in aortic tissue from PAH exposed animals and the controls. (**A**) Ahr ($p = 0.789$) ‡. (**B**) Keap1 ($p = 0.507$) ‡. (**C**) RelA ($p = 0.679$) ‡. (**D**) IKK-β ($p = 0.450$) †. (**E**) IL-6 ($p = 0.878$) ‡. (**F**) TNF-α ($p = 0.760$) †. Gene expression was normalized using the RPL32 and ACTB as reference genes. Data are presented as mean ± SEM. † Welch's ANOVA test. ‡ Kruskal–Wallis test (Control, $n = 4$; 10 μg, $n = 4$; 30 μg, $n = 4$; 50 μg, $n = 4$).

3.4. Protein Expression

The protein expression of ICAM-1 ($p = 0.117$) and VCAM-1 ($p = 0.210$) did not show significant differences in the aortic tissue, although we observed an elevated expression in the intervention groups compared to the control group (Figure 5).

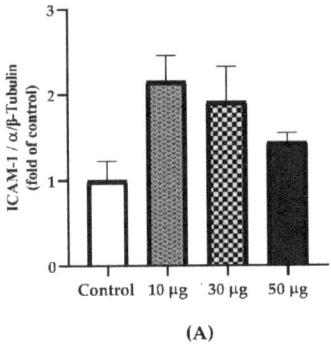
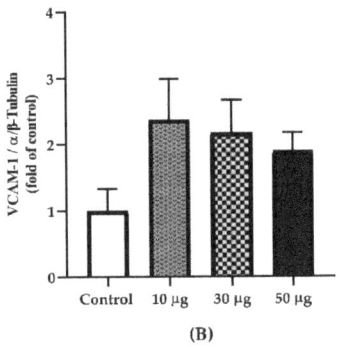
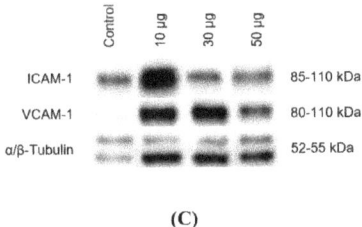

Figure 5. The effect of exposure to PAHs on the protein expression of adhesion molecules in aortic tissue. (**A**) Relative protein expression of ICAM-1 ($p = 0.117$). (**B**) Relative protein expression of VCAM-1 ($p = 0.210$). (**C**) Representative Western blots are shown for ICAM-1, VCAM-1, and α/β-tubulin. Data are presented as the mean ± SEM. Welch's ANOVA test. (Control, $n = 4$; 10 μg, $n = 4$; 30 μg, $n = 4$; 50 μg, $n = 4$).

4. Discussion

The concentrations and doses of PAHs used for this protocol were established according to previous studies using PM [26] and pollution generated by diesel combustion [27] as we did not find studies using PAH nasal instillation. Some studies have reported that exposure to PAH increases circulating pro-inflammatory cytokines, IL-6, IL-8, and TNF-α being the most studied markers [28,29]. In this study, a significant increase in serum IL-6 and IFN-γ was identified. Another report carried out on workers at a coal plant showed an increased concentration of IL-6 in plasma, demonstrating a dose-dependent relationship with PAH metabolites in urine [28]. IL-6 represents a good indicator of cytokine cascade activation, accurately reflecting the inflammatory state, in addition to its high stability since the half-life of IL-6 is longer than that of other pro-inflammatory cytokines [30]. On the other hand, IFN-γ induces the overexpression of additional pro-inflammatory cytokines such as IL-12, IL-15, TNF-α, IFN-γ-inducible protein-10 (IP-10), inducible nitric oxide synthase (iNOS), among others, inducing the activation of pro-inflammatory transcription factors such as the nuclear factor kappa light chain enhancer of activated B cells (NF-κB) [31]. However, in a study carried out on asthmatic and non-asthmatic children exposed to air pollution from traffic and followed for 6 years, there were no differences in circulating IFN-γ concentrations [32]. However, a study evaluating three different areas of environmental pollution according to their volatile components identified increased IFN-γ and TNF-α concentrations in industrialized and high-traffic areas compared to low-traffic areas [33]. Furthermore, a study evaluating different sources of pollutants derived from wood combustion identified a significant increase in blood TNF-α [34], showing that exposure to particles derived from wood combustion containing PAH can upregulate pro-inflammatory cytokines including IL-6 and TNF-α.

IL-10 has pleiotropic effects on immunoregulation and inflammation, downregulating the expression of Th1 cytokines, class II MHC, and co-stimulatory molecules in macrophages. IL-10 also improves B cell survival, proliferation, and antibody production [35]. This cytokine can block the activity of NF-kB, participating in the regulation of the JAK-STAT signaling pathway. By comparing different pro-inflammatory and anti-inflammatory cytokines associated with different levels of environmental pollution, Dobreva et al. showed that air pollutants, mostly $PM_{2.5}$, modulated cytokine production by altering the TNF-α (pro-inflammatory) and IL-10 (anti-inflammatory) [36].

An increase in the pro-inflammatory cytokines affects the regulation of vascular tone, cell adhesion, inflammation, proliferation, and the phenotype of smooth muscle cells as well as the formation of atheroma plaques [16]. Endothelial activation is characterized by an increase in the expression of adhesion molecules, leukocyte diapedesis, increased vascular tone due to decreased nitric oxide production, and reduced resistance to thrombosis [18]. The process of endothelial activation has been described as the factor initiating atheroma plaques in the vascular tissue. Thus, TNF-α enhances the expression of adhesion molecules in vascular endothelial cells. An in vitro study determined that stimulation of human coronary artery endothelial cells exposed to TNF-α increased ICAM-1 expression [37]. Our data indicate increased expression of the ICAM-1, VCAM-1 and E-Selectin genes, showing significant differences in the group exposed to 50 µg PAHs. Additionally, ICAM-1 and VCAM-1 protein expression was elevated in the PAH-exposed groups, although it did not reach statistical significance, being able to explain this by post-transcriptional regulations that should be studied in more depth.

We also observed a nonsignificant increase in IL-6 and TNF-α. Endothelial activation by TNF-α is carried out by two main mechanisms: activation of NF-κB and MAPK. The activation of NF-kB plays a central role in the regulation of multiple cellular processes such as inflammation, immune response, differentiation, proliferation, apoptosis, and cancer, thus it is considered as a master regulator of inflammatory responses [38]. Furthermore, TNF-α, IL-1β, IL-6, and IFN-γ expression are elevated within the great elastic arteries of old mice and humans [39]. This pro-inflammatory arterial phenotype is associated with increased NF-κB activity. When translocated to the nucleus, NF-κB activates the transcription of genes involved in the production of pro-inflammatory cytokines [40]. As we did not observe an increase in the gene expression of RelA and IKK-β, it becomes necessary to identify the mechanisms by which exposure to PAHs stimulates the increased expression of adhesion molecules in vascular tissue.

Based on the findings of this study, it is necessary to expand the studies that can investigate the mechanisms by which PAHs can generate deleterious effects on the cardiovascular system, being able to speculate that these compounds, due to their nature, manage to enter the cardiovascular system directly via bloodstream, affecting the vascular endothelium manage to enter the cardiovascular system directly via bloodstream, affecting the vascular endothelium. Thus, evidence shows that the passage of small molecules ($PM_{0.1}$) into the blood directly affects the vascular system. Within this group of particles, we can find particles derived from fossil fuels and wood combustion [7,41–43]. In this sense, reports have determined that PAHs bind to AhR, leading to the release of the latter from the multiprotein complex and its consequent translocation to the nucleus, where it dimerizes with the nuclear translocator AhR (ARNT), leading to binding to the xenobiotic response element (XRE) in the promoter region of target genes to stimulate transcription [44]. Furthermore, it has been proposed that AhR-mediated pathways are linked to responses to oxidative stress through the dissociation of the nuclear factor erythroid 2-related factor 2 (Nrf2) and the inhibitory protein keap1 [45].

Regarding the behavior of the variables studied, it was originally expected that there would be a dose–response relationship, a situation that was not observed in this investigation. In this regard, it is important to point out that the responses to the different pollutants did not always maintain this behavior, finding little evidence indicating that exposure to increasing doses of PM leads to vasomotor dysfunction and the progression of atherosclerotic plaque [46]. Furthermore, it has been suggested that systemic or pulmonary inflammation is not a prerequisite for dysfunction in the vasomotor response and accelerated the progression of atherosclerosis in animals exposed to PM [46]. Therefore, in the investigation, we wanted to review both the markers of systemic inflammation and the specific effect on tissue, particularly aortic tissue, evaluating markers of endothelial dysfunction that are recognized as potent factors for vasomotor dysfunction and atherosclerotic plaque formation. However, it has been documented that different types of PAH generate effects through different pathways in the tissues. An example of this is benzo[a]pyrene (B[a]P), which is considered to have a low affinity for AhR, but with potent effects on Ca^{2+} induction, a mechanism related to endothelial dysfunction. In contrast, pyrene, which seems to have an even greater effect on Ca^{2+} induction, but a non-nuclear Ahr stimulation pathway [47], showed differences in the effects of various PAHs in their pathophysiological mechanism of action. This is relevant to exemplify that the effect observed in tissue may be influenced by several metabolic pathways, which requires further investigation.

The PAH doses used in this research are within the ranges published in various studies and are adequately summarized in the review by Møller et al. [46]. However, it is important to point out that there is a great variation in the representation of PAHs in the particulate matter in the air, which depends on the concentrations of its different types, emission sources, time of year, place of measurement, and PM level, among others. These factors make direct extrapolation somewhat complex to perform. Thus, for example, residents living in rural areas generally inhale higher concentrations of PM-bound PAHs (4.2–655 ng/m^3) [48] than residents living in urban areas (0.4–11, 9 ng/m^3) [49]. In this study, a mixture of phenanthrene, fluoranthene, and pyrene was obtained, which are characteristic of the winter season associated with the combustion of wood for heating and cooking.

Although we have reported interesting findings regarding the role of exposure to PAHs in pro-inflammatory states and cardiovascular health, this study had limitations of a small number of animals per group, considering that no previous data were found regarding the model used for PAH management. In addition, the intervention contemplated 5 weeks of exposure, which could be a bit limited considering the long-term deleterious effects that people exposed to high levels of air pollution have been shown to manifest.

5. Conclusions

Our results suggest that PAHs of phenanthrene, fluoranthene, and pyrene, present in PM, partially stimulate the production of serum inflammatory cytokines, which have been associated with the development of various diseases related to high exposure to air pollution, in addition to being a relevant factor for the development of endothelial dysfunction and atherosclerotic disease. Furthermore, an increase in the expression of adhesion molecules related to endothelial dysfunction was found, an initial mechanism in the atherogenesis process that contributes to the formation, progression, and complications of the atherosclerotic plaque, alterations that are usually subclinical and poorly diagnosed. In this studied murine model, we showed that both mechanisms associated with the development of cardiovascular disease were manifested and may represent a model that allows for investigating the cellular and molecular mechanisms associated with exposure to PAHs present in PM.

Author Contributions: Conceptualization, G.A.R., N.S., K.S., F.L. and L.A.S.; Methodology, G.A.R., N.S. and L.A.S.; Software, G.A.R., M.H., C.M., K.S. and N.S.; Validation, G.A.R., M.H. and N.S.; Formal analysis, G.A.R. and N.S.; Investigation, G.A.R., M.H. and C.M.; Resources, N.S., F.L. and L.A.S.; Data curation, G.A.R. and N.S.; Writing—original draft preparation, G.A.R., N.S., M.H., C.M. and K.S.; Writing—review and editing, G.A.R., N.S. and L.A.S.; Visualization, G.A.R. and N.S.; Supervision, N.S., F.L. and L.A.S.; Project administration, N.S., F.L. and L.A.S.; Funding acquisition, N.S., K.S., F.L. and L.A.S. All authors have read and agreed to the published version of the manuscript.

Funding: This research was funded by FONDECYT-Chile [Grant numbers 1171618 and 1171765].

Institutional Review Board Statement: The Scientific Ethics Committee of the Universidad de La Frontera (No 105_18) approved the experimental protocol.

Informed Consent Statement: Not applicable.

Data Availability Statement: All data are described in the manuscript.

Acknowledgments: The authors are grateful to the Bioterio of the University of La Frontera, especially its manager, Patricio Mena Toboada.

Conflicts of Interest: The authors declare no conflict of interest.

References

1. *State of Global Air 2019*; Health Effects Institute: Boston, MA, USA, 2019. Available online: www.stateofglobalair.org (accessed on 30 March 2022).
2. Brook, R.D.; Rajagopalan, S. Stressed About Air Pollution: Time for Personal Action. *Circulation* **2017**, *136*, 628–631. [CrossRef] [PubMed]
3. Wyzga, R.E.; Rohr, A.C. Long-term particulate matter exposure: Attributing health effects to individual PM components. *J. Air Waste Manag. Assoc.* **2015**, *65*, 523–543. [CrossRef] [PubMed]
4. Jankowska-Kieltyka, M.; Roman, A.; Nalepa, I. The Air We Breathe: Air Pollution as a Prevalent Proinflammatory Stimulus Contributing to Neurodegeneration. *Front. Cell. Neurosci.* **2021**, *15*, 647643. [CrossRef] [PubMed]
5. Oliveira, M.; Slezakova, K.; Delerue-Matos, C.; Pereira, M.C.; Morais, S. Children environmental exposure to particulate matter and polycyclic aromatic hydrocarbons and biomonitoring in school environments: A review on indoor and outdoor exposure levels, major sources and health impacts. *Environ. Int.* **2019**, *124*, 180–204. [CrossRef] [PubMed]
6. IARC Working Group on the Evaluation of Carcinogenic Risks to Humans. Some non-heterocyclic polycyclic aromatic hydrocarbons and some related exposures. *IARC Monogr. Eval. Carcinog. Risks Hum.* **2010**, *92*, 1–853.
7. Schulz, H.; Harder, V.; Ibald-Mulli, A.; Khandoga, A.; Koenig, W.; Krombach, F.; Radykewicz, R.; Stampfl, A.; Thorand, B.; Peters, A. Cardiovascular effects of fine and ultrafine particles. *J. Aerosol. Med.* **2005**, *18*, 1–22. [CrossRef]
8. Brook, R.D.; Rajagopalan, S.; Pope, C.A., 3rd; Brook, J.R.; Bhatnagar, A.; Diez-Roux, A.V.; Holguin, F.; Hong, Y.; Luepker, R.V.; Mittleman, M.A.; et al. Particulate matter air pollution and cardiovascular disease: An update to the scientific statement from the American Heart Association. *Circulation* **2010**, *121*, 2331–2378. [CrossRef]
9. Lee, K.K.; Miller, M.R.; Shah, A.S.V. Air Pollution and Stroke. *J. Stroke* **2018**, *20*, 2–11. [CrossRef]
10. van Eeden, S.F.; Tan, W.C.; Suwa, T.; Mukae, H.; Terashima, T.; Fujii, T.; Qui, D.; Vincent, R.; Hogg, J.C. Cytokines involved in the systemic inflammatory response induced by exposure to particulate matter air pollutants (PM(10)). *Am. J. Respir. Crit. Care Med.* **2001**, *164*, 826–830. [CrossRef]
11. Yan, Z.; Jin, Y.; An, Z.; Liu, Y.; Samet, J.M.; Wu, W. Inflammatory cell signaling following exposures to particulate matter and ozone. *Biochim. Biophys. Acta* **2016**, *1860*, 2826–2834. [CrossRef]
12. Zhao, C.N.; Xu, Z.; Wu, G.C.; Mao, Y.M.; Liu, L.N.; Qian, W.; Dan, Y.L.; Tao, S.S.; Zhang, Q.; Sam, N.B.; et al. Emerging role of air pollution in autoimmune diseases. *Autoimmun. Rev.* **2019**, *18*, 607–614. [CrossRef]
13. Fiorito, G.; Vlaanderen, J.; Polidoro, S.; Gulliver, J.; Galassi, C.; Ranzi, A.; Krogh, V.; Grioni, S.; Agnoli, C.; Sacerdote, C.; et al. Oxidative stress and inflammation mediate the effect of air pollution on cardio- and cerebrovascular disease: A prospective study in nonsmokers. *Environ. Mol. Mutagenesis* **2018**, *59*, 234–246. [CrossRef] [PubMed]
14. Zhang, S.; Breitner, S.; Cascio, W.E.; Devlin, R.B.; Neas, L.M.; Ward-Caviness, C.; Diaz-Sanchez, D.; Kraus, W.E.; Hauser, E.R.; Schwartz, J.; et al. Association between short-term exposure to ambient fine particulate matter and myocardial injury in the CATHGEN cohort. *Environ. Pollut.* **2021**, *275*, 116663. [CrossRef] [PubMed]
15. Chen, M.; Zhao, J.; Zhuo, C.; Zheng, L. The Association Between Ambient Air Pollution and Atrial Fibrillation A Systematic Review and Meta-Analysis. *Int. Heart J.* **2021**, *62*, 290–297. [CrossRef] [PubMed]
16. Boulanger, C.M. Endothelium. *Arterioscler. Thromb. Vasc. Biol.* **2016**, *36*, e26–e31. [CrossRef] [PubMed]
17. Gimbrone, M.A., Jr.; García-Cardeña, G. Endothelial Cell Dysfunction and the Pathobiology of Atherosclerosis. *Circ. Res.* **2016**, *118*, 620–636. [CrossRef] [PubMed]
18. Steyers, C.M., 3rd; Miller, F.J., Jr. Endothelial dysfunction in chronic inflammatory diseases. *Int. J. Mol. Sci.* **2014**, *15*, 11324–11349. [CrossRef]
19. Sitia, S.; Tomasoni, L.; Atzeni, F.; Ambrosio, G.; Cordiano, C.; Catapano, A.; Tramontana, S.; Perticone, F.; Naccarato, P.; Camici, P.; et al. From endothelial dysfunction to atherosclerosis. *Autoimmun. Rev.* **2010**, *9*, 830–834. [CrossRef]
20. Zhang, Y.; Dong, S.; Wang, H.; Tao, S.; Kiyama, R. Biological impact of environmental polycyclic aromatic hydrocarbons (ePAHs) as endocrine disruptors. *Environ. Pollut.* **2016**, *213*, 809–824. [CrossRef]
21. Pozo, K.; Estellano, V.H.; Harner, T.; Diaz-Robles, L.; Cereceda-Balic, F.; Etcharren, P.; Pozo, K.; Vidal, V.; Guerrero, F.; Vergara-Fernandez, A. Assessing Polycyclic Aromatic Hydrocarbons (PAHs) using passive air sampling in the atmosphere of one of the most wood-smoke-polluted cities in Chile: The case study of Temuco. *Chemosphere* **2015**, *134*, 475–481. [CrossRef]

22. Hanson, L.R.; Fine, J.M.; Svitak, A.L.; Faltesek, K.A. Intranasal administration of CNS therapeutics to awake mice. *J. Vis. Exp.* **2013**, *74*, e4440. [CrossRef] [PubMed]
23. Schaar, K.L.; Brenneman, M.M.; Savitz, S.I. Functional assessments in the rodent stroke model. *Exp. Transl. Stroke Med.* **2010**, *2*, 13. [CrossRef] [PubMed]
24. Morton, D.B.; Griffiths, P.H. Guidelines on the recognition of pain, distress and discomfort in experimental animals and an hypothesis for assessment. *Vet. Rec.* **1985**, *116*, 431–436. [CrossRef] [PubMed]
25. Ruijter, J.M.; Lorenz, P.; Tuomi, J.M.; Hecker, M.; van den Hoff, M.J. Fluorescent-increase kinetics of different fluorescent reporters used for qPCR depend on monitoring chemistry, targeted sequence, type of DNA input and PCR efficiency. *Mikrochim. Acta* **2014**, *181*, 1689–1696. [CrossRef]
26. Silva-Renno, A.; Baldivia, G.C.; Oliveira-Junior, M.C.; Brandao-Rangel, M.A.R.; El-Mafarjeh, E.; Dolhnikoff, M.; Mauad, T.; Britto, J.M.; Saldiva, P.H.N.; Oliveira, L.V.F.; et al. Exercise Performed Concomitantly with Particulate Matter Exposure Inhibits Lung Injury. *Int. J. Sports Med.* **2018**, *39*, 133–140. [CrossRef]
27. Avila, L.C.; Bruggemann, T.R.; Bobinski, F.; da Silva, M.D.; Oliveira, R.C.; Martins, D.F.; Mazzardo-Martins, L.; Duarte, M.M.; de Souza, L.F.; Dafre, A.; et al. Effects of High-Intensity Swimming on Lung Inflammation and Oxidative Stress in a Murine Model of DEP-Induced Injury. *PLoS ONE* **2015**, *10*, e0137273. [CrossRef]
28. Ye, J.; Zhu, R.; He, X.; Feng, Y.; Yang, L.; Zhu, X.; Deng, Q.; Wu, T.; Zhang, X. Association of plasma IL-6 and Hsp70 with HRV at different levels of PAHs metabolites. *PLoS ONE* **2014**, *9*, e92964. [CrossRef]
29. Totlandsdal, A.I.; Ovrevik, J.; Cochran, R.E.; Herseth, J.I.; Bolling, A.K.; Lag, M.; Schwarze, P.; Lilleaas, E.; Holme, J.A.; Kubatova, A. The occurrence of polycyclic aromatic hydrocarbons and their derivatives and the proinflammatory potential of fractionated extracts of diesel exhaust and wood smoke particles. *J. Environ. Sci. Health A Tox. Hazard. Subst. Environ. Eng.* **2014**, *49*, 383–396. [CrossRef]
30. Tateishi, Y.; Oda, S.; Nakamura, M.; Watanabe, K.; Kuwaki, T.; Moriguchi, T.; Hirasawa, H. Depressed Heart Rate Variability Is Associated with High Il-6 Blood Level and Decline in the Blood Pressure in Septic Patients. *Shock* **2007**, *28*, 549–553. [CrossRef]
31. Mata-Espinosa, D.; Hernández-Pando, R. Interferón gamma aspectos básicos, importancia clínica y usos terapéuticos. *Rev. Investig. Clínica* **2008**, *60*, 421–431.
32. Klumper, C.; Kramer, U.; Lehmann, I.; von Berg, A.; Berdel, D.; Herberth, G.; Beckmann, C.; Link, E.; Heinrich, J.; Hoffmann, B.; et al. Air pollution and cytokine responsiveness in asthmatic and non-asthmatic children. *Environ. Res.* **2015**, *138*, 381–390. [CrossRef] [PubMed]
33. Samadi, M.T.; Shakerkhatibi, M.; Poorolajal, J.; Rahmani, A.; Rafieemehr, H.; Hesam, M. Association of long term exposure to outdoor volatile organic compounds (BTXS) with pro-inflammatory biomarkers and hematologic parameters in urban adults: A cross-sectional study in Tabriz, Iran. *Ecotoxicol. Environ. Saf.* **2019**, *180*, 152–159. [CrossRef] [PubMed]
34. Uski, O.J.; Happo, M.S.; Jalava, P.I.; Brunner, T.; Kelz, J.; Obernberger, I.; Jokiniemi, J.; Hirvonen, M.R. Acute systemic and lung inflammation in C57Bl/6J mice after intratracheal aspiration of particulate matter from small-scale biomass combustion appliances based on old and modern technologies. *Inhal. Toxicol.* **2012**, *24*, 952–965. [CrossRef] [PubMed]
35. Mosser, D.M.; Zhang, X. Interleukin-10: New perspectives on an old cytokine. *Immunol. Rev.* **2008**, *226*, 205–218. [CrossRef]
36. Dobreva, Z.G.; Kostadinova, G.S.; Popov, B.N.; Petkov, G.S.; Stanilova, S.A. Proinflammatory and anti-inflammatory cytokines in adolescents from Southeast Bulgarian cities with different levels of air pollution. *Toxicol. Ind. Health* **2015**, *31*, 1210–1217. [CrossRef]
37. Xue, M.; Qiqige, C.; Zhang, Q.; Zhao, H.; Su, L.; Sun, P.; Zhao, P. Effects of Tumor Necrosis Factor alpha (TNF-alpha) and Interleukina 10 (IL-10) on Intercellular Cell Adhesion Molecule-1 (ICAM-1) and Cluster of Differentiation 31 (CD31) in Human Coronary Artery Endothelial Cells. *Med. Sci. Monit.* **2018**, *24*, 4433–4439. [CrossRef]
38. Li, R.; Zhou, R.; Zhang, J. Function of $PM_{2.5}$ in the pathogenesis of lung cancer and chronic airway inflammatory diseases. *Oncol. Lett.* **2018**, *15*, 7506–7514. [CrossRef]
39. Donato, A.J.; Morgan, R.G.; Walker, A.E.; Lesniewski, L.A. Cellular and molecular biology of aging endothelial cells. *J. Mol. Cell. Cardiol.* **2015**, *89*, 122–135. [CrossRef]
40. Brown, J.D.; Lin, C.Y.; Duan, Q.; Griffin, G.; Federation, A.; Paranal, R.M.; Bair, S.; Newton, G.; Lichtman, A.; Kung, A.; et al. NF-kappaB directs dynamic super enhancer formation in inflammation and atherogenesis. *Mol. Cell* **2014**, *56*, 219–231. [CrossRef]
41. Ntziachristos, L.; Ning, Z.; Geller, M.D.; Sheesley, R.J.; Schauer, J.J.; Sioutas, C. Fine, ultrafine and nanoparticle trace element compositions near a major freeway with a high heavy-duty diesel fraction. *Atmos. Environ.* **2007**, *41*, 5684–5696. [CrossRef]
42. Lee, C.C.; Huang, S.H.; Yang, Y.T.; Cheng, Y.W.; Li, C.H.; Kang, J.J. Motorcycle exhaust particles up-regulate expression of vascular adhesion molecule-1 and intercellular adhesion molecule-1 in human umbilical vein endothelial cells. *Toxicol. In Vitro* **2012**, *26*, 552–560. [CrossRef] [PubMed]
43. Nemmar, A.; Hoet, P.M.; Vanquickenborne, B.; Dinsdale, D.; Thomeer, M.; Hoylaerts, M.; Vanbilloen, H.; Mortelmans, L.; Nemery, B.J.C. Passage of inhaled particles into the blood circulation in humans. *Circulation* **2002**, *105*, 411–414. [CrossRef] [PubMed]
44. Haarmann-Stemmann, T.; Abel, J.; Fritsche, E.; Krutmann, J. The AhR–Nrf2 pathway in keratinocytes: On the road to chemoprevention? *J. Investig. Dermatol.* **2012**, *132*, 7–9. [CrossRef] [PubMed]
45. Lawal, A.O. Air particulate matter induced oxidative stress and inflammation in cardiovascular disease and atherosclerosis: The role of Nrf2 and AhR-mediated pathways. *Toxicol. Lett.* **2017**, *270*, 88–95. [CrossRef]

46. Møller, P.; Christophersen, D.V.; Jacobsen, N.R.; Skovmand, A.; Gouveia, A.C.; Andersen, M.H.; Kermanizadeh, A.; Jensen, D.M.; Danielsen, P.H.; Roursgaard, M.; et al. Atherosclerosis and vasomotor dysfunction in arteries of animals after exposure to combustion-derived particulate matter or nanomaterials. *Crit. Rev. Toxicol.* **2016**, *46*, 437–476. [CrossRef]
47. Brinchmann, B.C.; Le Ferrec, E.; Bisson, W.H.; Podechard, N.; Huitfeldt, H.S.; Gallais, I.; Sergent, O.; Holme, J.A.; Lagadic-Gossmann, D.; Øvrevik, J. Evidence of selective activation of aryl hydrocarbon receptor nongenomic calcium signaling by pyrene. *Biochem. Pharm.* **2018**, *158*, 1–12. [CrossRef]
48. Orakij, W.; Chetiyanukornkul, T.; Chuesaard, T.; Kaganoi, Y.; Uozaki, W.; Homma, C.; Boongla, Y.; Tang, N.; Hayakawa, K.; Toriba, A. Personal inhalation exposure to polycyclic aromatic hydrocarbons and their nitro-derivatives in rural residents in northern Thailand. *Environ. Monit. Assess.* **2017**, *189*, 510. [CrossRef]
49. Mu, G.; Fan, L.; Zhou, Y.; Liu, Y.; Ma, J.; Yang, S.; Wang, B.; Xiao, L.; Ye, Z.; Shi, T.; et al. Personal exposure to PM(2.5)-bound polycyclic aromatic hydrocarbons and lung function alteration: Results of a panel study in China. *Sci. Total Environ.* **2019**, *684*, 458–465. [CrossRef]

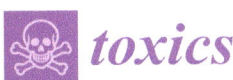

Article

Association of 3-Phenoxybenzoic Acid Exposure during Pregnancy with Maternal Outcomes and Newborn Anthropometric Measures: Results from the IoMum Cohort Study

Juliana Guimarães [1], Isabella Bracchi [1], Cátia Pinheiro [1], Nara Xavier Moreira [2,3], Cláudia Matta Coelho [1], Diogo Pestana [4], Maria do Carmo Prucha [5], Cristina Martins [5], Valentina F. Domingues [6], Cristina Delerue-Matos [6], Cláudia C. Dias [7], Luís Filipe R. Azevedo [7], Conceição Calhau [4], João Costa Leite [2], Carla Ramalho [5,8,9,*], Elisa Keating [1,*] and Virgínia Cruz Fernandes [6,*]

1 CINTESIS@RISE, Department of Biomedicine, Unit of Biochemistry, Faculty of Medicine, University of Porto, 4200-319 Porto, Portugal
2 CINTESIS@RISE, Faculty of Medicine, University of Porto, 4200-319 Porto, Portugal
3 Department of Nutrition and Dietetics (MND), Faculty of Nutrition Emília de Jesus Ferreiro (FNEJF), Fluminense Federal University (UFF), Niterói 20010-010, RJ, Brazil
4 CINTESIS@RISE, Nutrition and Metabolism, NOVA Medical School | FCM, Universidade Nova de Lisboa, 1169-056 Lisboa, Portugal
5 Department of Obstetrics, Centro Hospitalar Universitário S. João, 4200-319 Porto, Portugal
6 REQUIMTE/LAQV, Instituto Superior de Engenharia, Politécnico do Porto, 4249-015 Porto, Portugal
7 CINTESIS@RISE, Department of Community Medicine, Information and Health Decision Sciences (MEDCIDS), Faculty of Medicine, University of Porto, 4200-319 Porto, Portugal
8 Department of Ginecology-Obstetrics and Pediatrics, Faculty of Medicine, University of Porto, 4200-319 Porto, Portugal
9 Instituto de Investigação e Inovação em Saúde, i3S, Universidade do Porto, 4200-135 Porto, Portugal
* Correspondence: carlaramalho@med.up.pt (C.R.); keating@med.up.pt (E.K.); vircru@gmail.com (V.C.F.)

Abstract: The aims of this study were to characterize the exposure of pregnant women living in Portugal to 3-phenoxybenzoic acid (3-PBA) and to evaluate the association of this exposure with maternal outcomes and newborn anthropometric measures. We also aimed to compare exposure in summer with exposure in winter. Pregnant women attending ultrasound scans from April 2018 to April 2019 at a central hospital in Porto, Portugal, were invited to participate. Inclusion criteria were: gestational week between 10 and 13, confirmed fetal vitality, and a signature of informed consent. 3-PBA was measured in spot urine samples by gas chromatography with mass spectrometry (GC-MS). The median 3-PBA concentration was 0.263 (0.167; 0.458) µg/g creatinine (n = 145). 3-PBA excretion was negatively associated with maternal pre-pregnancy body mass index (BMI) (p = 0.049), and it was higher during the summer when compared to winter ($p < 0.001$). The frequency of fish or yogurt consumption was associated positively with 3-PBA excretion, particularly during the winter (p = 0.002 and p = 0.015, respectively), when environmental exposure is low. Moreover, 3-PBA was associated with levothyroxine use (p = 0.01), a proxy for hypothyroidism, which could be due to a putative 3-PBA—thyroid hormone antagonistic effect. 3-PBA levels were not associated with the anthropometric measures of the newborn. In conclusion, pregnant women living in Portugal are exposed to 3-PBA, particularly during summer, and this exposure may be associated with maternal clinical features.

Keywords: 3-PBA; pyrethroid pesticides; pregnancy; newborn; anthropometry

Citation: Guimarães, J.; Bracchi, I.; Pinheiro, C.; Moreira, N.X.; Coelho, C.M.; Pestana, D.; Prucha, M.d.C.; Martins, C.; Domingues, V.F.; Delerue-Matos, C.; et al. Association of 3-Phenoxybenzoic Acid Exposure during Pregnancy with Maternal Outcomes and Newborn Anthropometric Measures: Results from the IoMum Cohort Study. *Toxics* **2023**, *11*, 125. https://doi.org/10.3390/toxics11020125

Academic Editor: Sunmi Kim

Received: 19 December 2022
Revised: 16 January 2023
Accepted: 19 January 2023
Published: 27 January 2023

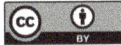

Copyright: © 2023 by the authors. Licensee MDPI, Basel, Switzerland. This article is an open access article distributed under the terms and conditions of the Creative Commons Attribution (CC BY) license (https://creativecommons.org/licenses/by/4.0/).

1. Introduction

Pesticides belong to a large family of compounds used to control insect (insecticides, insect repellents), weeds (herbicides), microbe (fungicides, disinfectants), or mouse and rat (rodenticides) pests [1].

Synthetic pyrethroids (SPs) belong to the class of insecticides and are commonly used. These insecticides derive from natural compounds produced by some species of chrysanthemum flowers, the so-called pyrethrins, and they are used to manage pests both in agriculture and in residences and to reduce the transmission of diseases acquired by insects [2,3].

3-phenoxybenzoic acid (3-PBA) is a general metabolite of several SPs, which is used as a biomarker of SP exposure [4].

In northern Portugal, three studies were carried out to characterize agricultural soil sample contamination with 3-PBA. Those studies showed that 3-PBA was detectable at the range of ng per g of soil, in samples of the north of Portugal [2,5,6]. One other study showed that pyrethroids interfere with the germination and development of plants since their phototoxicity can alter the levels of chlorophyll and carotenoids [4]. The presence of pyrethroids in agricultural soils indicates the relevance of extending monitoring programs for the analysis of these compounds in soils and soil-borne foods [2,5,6].

For example, 75% of fruits and vegetable samples labelled as 'organic' (including tomatoes, oranges, grapes, apples, bananas, onions, lettuce, green peppers, carrots, and broccoli) collected from grocery stores in North Carolina, USA, had measurable levels of at least one pyrethroid [7].

The 2018 European Union (EU) report on pesticide residues in food showed that Portugal was one of the countries with the highest maximum residue levels (MRLs) exceeding rates, but none of the residues detected to exceed MRLs were pyrethroids [8]. The overall results of this report suggest that the levels of pesticides assessed in the food products analyzed are unlikely to pose a concern for the health of the consumer [8].

Besides food, pyrethroids are also found in pet shampoos, medication used for treating scabies, and topical louse treatments [9].

Exposure to pesticides in the population is widespread, especially via dermal, ingestion, and inhalation routes, and consequently, SPs may enter the food chain, affecting the environment and human health [10].

3-PBA found in the human body may result from absorption of 3-PBA resulting from environmental degradation of several SPs [2], or it may result from the endogenous hydrolysis of SPs by mammalian carboxylesterases (CEs) [11].

Once in the human body, pyrethroid compounds, including 3-PBA, are known to be transported by the placenta, since detectable levels of permethrin were found in cord blood samples collected upon delivery [12].

The developing nervous system is highly susceptible to the neurotoxicity of pesticides, as well as to many types of environmental toxicants. This heightened sensitivity occurs not only during prenatal but also postnatal development, extending into adolescence [13]. Impacts on the developing nervous system can have deleterious effects that last a lifetime, long after exposure has ended, as the toxicant causes alterations of development of the nervous system [14].

Like many other insecticide compounds, pyrethroids are known to be neurotoxic [15]. In fact, intraperitoneal injection of 3-PBA in mice daily for 2 months has shown to induce synuclein aggregation in dopaminergic neurons, which may contribute to dopaminergic neurodegeneration [11]. Given its high lipophilicity, 3-PBA can cross the blood-brain barrier (BBB) and bioaccumulate in the brain, which is rich in lipids [11]. This increases the plausibility of its neurotoxic effects.

Additionally, a recent review provides relevant evidence which confirms that pyrethroids exposure during pregnancy may impact neurodevelopment for example by interference with thyroid hormone (TH) function [15].

Adverse effects on thyroid function warrant caution because THs play an important role in many aspects of human physiology including growth, development, energy metabolism, and reproduction [16,17]. Across vertebrates, particularly during pregnancy and the neonatal period, THs orchestrate metamorphosis, brain development, and metabolism. SPs and their metabolites have structural similarities with THs [18]. These similarities are believed to underlie SPs and 3-PBA interference with nuclear receptors of TH. In fact these compounds have been shown to inhibit TR-mediated gene expression [19]. A study evaluating environmental exposure to pyrethroids and thyroid hormones of pregnant women in Shandong, China, indicated that exposure to pyrethroids was widespread and negatively associated with serum concentrations of free triiodothyronine (FT3) [20]. Nevertheless, Zang et al., in a cohort of women in the first trimester of pregnancy, could not show an association between chemical exposure to pyrethroid pesticides during the early gestation period and maternal thyroid function [21]. There is a need to further explore the effects of pyrethroid exposure on thyroid function in pregnant women.

Some studies have evaluated urinary pyrethroid levels among pregnant women in different regions of the globe. In a randomized trial carried out in Idaho, USA, levels of 3-PBA were measured in 1st trimester pregnant women who received either organic or conventional fruits and vegetables for consumption for 24 weeks. 3-PBA concentrations were significantly higher in urine samples collected from women in the conventional produce group compared to the organic produce group (0.95 vs 0.27 µg/L, p = 0.03) [22]. A study carried out in French pregnant women showed that among 5 pyrethroid metabolites, the urinary concentrations of 3-PBA were the highest with a mean concentration of 0.36 µg/L (0.50 µg/g creatinine) [23]. In China, a study carried out in pregnant women living in a rural area of the Jiangsu Province showed that median urinary 3-PBA concentration was 1.01 g/L (1.55 µg/g creatinine) [24].

A biomonitoring study conducted in the US has indicated that in recent decades, there has been an increase in pyrethroid insecticides home usage and a decrease in the use of organophosphorus pesticides (OP), resulting in detectable amounts of pyrethroid metabolites in population samples [25].

Human fertility rates are known to be decreasing both in developed and developing countries [26]. This reduction has been associated with socioeconomic changes and adverse lifestyle factors [27]. However, pesticide environmental contaminants have attracted international attention and recently came to be considered as possible contributors to human infertility [28].

Environmental exposure to pyrethroids can also adversely impact on pregnancy outcomes and offspring health, including newborn anthropometry, neurodevelopment, and behavioral problems [18]. A study of exposure to pyrethroid sprays during pregnancy has shown associations of this exposure with autism spectrum disorders (ASD) and developmental delay [29]. Cross-sectional studies also implicate pyrethroids in ASD [30] and Attention Deficit Hyperactivity Disorder (ADHD) [31].

Several previous studies of pyrethroid biomarkers and behavior have reported associations between pyrethroid levels and adverse behavioral problems in children. Although detection frequencies of pyrethroid metabolites were low, suggestive evidence that prenatal exposure to 3-PBA may be associated with a variety of behavioral and executive functioning deficits was found [32].

However, to date, there have been no studies evaluating the levels of exposure of Portuguese pregnant women to this pesticide neither its impact on maternal nor neonatal outcomes. So, the aims of this study were to characterize the exposure of pregnant women living in Portugal to 3-PBA and to evaluate the association of this exposure with maternal outcomes and newborn anthropometric measures. Additionally, considering that the exposure of the global population to 3-PBA is expected to vary with the seasons [24,33–35], with the maximum likelihood of exposure in summer [36], we decided to compare samples collected in summer with those collected in winter.

2. Materials and Methods

2.1. Ethical Approval

This study was performed according to the protocol approved by the Ethics Committee of São João University Hospital Center (CHUSJoão)/Faculty of Medicine of the University of Porto. Informed written consent was obtained from all study participants.

2.2. Study Design and Participants

A prospective observational study was carried out from the IoMum cohort (Monitoring iodine status in Portuguese pregnant women and the impact of supplementation—trial registration number NCT04010708) according to the guidelines laid down in the Declaration of Helsinki. Pregnant women attending their first trimester routine ultrasound scan at Centro Hospitalar Universitário de São João (CHUSJ), Porto, between April 2018 and April 2019 were invited to participate as described previously [37–39]. All women who had a routine ultrasound scan between 10 and 13 weeks of gestation with confirmed fetal vitality, who signed the informed consent form, and who provided a urine sample at recruitment in summer or in the winter were included in the study. Exclusion criteria were twin pregnancy, declaration of informed consent for use of the data of the newborn not being signed by the mother, and urine sample collection in spring or autumn (Figure 1).

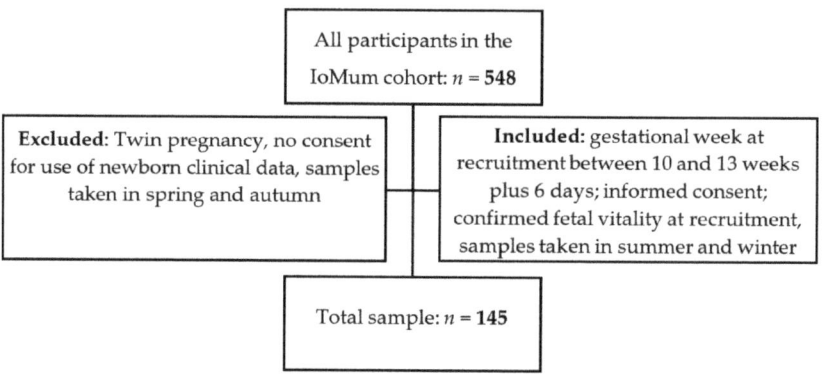

Figure 1. Recruitment and inclusion flowchart of the study.

Gestational age was determined from the measurement of the fetal crown-rump length.

At the time of enrollment between 10 and 13 weeks plus 6 days (timepoint 1, T1) and after informed consent, information was collected on various demographic and lifestyle factors, including age, area of residence, education, weight, and height of the pregnant, gestational age, smoking habits, and use of medicines. In the lifestyle questionnaire, food frequency information was obtained from a semi-quantitative food intake assessment questionnaire, where we verified the frequency of consumption of cow's milk, yogurt, cheese, eggs, and fish.

At this time point (T1), a spot urine sample was also collected, and women were invited to a second contact with the IoMum team from 35 weeks until the end of gestation (time point 2, T2) for additional demographic and lifestyle information collection, spot urine collection and a finger prick blood spot. The urine samples were refrigerated upon collection and transported to the laboratory within the following 24 h for aliquot creation and freezing at $-80\ °C$ for future analysis.

Information collected at T2 falls outside the scope of this work, and so, it will not be further detailed. Information regarding both maternal and the newborn's clinical details were obtained from the clinical records, including pregnancy outcomes and complications, mode of delivery, gestational age at delivery, and newborn's anthropometric and vitality parameters.

2.3. Biochemical Analysis

2.3.1. Chemical Elements Quantification

The analysis of 3-PBA was performed by gas chromatography with mass spectrometry (GC/MS), as described [2] 1 µL of sample was injected onto a Thermo Trace-Ultra gas chromatography, coupled to an ion trap mass detector Thermo Polaris, operated in the electron impact ionization at 70 eV. The ion source and the MS transfer temperature were set at 250 °C. Operating in the splitless mode (0.5 min), the helium was used as carrier gas at a constant flow rate of 1.3 mL min^{-1}. The temperature of the injector was 240 °C. The column was a 30 m ZB-5MSi (0.25 mm i.d., 0.25 µm film thickness Zebron-Phenomenex), and oven temperature was programmed as described [2]. The analysis was developed in the SIM mode, based on the detection of selected ions for 3-PBA (141, 196, and 364).

Sample preparation was performed by solid-phase extraction (SPE). Briefly, the urine samples were thawed at room temperature. Then, a solution of urine in 1.5 mL of deionized water (H_2O), 150 µL of sodium hydroxide (NaOH) (Merck), and 100 µL of the internal standard 2-phenoxy benzoic acid (2-PBA) (Sigma Aldrich) (1.5 mL + 1.5 mL + 150 µL + 100 µL, respectively) of were incubated at 37 °C for 15 min. After chemical deconjugation, the samples were transferred to the preconditioned SPE columns (Strata-X) (Phenomenex) with 5 mL methanol (MeOH) (Riedel de Haen) and 5 mL ammonium acetate (Merck). The columns were then immediately washed with 5 mL (MeOH): (H_2O) (30/70 V/V). Following a short vacuum pulse to remove excess wash solution, the columns were dried under vacuum for 40 min using the SPE vacuum manifold. Elution was carried out with 5 mL of acidified MeOH (2% formic acid) (Carlo Erba), directly into a glass vial. Subsequently, the eluates were concentrated to 50 µL under a gentle stream of nitrogen.

3-PBA derivatization procedure was necessary prior to GC/MS analysis. The derivatization was performed by addition of 30 µL hexafluoro-2-propanol (HFIP) (Sigma Aldrich Darmstadt, Germany), 20 µL (N, N'-Diisopropylcarbodiimide (DIC) (Sigma Aldrich Darmstadt, Germany) and 400 µL of n-hexane (Merck, Darmstadt, Germany) to the 50 µL of the eluate obtained from the SPE extraction and vortex at room temperature during 10 min. In the final step, liquid-liquid extraction was performed with 1 mL of a 5% aqueous potassium carbonate solution (Panreac, Darmstadt, Germany) (to neutralize the excess derivatizing agent), shaken 5 min in the vortex, and finally, the supernatant was removed and placed in a vial with insert for injecting into GC/MS. The calibration curves and linear ranges of the detector response for 3-PBA were evaluated by analyzing the working standard solutions (15–200 µg L^{-1}, 8 concentrations) in triplicate. In this study, the linearity, selectivity, the limit of detection (LOD) and limit of quantification (LOQ) were evaluated and the determinations that were below the LOD have been replaced by the constant LOD/2, according to Richardson, and Ciampi and Schisterman et al. [40–42]. LOD (0.364 µg/L) and LOQ (1.212 µg/L) were calculated as the minimum amount of analyte detectable with a signal-to-noise ratio (S/N) of 3 and 10, respectively; the linearity of the method was established by setting calibration curves using linear regression analysis over the concentration range. Selectivity was verified by comparing the chromatograms of the standards dissolved in n-hexane, the standards extracted from the spiked urine and the matrix blanks.

2.3.2. Creatinine Quantification

Urine-based biomarkers are useful for assessing individuals' exposure to environmental factors. However, inter-individual variations in urine concentration (which can be assessed by urinary creatinine) can directly affect urinary levels of contaminants. So, urinary creatinine was used to adjust 3-PBA urinary levels to urine concentration [43].

Measurements were performed using an ADVIA 1800 instrument according to the manufacturer's instructions, based on the enzymatic reaction described by Fossati, Prencipe, and Berti [44].

Briefly, urinary creatinine was quantified by enzymatic conversion (creatininase) to creatine, which was then hydrolyzed by creatinase to produce sarcosine, and this decomposed by the sarcosine oxidase to form glycine, formaldehyde and hydrogen peroxide. The hydrogen peroxide formed produces a blue pigment through the action of peroxidase and by quantitative oxidative condensation with N-(3-sulfopropyl)-3-methoxy-5-methylaniline (HMMPS) and 4-aminoantipyrine. The creatinine concentration was obtained by measuring the absorbance of the blue color at 596/694 nm.

2.4. Maternal Outcomes and Newborn Anthropometric Measures

Maternal outcomes considered for association analyses with levels of 3-PBA were: medication for thyroid disease (as a proxy for hypothyroidism), glycemia in the first trimester, and type of delivery (women who had cesarean delivery, women who had a vaginal delivery).

For the categorization of variables of weight, head circumference and length of the newborn, percentile classification was used [45]. As a result, the newborns were classified into 3 categories regarding weight, head circumference, and length at birth:

- SGA: small for gestational age (below 10th percentile)
- AGA: appropriate for gestational age (between 10th percentile and 90th percentile)
- LGA: large for gestational age (above the 90th percentile)

2.5. Statistical Analysis

Descriptive statistics are presented as absolute and relative frequencies for categorical variables, mean and standard deviation (SD), or median and interquartile range (25th percentile (*P25*); 75th percentile (*P75*)) for continuous variables, depending on the symmetry of their distribution.

When testing hypotheses about continuous variables we used non-parametric tests (Mann-Whitney and Kruskal-Wallis tests) considering the hypotheses of non-normality and number of groups. When testing hypotheses on categorical variables, the chi-square test and the Fisher's exact test were used, as appropriate.

The level of statistical significance was set at 5%, so the differences were considered statistically significant whenever $p < 0.05$. Statistical analyses were performed using SPSS® v.28.0 (Statistical Package for the Social Sciences: Armonk, NY, USA).

3. Results

3.1. Sociodemographic Data

The sociodemographic characteristics of the study population are presented in Table 1. Most of the population resides in the municipalities corresponding to the coverage areas of CHUSJ (Maia (30%), Valongo (26%), and Porto (18%)), and a minority resides in other municipalities of the North of Portugal, including Matosinhos ($n = 5$ (4%)), Vila Nova de Gaia ($n = 4$ (3%)), and Vila do Conde ($n = 3$ (2%)). Forty five percent of the population has a low level of education ($\leq$12 years), while around 19% of the population has higher degrees of education equivalent to a Master or PhD degree. The median age of the participants was 31.7 years old, with the youngest and the oldest participants being 19 and 40 years old, respectively. The median pre-pregnancy body mass index (BMI) was 23.6 kg/m², and 65% of women were within the normal weight range (18.5–24.9 kg/m²). Calculation of BMI was based on the self-reported weights and heights of pregnant women 6 months before the day of recruitment. Regarding the number of pregnancies, 52% of women were primiparous. Only 7% of the pregnancies resulted in preterm births, and in total, this sample gave birth to 68 boys and 73 girls.

The mean (SD) weight at birth was 3152 (478) g, and 86% of newborns had adequate weights for their gestational ages. The median (*P25*; *P75*) urinary 3-PBA concentration was 0.182 (0.182; 0.372) µg/L, which is above the detection limit (LOD, 0.364 µg/L). To account for the urine concentration, we adjusted 3-PBA urinary excretion for creatinine concentration (median (*P25*; *P72*) of 0.263 (0.167; 0.458) µg/g and used this variable in all the remaining analyses.

Table 1. General characteristics of the study sample ($n = 145$).

Residence Area, n (%)			
	Maia	41	(30)
	Porto	25	(18)
	Valongo	35	(26)
	Outros	35	(26)
Maternal education level, n (%)			
	Low ($\leq$12 years)	62	(45)
	Medium (13–15 years)	50	(36)
	High ($\geq$16 years)	26	(19)
Age (years), n		145	
	Mean	32	
	SD	5.2	
Pre-pregnancy BMI (kg/m^2), n		142	
	Median	24	
	P25; P75	21; 26	
	Minimum	16	
	Maximum	36	
Pre-pregnancy BMI categories, n (%)			
	Low weight	11	(8)
	Normal weight	92	(65)
	Overweight	24	(17)
	Obesity	15	(10)
Gestational age at recruitment (weeks), n		145	
	Median	12	
	P25; P75	12; 13	
Primiparous, n (%)			
	No	70	(48)
	Yes	75	(52)
Preterm (37 weeks), n (%)			
	No	131	(93)
	Yes	10	(7)
Newborn sex, n (%)			
	Male	68	(48)
	Female	73	(52)
Birth weight (grams), n		141	
	Mean	3152	
	SD	477	
Birth weight classification, n (%)			
	SGA	12	(9)
	AGA	122	(86)
	LGA	7	(5)
3-PBA (µg/L), n		145	
	Median	0.182	
	P25; P75	0.182; 0.372	
	<LOD, n (%)	103	(71)
	$\geq$LOD, n (%)	42	(29)
3-PBA (µg/g), n		145	
	Median	0.263	
	P25; P75	0.167; 0.458	

SGA, small for gestational age; AGA, appropriate for gestational age; LGA, large for gestational age. LOD, limit of detection. Missing's: between 2 and 6%.

Table 2 explores the association between urinary concentration of the pyrethroid metabolite 3-PBA with sociodemographic characteristics. The median concentration was the lowest in Porto, although the differences observed were not statistically significant. Maternal education level or smoking habits did not appear to be consistently associated with 3-PBA status. Regarding the BMI categories, a statistically significant difference was observed ($p = 0.049$), where the lowest medians were found in mothers with obesity.

Table 2. Urinary levels of 3-PBA (µg/g) by participant characteristics.

	n	(%)	P25	Median	P75	p
Residence Area						
Maia	41	(30)	0.174	0.274	0.450	
Porto	25	(18)	0.131	0.174	0.294	0.056 [a]
Valongo	35	(26)	0.172	0.278	0.368	
Other	35	(26)	0.172	0.333	0.507	
Maternal education level						
Low (≤12 years)	62	(45)	0.166	0.278	0.525	
Medium (13–15 years)	50	(36)	0.172	0.310	0.410	0.242 [a]
High (≥16 years)	26	(19)	0.139	0.189	0.368	
Smoking habits						
Non-Smoker	94	(66)	0.172	0.276	0.497	
Smoker	23	(16)	0.169	0.254	0.309	0.185 [a]
Former smoker	26	(18)	0.142	0.206	0.334	
Pre-pregnancy BMI categories						
Underweight	11	(8)	0.152	0.291	0.328	
Normal weight	92	(65)	0.188	0.293	0.507	0.049 [a]
Overweight	24	(17)	0.165	0.241	0.340	
Obesity	15	(11)	0.103	0.155	0.346	

Classification of the residence Area based on Instituto Nacional de Estatística de Portugal I.P., 2014. [a] Kruskal-Wallis. Missing's: between 2 and 6%.

3.2. 3-PBA Exposure by Seasons

Table 3 presents the distribution of the population by season of urine collection and the corresponding 3-PBA urinary excretion, illustrated in Figure 2. 3-PBA with or without the adjustment for creatinine levels was higher in summer-collected urine ($p < 0.001$). In addition, we observed that 3-PBA detection rate was much higher in summer when compared with winter samples (53% ($n = 39$) versus 4% ($n = 3$); $p < 0.001$).

Table 3. Levels of creatinine and 3-PBA with and without adjustment of creatinine in winter and summer samples.

			Creatinine (mg/dL)				3-PBA (µg/L)					3-PBA (µg/g)				
Seasons	n	(%)	P25	Median	P75	p	P25	Median	P75	(Min; Max)	p	P25	Median	P75	(Min; Max)	p
Summer	74	51	46.06	79.61	121.81	0.397 [a]	0.182	0.371	0.394	(0.182; 0.553)	<0.001 [a]	0.209	0.331	0.556	(0.082; 2.166)	<0.001 [a]
Winter	71	49	58.47	85.35	133.75		0.182	0.182	0.182	(0.182; 0.390)		0.139	0.218	0.311	(0.780; 1.064)	

[a] Mann-Whitney.

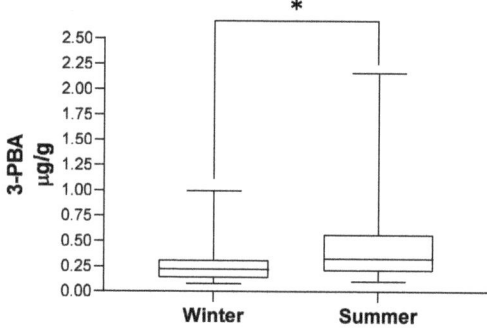

Figure 2. 3-PBA urinary excretion according to season of urine collection. In each box, the central horizontal line marks the median value. * $p < 0.001$.

3.3. 3-PBA Exposure in Association with Food Intake

Table 4 shows the variation of urinary levels of 3-PBA, separated by seasons (summer and winter) with consumption of fish or yogurt. 3-PBA levels were found to be positively associated with the frequency of consumption of these foods in winter but not in summer. The frequency of consumption of other foods, such as cow's milk, eggs, and cheese was not associated with 3-PBA levels (data not shown).

Table 4. 3-PBA levels in association with food intake.

Food Intake	3-PBA Summer (µg/g)					3-PBA Winter (µg/g)				
	n	(%)	Median	(P25; P75)	p	n	(%)	Median	(P25; P75)	p
Fish										
≤3 times a week	41	(32)	0.318	(0.228; 0.608)	0.533 [a]	67	(52)	0.213	(0.139; 0.301)	0.002 [a]
>3 times a week	17	(13)	0.325	(0.155; 0.650)		3	(2)	0.976	(0.343; 1.064)	
Yogurt										
≤6 times a week	40	(28)	0.350	(0.236; 0.521)	0.938 [a]	40	(28)	0.180	(0.133; 0.270)	0.015 [a]
≥1 time a day	33	(23)	0.328	(0.174; 0.618)		30	(21)	0.269	(0.170; 0.462)	

[a] Mann-Whitney. Missing's: between 1 and 23%.

3.4. 3-PBA Levels and Maternal Outcomes

The association between 3-PBA levels and maternal and pregnancy clinical characteristics was studied.

Considering the structural similarities found between pyrethroids and THs and the consequent suspicion that they could antagonize thyroid hormone activities [19,21,46], levels of 3-PBA in our sample were analyzed according to medication for thyroid disease (as a proxy for hypothyroidism). We found that women who reported taking levothyroxine had higher median (P25; P75) urinary 3-PBA levels when compared to women who reported not having thyroid disease (0.534 (0.333; 0.976) µg/g, n = 9, and 0.266 (0.168; 0.430) µg/g, n = 124, respectively, $p = 0.010$).

Additionally, 1st trimester 3-PBA levels had a weak positive correlation with maternal fasting glycemia in the first trimester ($r = 0.256$; $p = 0.011$, Spearmen correlation), and women who had cesarean delivery had higher median (P25; P75) first trimester 3-PBA levels when compared with women who had vaginal delivery (0.302 (0.206; 0.528) µg/g versus 0.255 (0.153; 0.410) µg/g, respectively, $p = 0.041$).

3.5. Neonatal Outcomes

Median 3-PBA concentrations were very similar between male and female offspring (Table 5).

Table 5. 3-PBA levels and newborn sex.

Newborn Sex	n	(%)	P25	Median	P75	(Min; Max) µg/g	p
Male	68	(48)	0.161	0.271	0.401	(0.078; 1.428)	0.463 [a]
Female	73	(52)	0.170	0.270	0.507	(0.780; 2.166)	

[a] Mann-Whitney. Missing's: 3%.

Table 6 shows the variation of urinary 3-PBA levels with neonatal outcomes; the described pyrethroid pesticide metabolite was not associated with anthropometric categories at birth.

Table 6. Maternal first trimester urinary 3-PBA levels and newborn outcomes.

Birth Size Categories		n	(%)	P25	Median	P75	p
Birth weight							
	SGA	12	(8)	0.196	0.303	0.356	
	AGA	122	(87)	0.167	0.261	0.462	0.786 [a]
	LGA	7	(5)	0.174	0.301	0.497	
Birth head circumference							
	SGA	13	(10)	0.203	0.278	0.333	
	AGA	112	(83)	0.166	0.263	0.463	0.973 [a]
	LGA	10	(7)	0.168	0.257	0.456	
Birth length							
	SGA	9	(6)	0.221	0.263	0.291	
	AGA	131	(93)	0.168	0.274	0.476	0.171 [a]
	LGA	1	(1)	0.101	0.101	0.101	

SGA, small for gestational age; AGA, adequate for gestational age; LGA, large for gestational age. [a] Kruskal-Wallis. Missing's: between 3 and 7%.

4. Discussion

Analysis of results for 3-PBA urinary excretion in pregnant women showed concentrations above LOD in 29% of the sample population.

3-PBA urinary excretion tended to associate with residence area, being lower in Porto, when compared to other municipalities. The fact that Porto is a predominantly urban city when compared with Valongo [47], for example, which has a great amount of rural territory, could account for this trend. In line with this rationale, Wielgomas et al. found that the detection of metabolites of SPs in preschool and school children and their parents was more frequent and with higher urinary excretion in rural when compared with urban areas in Poland [48]. In that study, 3-PBA was detected in 77% and 94% of samples from urban and rural areas, respectively, and curiously, 3-PBA urinary levels found in rural and urban areas were very similar to those found in our study (0.272 vs 0.155 µg/g for rural vs urban areas in Poland [48], respectively; 0.278 vs 0.174 µg/g for Porto vs Valongo in Portugal, respectively). Concerning frequency of exposure to 3-PBA, our study revealed a low detection rate (29%) when compared, for example, with reports for Polish, American, French, or Chinese population samples [22–24,48]. On the other hand, the 3-PBA detection rate herein described is comparable or higher than those obtained in studies from Germany [49–51], Spain [52,53], or France [54,55]. The variation in concentration 3-PBA medians, LOD/LOQ values or rates of detection across studies can be attributable to local exposure characteristics but, importantly, to heterogeneity in urine sampling, sample preparation, quantification methods, and reporting [56]. Altogether, these findings corroborate the claim recently published by Andersen et al. [56] for the need for guidelines to harmonize quantification methods and reporting in human biomonitoring studies.

Regarding pre-gestational BMI categories, 3-PBA levels were the lowest in mothers with obesity. Being highly lipophilic, 3-PBA conjugates with lipids such as cholesterol, bile acids, and triglycerides, which results in 3-PBA retention in organs particularly rich in lipid content [57] such as adipose tissue. This retention could result in the observed decrease in 3-PBA urinary excretion with increasing BMI (and fat mass).

Yoo M et al. also reported a negative association between 3-PBA levels and BMI for high levels of exposure in Korean adults [58]. Despite this, other studies have shown either a positive or no association between 3-PBA urinary excretion and BMI in pregnant women [59] or in the elder, respectively. We cannot currently explain the disparity of these results when compared to ours.

Importantly, 3-PBA exposure was found to be higher in the summer, when compared to winter-collected urine samples. Several studies have shown that urinary pyrethroid metabolite levels of pregnant women follow trends of seasonal insecticide use related to pest management practice [24,33–36]. A study carried out in China also observed a trend of seasonal variation, with levels of urinary metabolites in the summer significantly higher than those in the winter. These data indicate the need to assess the potential adverse effects of exposure to pyrethroid pesticides on fetuses and infants, in order to take appropriate measures to protect pregnant women from higher exposure to pesticides in more susceptible seasons [24]. Despite this, we cannot exclude that seasonal variations in 3-PBA levels could also be due to seasonal variations in fruits or vegetables consumption. In fact, a systematic review with metanalysis has shown that fruit consumption across the world tends to be higher in autumn and winter, but vegetable consumption tends to be higher in spring and summer [60]. This may, in all probability, result in differential SPs exposure according to seasons.

In relation to food consumption, 3-PBA levels were associated with a higher consumption of fish and yogurt in winter-collected samples; the lack of association between food consumption and 3-PBA urinary levels in summer-collected samples could be due to a greater exposure to environmental 3-PBA in the summer, which could mask the foodborne exposure.

Although the available evidence regarding associations between dairy or fish consumption and 3-PBA urinary levels is currently weak, 3-PBA-parent pesticides, such as cypermethrin, bifenthrin, and cyhalothrin have been detected both in fish and in dairy samples [61,62] and our data show that these foods could act as vehicles for 3-PBA exposure. In fact, 3-PBA levels were 4.5 times higher in the group of people consuming fish more than 3 times a week and 1.5 times higher in the group of people consuming at least one yogurt a day. Despite the magnitude of the difference and the statistical significance, association of 3-PBA levels with fish consumption should be interpreted with caution, because of the small sample size in the category of fish consumption >3 times/week.

In addition, we cannot explain the reason why yogurt was the only dairy food which consumption associated with 3-PBA levels. Despite this, our data suggest that fish and yogurt may represent a form of pyrethroid bioaccumulation.

With respect to the association of 3-PBA with maternal clinical characteristics, we observed higher levels of 3-PBA in women medicated for hypothyroidism, which corroborates the idea that pyrethroids, whose structure is similar to THs, could associate with thyroid dysfunction, as suggested by others [19,46]. However, in our study, only 9 women are included in the hypothyroidism medicated group, and so, these results should be read with caution.

It is estimated that at least 10% of approved pesticides in the European Union (EU) possess endocrine disruption (ED) properties [63,64]. Experimental studies have reported that many currently used pesticides (or their metabolites) may interfere with the hypothalamic-pituitary-gonadal and hypothalamic-pituitary-thyroid axes [46,65]. Especially among vulnerable human populations, such as developing fetuses and infants, changes in THs beyond the reference range may cause a significant adverse impact on health, including the development of neurodevelopmental problems [16,66]. However, the effects of current human pyrethroid exposure levels on reproductive and thyroid function are poorly understood.

Still, with regard to maternal clinical characteristics, there was a weak but statistically significant correlation between 3-PBA levels and maternal fasting glycemia in the first trimester. This result is in line with a study conducted in China that studied the association between serum levels of pyrethroid insecticides and risk of type 2 diabetes which found that high concentrations of serum pyrethroid insecticides were significantly associated with an increased risk of type 2 diabetes [67]. A US study suggests that exposure to pyrethroids, as estimated by urinary 3-PBA concentrations, was associated with an increased risk of diabetes in the general adult population [68]. Hansen et al. found a severely increased prevalence of prediabetes among Bolivian pesticide sprayers compared with a control group. Within the sprayer group, an association between cumulative exposure to pyrethroids and abnormal glucose regulation was seen [69].

Finally, in our study, we found no associations between pyrethroid pesticide metabolite levels and the anthropometric profile of newborns at birth. Like us, Berkowitz et al., found no significant association between newborn anthropometric measures (birth weight, length, and head circumference) and maternal 3-PBA urinary in early pregnancy [70]. In a prospective birth cohort in rural northern China between September 2010 and 2012, no associations were found between 3-PBA levels and birth length, head circumference, or gestational duration [18]. Contrarily, a study conducted in New York City aimed to investigate the association between delivery outcomes and urinary biomarkers of pyrethroids among healthy pregnant women and found that 3-PBA concentrations were positively associated with head circumference in boys (p = 0.53, 95% CI: 0.03, 1.04) [3]. Also, in a study carried out in northern China, aimed at linking pesticides and other environmental exposures with the health of pregnant women and their children, it was observed that the total levels of pyrethroid metabolites in the mother's urine maternal urine were positively associated with birth weight and head circumference [71].

One main limitation of this study was the small sample size, which resulted from the selection of samples collected during the summer and winter and exclusion of spring- or autumn-collected samples. In addition, the initial questionnaire did not ask pregnant women about the frequency of consumption of other foods, such as fruits and vegetables, and exposure to additional agents that may contain environmental pollutants.

Another limitation was that we could not analyze occupational exposure to 3-PBA due to lack of detailed information regarding the profession of the participants. In fact, information regarding professional occupations was extracted from clinical registries with no possible association with the likelihood of exposure.

A strong point of our study was that, although the recruitment was carried out at central hospital, we could invite pregnant women undergoing routine prenatal surveillance, not being restricted to pregnant women in hospital consultation, and therefore, we included women with and without pathology.

5. Conclusions

In conclusion, the present study characterized 3-PBA status in a sample of pregnant women living in the Porto metropolitan area. Nonetheless, 3-PBA excretion associated negatively with maternal pre-pregnancy BMI, suggesting 3-PBA adipose tissue retention. Our data also suggest that 3-PBA exposure is higher during the summer, and food such as fish and yogurt may be a source of 3-PBA dietary exposure, particularly when environmental exposure is low.

As to clinical features, our data suggest that 3-PBA may be associated with thyroid dysfunction, which could be due to a thyroid hormone antagonistic effect, as previously described by other authors. This conclusion should be considered cautiously given the small sample size of the hypothyroidism medicated group in our study.

In fact, this data, together with the association herein found between 3-PBA and fasting glycemia, deserve future attention.

Finally, in this work, we did not find an association between 3-PBA maternal urinary excretion in the first trimester and anthropometric measures of the newborn.

This study highlights that pregnant women living in Portugal may be exposed to 3-PBA and that this exposure may associate with maternal clinical features during pregnancy. More studies are needed to confirm data regarding association of 3-PBA exposure and newborn outcomes and to analyze the impact of these exposures on long-term maternal or childhood outcomes.

Author Contributions: J.G.: conceptualization, methodology, investigation, formal analysis, writing—original draft, visualization, funding acquisition; I.B.: investigation, writing—review and editing; C.P.: investigation, writing—review and editing; N.X.M.: investigation; C.M.C.: conceptualization, D.P.: investigation, methodology; M.d.C.P.: resources; C.M.: resources; V.F.D.: resources; C.D.-M.: investigation; C.C.D.: formal analysis; L.F.R.A.: conceptualization, methodology; C.C.: conceptualization, methodology, funding acquisition; J.C.L.: conceptualization, methodology; C.R.: methodology, resources, investigation, methodology, supervision, writing—review and editing; E.K.: conceptualization, methodology, supervision, project administration, funding acquisition, writing—review and editing. V.C.F.: investigation, formal analysis, methodology, supervision, writing—review and editing, funding acquisition. All authors have read and agreed to the published version of the manuscript.

Funding: This article was supported by national funds through the FCT Foundation for Science and Technology, I.P., within the scope of the projects RISE - LA/P/0053/2020; CINTESIS, R&D UNIT (reference UIDB/4255/2020) and LAQV (references: UIDB/50006/2020 AND UIDP/50006/2020). Virgínia Cruz Fernandes was funded by FCT/MCTES (Foundation for Science and Technology and Ministry of Science, Technology and Higher Education) and the ESF (European Social Fund) through NORTE 2020 (North Region Operational Program) through a grant of Post-Doc (reference SFRH/BPD/109153/2015). Juliana Guimarães was funded by FCT/MCTES (Foundation for Science and Technology and Ministry of Science, Technology and Higher Education) under CINTESIS by a PhD scholarship (reference UI/BD/152087/2021).

Institutional Review Board Statement: This study was performed according to the protocol approved by the Ethics Committee of São João University Hospital Center (CHUSJoão)/Faculty of Medicine of the University of Porto.

Informed Consent Statement: Informed consent was obtained from all subjects involved in the study.

Data Availability Statement: The data sets generated during and/or analyzed during the current study are available from the corresponding author on reasonable request.

Acknowledgments: The authors would like to thank the kind participation of all pregnant women and the support of the recruitment activities by the health professionals of the Department of Obstetrics, Centro Hospitalar Universitário S. João, Porto, Portugal and also to the professionals of REQUIMTE/LAQV, Instituto Superior de Engenharia, Politécnico do Porto, for their collaboration in carrying out the analyzes of the 3-PBA metabolite. This work received support from PT national funds (FCT/MCTES, Fundação para a Ciência e Tecnologia and Ministério da Ciência, Tecnologia e Ensino Superior) through the projects LA/P/0053/2020; UIDB/4255/2020; UIDB/5006/2020 and UIDP/50006/2020. Virgínia Cruz Fernandes thanks FCT/MCTES (Fundação para a Ciência e Tecnologia and Ministério da Ciência, Tecnologia e Ensino Superior) and ESF (European Social Fund) through NORTE 2020 (Programa Operacional Região Norte) for his/her Post-Doc grant ref. SFRH/BPD/109153/2015. Juliana Guimarães was funded by FCT/MCTES (Foundation for Science and Technology and Ministry of Science, Technology and Higher Education) under CINTESIS by a PhD scholarship (reference UI/BD/152087/2021).

Conflicts of Interest: The authors have no relevant financial or non-financial interests to disclose. The authors have no competing interests to declare that are relevant to the content of this article. All authors certify that they have no affiliations with or involvement in any organization or entity with any financial interest or non-financial interest in the subject matter or materials discussed in this manuscript. The authors have no financial or proprietary interests in any material discussed in this article.

References

1. Lewis, R.C.; Cantonwine, D.E.; Anzalota Del Toro, L.V.; Calafat, A.M.; Valentin-Blasini, L.; Davis, M.D.; Baker, S.E.; Alshawabkeh, A.N.; Cordero, J.F.; Meeker, J.D. Urinary biomarkers of exposure to insecticides, herbicides, and one insect repellent among pregnant women in Puerto Rico. *Environ. Health* **2014**, *13*, 97. [CrossRef] [PubMed]
2. Bragança, I.; Lemos, P.C.; Delerue-Matos, C.; Domingues, V.F. Pyrethroid pesticide metabolite, 3-PBA, in soils: Method development and application to real agricultural soils. *Environ. Sci. Pollut. Res. Int.* **2019**, *26*, 2987–2997. [CrossRef]
3. Balalian, A.A.; Liu, X.; Herbstman, J.B.; Daniel, S.; Whyatt, R.; Rauh, V.; Calafat, A.M.; Wapner, R.; Factor-Litvak, P. Prenatal exposure to organophosphate and pyrethroid insecticides and the herbicide 2,4-dichlorophenoxyacetic acid and size at birth in urban pregnant women. *Environ. Res.* **2021**, *201*, 111539. [CrossRef] [PubMed]
4. EPA. Evironmental Protection Agency. *Pesticide Science and Assessing Pesticide Risks*; epa.gov/; EPA: Springfield, IL, USA, 2022.
5. Bragança, I.; Lemos, P.C.; Barros, P.; Delerue-Matos, C.; Domingues, V.F. Phytotoxicity of pyrethroid pesticides and its metabolite towards Cucumis sativus. *Sci. Total Environ.* **2018**, *619–620*, 685–691. [CrossRef]
6. Bragança, I.; Mucha, A.P.; Tomasino, M.P.; Santos, F.; Lemos, P.C.; Delerue-Matos, C.; Domingues, V.F. Deltamethrin impact in a cabbage planted soil: Degradation and effect on microbial community structure. *Chemosphere* **2019**, *220*, 1179–1186. [CrossRef]
7. Li, W.; Morgan, M.K.; Graham, S.E.; Starr, J.M. Measurement of pyrethroids and their environmental degradation products in fresh fruits and vegetables using a modification of the quick easy cheap effective rugged safe (QuEChERS) method. *Talanta* **2016**, *151*, 42–50. [CrossRef]

8. European Food Safety Authority (EFSA); Medina-Pastor, P.; Triacchini, G. The 2018 European Union report on pesticide residues in food. *EFSA J.* **2020**, *18*, e06057. [PubMed]
9. Saillenfait, A.M.; Ndiaye, D.; Sabaté, J.P. Pyrethroids: Exposure and health effects—An update. *Int. J. Hyg. Environ. Health* **2015**, *218*, 281–292. [CrossRef] [PubMed]
10. Kim, K.H.; Kabir, E.; Jahan, S.A. Exposure to pesticides and the associated human health effects. *Sci. Total Environ.* **2017**, *575*, 525–535. [CrossRef]
11. Wan, F.; Yu, T.; Hu, J.; Yin, S.; Li, Y.; Kou, L.; Chi, X.; Wu, J.; Sun, Y.; Zhou, Q.; et al. The pyrethroids metabolite 3-phenoxybenzoic acid induces dopaminergic degeneration. *Sci. Total Environ.* **2022**, *838*, 156027. [CrossRef]
12. Personne, S.; Marcelo, P.; Pilard, S.; Baltora-Rosset, S.; Corona, A.; Robidel, F.; Lecomte, A.; Brochot, C.; Bach, V.; Zeman, F. Determination of maternal and foetal distribution of cis- and trans-permethrin isomers and their metabolites in pregnant rats by liquid chromatography tandem mass spectrometry (LC-MS/MS). *Anal. Bioanal. Chem.* **2019**, *411*, 8043–8052. [CrossRef]
13. Connors, S.L.; Levitt, P.; Matthews, S.G.; Slotkin, T.A.; Johnston, M.V.; Kinney, H.C.; Johnson, W.G.; Dailey, R.M.; Zimmerman, A.W. Fetal mechanisms in neurodevelopmental disorders. *Pediatr. Neurol.* **2008**, *38*, 163–176. [CrossRef]
14. Abreu-Villaça, Y.; Levin, E.D. Developmental neurotoxicity of succeeding generations of insecticides. *Environ. Int.* **2017**, *99*, 55–77. [CrossRef] [PubMed]
15. Andersen, H.R.; David, A.; Freire, C.; Fernández, M.F.; D'Cruz, S.C.; Reina-Pérez, I.; Fini, J.B.; Blaha, L. Pyrethroids and developmental neurotoxicity - A critical review of epidemiological studies and supporting mechanistic evidence. *Environ. Res.* **2022**, *214 Pt 2*, 113935. [CrossRef]
16. Hwang, M.; Lee, Y.; Choi, K.; Park, C. Urinary 3-phenoxybenzoic acid levels and the association with thyroid hormones in adults: Korean National Environmental Health Survey 2012-2014. *Sci. Total Environ.* **2019**, *696*, 133920. [CrossRef]
17. Casals-Casas, C.; Desvergne, B. Endocrine disruptors: From endocrine to metabolic disruption. *Annu. Rev. Physiol.* **2011**, *73*, 135–162. [CrossRef]
18. Zhang, J.; Yoshinaga, J.; Hisada, A.; Shiraishi, H.; Shimodaira, K.; Okai, T.; Koyama, M.; Watanabe, N.; Suzuki, E.; Shirakawa, M.; et al. Prenatal pyrethroid insecticide exposure and thyroid hormone levels and birth sizes of neonates. *Sci. Total Environ.* **2014**, *488–489*, 275–279. [CrossRef] [PubMed]
19. Du, G.; Shen, O.; Sun, H.; Fei, J.; Lu, C.; Song, L.; Xia, Y.; Wang, S.; Wang, X. Assessing hormone receptor activities of pyrethroid insecticides and their metabolites in reporter gene assays. *Toxicol. Sci.* **2010**, *116*, 58–66. [CrossRef] [PubMed]
20. Hu, Y.; Zhang, Z.; Qin, K.; Zhang, Y.; Pan, R.; Wang, Y.; Shi, R.; Gao, Y.; Tian, Y. Environmental pyrethroid exposure and thyroid hormones of pregnant women in Shandong, China. *Chemosphere* **2019**, *234*, 815–821. [CrossRef] [PubMed]
21. Zhang, J.; Hisada, A.; Yoshinaga, J.; Shiraishi, H.; Shimodaira, K.; Okai, T.; Noda, Y.; Shirakawa, M.; Kato, N. Exposure to pyrethroids insecticides and serum levels of thyroid-related measures in pregnant women. *Environ. Res.* **2013**, *127*, 16–21. [CrossRef]
22. Curl, C.L.; Porter, J.; Penwell, I.; Phinney, R.; Ospina, M.; Calafat, A.M. Effect of a 24-week randomized trial of an organic produce intervention on pyrethroid and organophosphate pesticide exposure among pregnant women. *Environ. Int.* **2019**, *132*, 104957. [CrossRef] [PubMed]
23. Dereumeaux, C.; Saoudi, A.; Goria, S.; Wagner, V.; De Crouy-Chanel, P.; Pecheux, M.; Berat, B.; Zaros, C.; Guldner, L. Urinary levels of pyrethroid pesticides and determinants in pregnant French women from the Elfe cohort. *Environ. Int.* **2018**, *119*, 89–99. [CrossRef]
24. Qi, X.; Zheng, M.; Wu, C.; Wang, G.; Feng, C.; Zhou, Z. Urinary pyrethroid metabolites among pregnant women in an agricultural area of the Province of Jiangsu, China. *Int. J. Hyg. Environ. Health* **2012**, *215*, 487–495. [CrossRef]
25. Baker, S.E.; Barr, D.B.; Driskell, W.J.; Beeson, M.D.; Needham, L.L. Quantification of selected pesticide metabolites in human urine using isotope dilution high-performance liquid chromatography/tandem mass spectrometry. *J. Expo. Anal. Environ. Epidemiol.* **2000**, *10*, 789–798. [CrossRef]
26. Skakkebaek, N.E.; Jørgensen, N.; Main, K.M.; Rajpert-De Meyts, E.; Leffers, H.; Andersson, A.M.; Juul, A.; Carlsen, E.; Mortensen, G.K.; Jensen, T.K.; et al. Is human fecundity declining? *Int. J. Androl.* **2006**, *29*, 2–11. [CrossRef] [PubMed]
27. Snijder, C.A.; te Velde, E.; Roeleveld, N.; Burdorf, A. Occupational exposure to chemical substances and time to pregnancy: A systematic review. *Hum. Reprod. Update* **2012**, *18*, 284–300. [CrossRef] [PubMed]
28. Mehrpour, O.; Karrari, P.; Zamani, N.; Tsatsakis, A.M.; Abdollahi, M. Occupational exposure to pesticides and consequences on male semen and fertility: A review. *Toxicol. Lett.* **2014**, *230*, 146–156. [CrossRef]
29. Shelton, J.F.; Geraghty, E.M.; Tancredi, D.J.; Delwiche, L.D.; Schmidt, R.J.; Ritz, B.; Hansen, R.L.; Hertz-Picciotto, I. Neurodevelopmental disorders and prenatal residential proximity to agricultural pesticides: The CHARGE study. *Environ. Health Perspect.* **2014**, *122*, 1103–1109. [CrossRef]
30. Domingues, V.F.; Nasuti, C.; Piangerelli, M.; Correia-Sa, L.; Ghezzo, A.; Marini, M.; Abruzzo, P.M.; Visconti, P.; Giustozzi, M.; Rossi, G.; et al. Pyrethroid Pesticide Metabolite in Urine and Microelements in Hair of Children Affected by Autism Spectrum Disorders: A Preliminary Investigation. *Int. J. Environ. Res. Public Health* **2016**, *13*, 388. [CrossRef] [PubMed]
31. Wagner-Schuman, M.; Richardson, J.R.; Auinger, P.; Braun, J.M.; Lanphear, B.P.; Epstein, J.N.; Yolton, K.; Froehlich, T.E. Association of pyrethroid pesticide exposure with attention-deficit/hyperactivity disorder in a nationally representative sample of U.S. children. *Environ. Health* **2015**, *14*, 44. [CrossRef] [PubMed]

32. Furlong, M.A.; Barr, D.B.; Wolff, M.S.; Engel, S.M. Prenatal exposure to pyrethroid pesticides and childhood behavior and executive functioning. *Neurotoxicology* **2017**, *62*, 231–238. [CrossRef] [PubMed]
33. Šulc, L.; Janoš, T.; Figueiredo, D.; Ottenbros, I.; Šenk, P.; Mikeš, O.; Huss, A.; Čupr, P. Pesticide exposure among Czech adults and children from the CELSPAC-SPECIMEn cohort: Urinary biomarker levels and associated health risks. *Environ. Res.* **2022**, *214*, 114002. [CrossRef] [PubMed]
34. Osaka, A.; Ueyama, J.; Kondo, T.; Nomura, H.; Sugiura, Y.; Saito, I.; Nakane, K.; Takaishi, A.; Ogi, H.; Wakusawa, S.; et al. Exposure characterization of three major insecticide lines in urine of young children in Japan-neonicotinoids, organophosphates, and pyrethroids. *Environ. Res.* **2016**, *147*, 89–96. [CrossRef] [PubMed]
35. English, K.; Li, Y.; Jagals, P.; Ware, R.S.; Wang, X.; He, C.; Mueller, J.F.; Sly, P.D. Development of a questionnaire-based insecticide exposure assessment method and comparison with urinary insecticide biomarkers in young Australian children. *Environ. Res.* **2019**, *178*, 108613. [CrossRef]
36. Wang, D.; Kamijima, M.; Imai, R.; Suzuki, T.; Kameda, Y.; Asai, K.; Okamura, A.; Naito, H.; Ueyama, J.; Saito, I.; et al. Biological monitoring of pyrethroid exposure of pest control workers in Japan. *J. Occup. Health* **2007**, *49*, 509–514. [CrossRef]
37. Matta Coelho, C.; Guimarães, J.; Bracchi, I.; Xavier Moreira, N.; Pinheiro, C.; Ferreira, P.; Pestana, D.; Barreiros Mota, I.; Cortez, A.; Prucha, C.; et al. Noncompliance to iodine supplementation recommendation is a risk factor for iodine insufficiency in Portuguese pregnant women: Results from the IoMum cohort. *J. Endocrinol. Investig.* **2022**, *45*, 1865–1874. [CrossRef] [PubMed]
38. Pinheiro, C.; Xavier Moreira, N.; Ferreira, P.; Matta Coelho, C.; Guimarães, J.; Pereira, G.; Cortez, A.; Bracchi, I.; Pestana, D.; Barreiros Mota, I.; et al. Iodine knowledge is associated with iodine status in Portuguese pregnant women: Results from the IoMum cohort study. *Br. J. Nutr.* **2021**, *126*, 1331–1339. [CrossRef]
39. Ferreira, P.; Pinheiro, C.; Matta Coelho, C.; Guimarães, J.; Pereira, G.; Xavier Moreira, N.; Cortez, A.; Bracchi, I.; Pestana, D.; Barreiros Mota, I.; et al. The association of milk and dairy consumption with iodine status in pregnant women in Oporto region. *Br. J. Nutr.* **2021**, *126*, 1314–1322. [CrossRef]
40. Richardson, D.B.; Ciampi, A. Effects of exposure measurement error when an exposure variable is constrained by a lower limit. *Am. J. Epidemiol.* **2003**, *157*, 355–363. [CrossRef]
41. Schisterman, E.F.; Vexler, A.; Whitcomb, B.W.; Liu, A. The limitations due to exposure detection limits for regression models. *Am. J. Epidemiol.* **2006**, *163*, 374–383. [CrossRef]
42. Govarts, E.G.L.; Rambaud, L.; Vogel, N.; Montazeri, P.; Berglund, M.; Santonen, T. *Deliverable Report; Statistical Analysis Plan for the Co-Funded Studies of WP8; WP10—Data Management and Analysis; Deadline: March 2020 Upload by Coordinator: 10 December 2020*; European Human Biomonitoring Initiative (HBM4EU) no.733032; 2020; Available online: https://www.hbm4eu.eu/work-packages/deliverable-10-12-update-statistical-analysis-plan-for-the-co-funded-studies-of-wp8/ (accessed on 18 December 2022).
43. O'Brien, K.M.; Upson, K.; Buckley, J.P. Lipid and Creatinine Adjustment to Evaluate Health Effects of Environmental Exposures. *Curr. Environ. Health Rep.* **2017**, *4*, 44–50. [CrossRef] [PubMed]
44. Fossati, P.; Prencipe, L.; Berti, G. Enzymic creatinine assay: A new colorimetric method based on hydrogen peroxide measurement. *Clin. Chem.* **1983**, *29*, 1494–1496. [CrossRef]
45. Alexander, G.R.; Kogan, M.D.; Himes, J.H. 1994-1996 U.S. singleton birth weight percentiles for gestational age by race, Hispanic origin, and gender. *Matern. Child Health J.* **1999**, *3*, 225–231. [CrossRef] [PubMed]
46. Leemans, M.; Couderq, S.; Demeneix, B.; Fini, J.B. Pesticides With Potential Thyroid Hormone-Disrupting Effects: A Review of Recent Data. *Front. Endocrinol.* **2019**, *10*, 743. [CrossRef] [PubMed]
47. Report, D. *Classification of Parishes on the Mainland into Rural and Non-Rural*; Rural Development Program (PRODER); Portugal, 2013; p. 81. Available online: https://enrd.ec.europa.eu/country/portugal_en (accessed on 18 December 2022).
48. Wielgomas, B.; Piskunowicz, M. Biomonitoring of pyrethroid exposure among rural and urban populations in northern Poland. *Chemosphere* **2013**, *93*, 2547–2553. [CrossRef] [PubMed]
49. Leng, G.; Ranft, U.; Sugiri, D.; Hadnagy, W.; Berger-Preiss, E.; Idel, H. Pyrethroids used indoors–biological monitoring of exposure to pyrethroids following an indoor pest control operation. *Int. J. Hyg. Environ. Health* **2003**, *206*, 85–92. [CrossRef]
50. Hardt, J.; Angerer, J. Biological monitoring of workers after the application of insecticidal pyrethroids. *Int. Arch. Occup. Environ. Health* **2003**, *76*, 492–498. [CrossRef]
51. Berger-Preiss, E.; Levsen, K.; Leng, G.; Idel, H.; Sugiri, D.; Ranft, U. Indoor pyrethroid exposure in homes with woollen textile floor coverings. *Int. J. Hyg. Environ. Health* **2002**, *205*, 459–472. [CrossRef] [PubMed]
52. Freire, C.; Suárez, B.; Vela-Soria, F.; Castiello, F.; Reina-Pérez, I.; Andersen, H.R.; Olea, N.; Fernández, M.F. Urinary metabolites of non-persistent pesticides and serum hormones in Spanish adolescent males. *Environ. Res.* **2021**, *197*, 111016. [CrossRef]
53. Roca, M.; Miralles-Marco, A.; Ferré, J.; Pérez, R.; Yusà, V. Biomonitoring exposure assessment to contemporary pesticides in a school children population of Spain. *Environ. Res.* **2014**, *131*, 77–85. [CrossRef] [PubMed]
54. Viel, J.F.; Warembourg, C.; Le Maner-Idrissi, G.; Lacroix, A.; Limon, G.; Rouget, F.; Monfort, C.; Durand, G.; Cordier, S.; Chevrier, C. Pyrethroid insecticide exposure and cognitive developmental disabilities in children: The PELAGIE mother-child cohort. *Environ. Int.* **2015**, *82*, 69–75. [CrossRef] [PubMed]
55. Viel, J.F.; Rouget, F.; Warembourg, C.; Monfort, C.; Limon, G.; Cordier, S.; Chevrier, C. Behavioural disorders in 6-year-old children and pyrethroid insecticide exposure: The PELAGIE mother-child cohort. *Occup. Environ. Med.* **2017**, *74*, 275–281. [CrossRef] [PubMed]

56. Andersen, H.R.; Rambaud, L.; Riou, M.; Buekers, J.; Remy, S.; Berman, T.; Govarts, E. Exposure Levels of Pyrethroids, Chlorpyrifos and Glyphosate in EU-An Overview of Human Biomonitoring Studies Published since 2000. *Toxics* **2022**, *10*, 789. [CrossRef]
57. Eljarrat, E. Pyrethroid Insecticides. In *The Handbook of Environmental Chemistry*; HEC: Paris, France, 2020; Volume 92.
58. Yoo, M.; Lim, Y.H.; Kim, T.; Lee, D.; Hong, Y.C. Association between urinary 3-phenoxybenzoic acid and body mass index in Korean adults: 1(st) Korean National Environmental Health Survey. *Ann. Occup. Environ. Med.* **2016**, *28*, 2. [CrossRef] [PubMed]
59. Dalsager, L.; Christensen, L.E.; Kongsholm, M.G.; Kyhl, H.B.; Nielsen, F.; Schoeters, G.; Jensen, T.K.; Andersen, H.R. Associations of maternal exposure to organophosphate and pyrethroid insecticides and the herbicide 2,4-D with birth outcomes and anogenital distance at 3 months in the Odense Child Cohort. *Reprod. Toxicol.* **2018**, *76*, 53–62. [CrossRef] [PubMed]
60. Stelmach-Mardas, M.; Kleiser, C.; Uzhova, I.; Peñalvo, J.L.; La Torre, G.; Palys, W.; Lojko, D.; Nimptsch, K.; Suwalska, A.; Linseisen, J.; et al. Seasonality of food groups and total energy intake: A systematic review and meta-analysis. *Eur. J. Clin. Nutr.* **2016**, *70*, 700–708. [CrossRef]
61. Farag, M.R.; Alagawany, M.; Bilal, R.M.; Gewida, A.G.A.; Dhama, K.; Abdel-Latif, H.M.R.; Amer, M.S.; Rivero-Perez, N.; Zaragoza-Bastida, A.; Binnaser, Y.S.; et al. An Overview on the Potential Hazards of Pyrethroid Insecticides in Fish, with Special Emphasis on Cypermethrin Toxicity. *Animals* **2021**, *11*, 1880. [CrossRef] [PubMed]
62. Riederer, A.M.; Hunter, R.E., Jr.; Hayden, S.W.; Ryan, P.B. Pyrethroid and organophosphorus pesticides in composite diet samples from Atlanta, USA adults. *Environ. Sci. Technol.* **2010**, *44*, 483–490. [CrossRef] [PubMed]
63. McKinlay, R.; Plant, J.A.; Bell, J.N.; Voulvoulis, N. Endocrine disrupting pesticides: Implications for risk assessment. *Environ. Int.* **2008**, *34*, 168–183. [CrossRef]
64. Lyssimachou, A.; Muilerman, H. *Impact Assessment of the Criteria for Endocrine Disrupting Pesticides*; Pesticide Action Network/PAN Europe: Brussels, Belgium, 2015–2016; p. 8.
65. Orton, F.; Rosivatz, E.; Scholze, M.; Kortenkamp, A. Widely used pesticides with previously unknown endocrine activity revealed as in vitro antiandrogens. *Environ. Health Perspect.* **2011**, *119*, 794–800. [CrossRef] [PubMed]
66. Berbel, P.; Mestre, J.L.; Santamaría, A.; Palazón, I.; Franco, A.; Graells, M.; González-Torga, A.; de Escobar, G.M. Delayed neurobehavioral development in children born to pregnant women with mild hypothyroxinemia during the first month of gestation: The importance of early iodine supplementation. *Thyroid* **2009**, *19*, 511–519. [CrossRef]
67. Jia, C.; Zhang, S.; Cheng, X.; An, J.; Zhang, X.; Li, P.; Li, W.; Wang, X.; Yuan, Y.; Zheng, H.; et al. Association between serum pyrethroid insecticide levels and incident type 2 diabetes risk: A nested case-control study in Dongfeng-Tongji cohort. *Eur. J. Epidemiol.* **2022**, *37*, 959–970. [CrossRef] [PubMed]
68. Park, J.; Park, S.K.; Choi, Y.H. Environmental pyrethroid exposure and diabetes in U.S. adults. *Environ. Res.* **2019**, *172*, 399–407. [CrossRef] [PubMed]
69. Hansen, M.R.; Jørs, E.; Lander, F.; Condarco, G.; Schlünssen, V. Is cumulated pyrethroid exposure associated with prediabetes? A cross-sectional study. *J. Agromed.* **2014**, *19*, 417–426. [CrossRef] [PubMed]
70. Berkowitz, G.S.; Wetmur, J.G.; Birman-Deych, E.; Obel, J.; Lapinski, R.H.; Godbold, J.H.; Holzman, I.R.; Wolff, M.S. In utero pesticide exposure, maternal paraoxonase activity, and head circumference. *Environ. Health Perspect.* **2004**, *112*, 388–391. [CrossRef] [PubMed]
71. Ding, G.; Cui, C.; Chen, L.; Gao, Y.; Zhou, Y.; Shi, R.; Tian, Y. Prenatal exposure to pyrethroid insecticides and birth outcomes in Rural Northern China. *J. Expo. Sci. Environ. Epidemiol.* **2015**, *25*, 264–270. [CrossRef]

Disclaimer/Publisher's Note: The statements, opinions and data contained in all publications are solely those of the individual author(s) and contributor(s) and not of MDPI and/or the editor(s). MDPI and/or the editor(s) disclaim responsibility for any injury to people or property resulting from any ideas, methods, instructions or products referred to in the content.

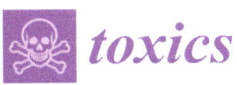

Systematic Review

Pesticide Exposure and Risk of Rheumatoid Arthritis: A Systematic Review and Meta-Analysis

Jiraporn Chittrakul, Ratana Sapbamrer * and Wachiranun Sirikul

Department of Community Medicine, Faculty of Medicine, Chiang Mai University, Chiang Mai 50200, Thailand; jerasooutch@gmail.com (J.C.); wachiranun.sir@gmail.com (W.S.)
* Correspondence: ratana.sapbamrer@cmu.ac.th; Tel.: +66-53-935-472

Abstract: Rheumatoid arthritis (RA) is a disease that affects people all over the world and can be caused by a variety of factors. Exposure to pesticides is one of the risk factors for the development of RA. However, the evidence of exposure to pesticides linked with the development of RA is still controversial. This study aimed to investigate the association between exposure to pesticides and RA by a systematic review of relevant literature and a meta-analysis. Full-text articles published in PubMed, Web of Science, Scopus, and Google Scholar between 1956 and 2021 were reviewed and evaluated. A total of eight studies were eligible for inclusion (two cohort studies, four case-control studies, and two cross-sectional studies). The adjusted odds ratio for pesticide exposure on RA was 1.20 for insecticides (95% CI = 1.12–1.28), 0.98 for herbicides (95% CI = 0.89–1.08), 1.04 for fungicides (95% CI = 0.86–1.27), and 1.15 in for non-specific pesticides (95% CI = 1.09–1.21). There is some evidence to suggest that exposure to insecticides (especially fonofos, carbaryl, and guanidines) contributes to an increased risk of RA. However, the evidence is limited because of a small number of studies. Therefore, further epidemiological studies are needed to substantiate this conclusion.

Keywords: pesticide; insecticide; herbicide; fungicide; rheumatoid arthritis; autoimmune disease

Citation: Chittrakul, J.; Sapbamrer, R.; Sirikul, W. Pesticide Exposure and Risk of Rheumatoid Arthritis: A Systematic Review and Meta-Analysis. *Toxics* **2022**, *10*, 207. https://doi.org/10.3390/toxics10050207

Academic Editors: Virgínia Cruz Fernandes and Michael Caudle

Received: 28 February 2022
Accepted: 20 April 2022
Published: 21 April 2022

Publisher's Note: MDPI stays neutral with regard to jurisdictional claims in published maps and institutional affiliations.

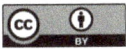

Copyright: © 2022 by the authors. Licensee MDPI, Basel, Switzerland. This article is an open access article distributed under the terms and conditions of the Creative Commons Attribution (CC BY) license (https://creativecommons.org/licenses/by/4.0/).

1. Introduction

Rheumatoid arthritis (RA), an autoimmune disease that causes joint inflammation, is a serious public health issue. Between 1980 and 2018, the global prevalence of RA was 460 per 100,000 people [1–4]. Genetics, smoking, infections, dietary behavior, chemical pollution, and autoimmune illnesses are risk factors for RA [3,5,6]. It has been reported that exposure to pesticides causes inflammation within the immune system that is directly toxic to that system, leading to chronic disease including RA [7]. It has also been found that RA affects not only the physical but also the socio-economic effects of the patient, including medical costs and the loss of disability income in work [8,9]. The focus of this study is to clearly identify the modifiable factors that cause RA, facilitating early intervention in those at risk of RA.

Despite increased awareness of the dangers associated with pesticide poisoning, it is still a major worldwide public health issue [10]. Pesticides are chemicals used in agriculture, gardening operations, and some house-cleaning products. Pesticides are usually classified by their pest target, for example, insecticides, herbicides, and fungicides [11]. Pesticides can enter the body by contact with skin, ingestion, and inhalation [12]. Doses and duration of exposure to pesticides are crucial factors in both acute and chronic health effects. Acute poisoning is caused by a single exposure to a high dosage of a pesticide, while chronic conditions are adverse health effects resulting from long-term exposure to pesticides [12,13]. Long term exposure to pesticides can disrupt organ functions such as those in the nervous system, endocrine system, respiratory system, reproductive system, kidney system, cardiovascular system, and immune system, resulting in conditions such as cancer, Parkinson's disease, Alzheimer's disease, multiple sclerosis, diabetes, coronary heart disease, chronic kidney disease, respiratory diseases, autoimmune diseases, and systemic lupus erythematosus [6,14–16]. RA is a major immune system disease, according to early studies suggesting that pesticides damage humans' immune system. Moreover, some studies have shown that occupational exposure to pesticides was linked with the development of RA [6], whereas other studies failed to confirm such an association [17,18]. As a consequence, the evidence available with regard to the link between pesticides and RA was inconsistent. As this is a contentious, rapidly changing field, the evidence needs to be continuously, systematically reviewed to update the state of knowledge. The aim of this study is to carry out a systematic review and meta-analysis of the existing literature specifically on the effects of pesticides on RA.

2. Materials and Methods

This review was performed in accordance with the PRISMA (Preferred Reporting Items for Systematic Reviews and Meta-Analyses) guidelines, and we have registered PROSPERO, registration number 4202299598.

2.1. Searching Strategy

This study aimed to review scientific evidence and carry out a meta-analysis of exposure to pesticides contributing to RA. The study was carried out in accordance with the Preferred Reporting Items for Systematic Reviews and Meta-Analysis (PRISMA). PubMed, Web of Science, Scopus, and Google Scholar were searched for full-text articles using the following keywords: "rheumatoid arthritis" OR "autoimmune disease" plus "pesticide" OR "herbicide" OR "insecticide" OR "fungicide". The study was registered under PROSPERO (registration number: CRD42022299598, 20 January 2022). The final search was completed on 14 February 2022. The search process was performed by all authors.

2.2. Inclusion Criteria

The inclusion criteria were as follows: (1) original article; (2) full-text article; (3) published between 1956 and 2021; (4) written in the English language; (5) assessed RA by a diagnosis of physicians or self-reported; (6) assessed the association between pesticide exposure and rheumatoid arthritis; and (7) data analysis was by regression analysis, or discriminant analysis for adjustment of confounding variables. The studies that were review articles, had irrelevant information, or were without variables of interest were excluded from the study.

The study selection process resulted in the following: 642 records identified through the databases; 274 records remained after duplicate removal; 36 articles remained after screening for full-text articles; finally resulting in 8 eligible articles for inclusion in the quantitative synthesis. A total of 28 articles were excluded because of being animal studies ($n = 2$), review articles ($n = 6$), biochemical studies ($n = 2$), and without variables of interest ($n = 18$) (Figure 1).

2.3. Data Extraction and Quality Assessment

The data from eligible articles were independently extracted by two investigators. The extracted data were as follows: the name of the first author, publication year, country, study design, number of the population, age, gender, name of the chemical, adjusted odds ratio (aOR), 95% confidence intervals (95% CI), and confounding variables.

The quality of the eligible articles was assessed using National Heart, Lung, and Blood Institute (NHLBI) Guidelines for reporting observational cohort, cross-sectional, and case-control studies [19]. The NHBLI checklist consisted of 14 items for reporting observational cohort and cross-sectional studies and 12 items for reporting case-control studies. The quality of the eligible articles was independently assessed by three reviewers (Tables S1 and S2).

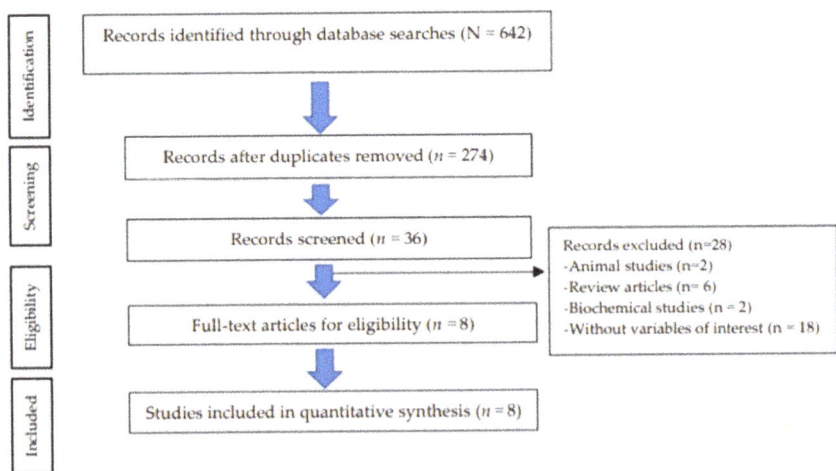

Figure 1. Flow chart of the study selection process (PRISMA).

2.4. Data Analysis

The eight studies selected were divided into four groups on the basis of the different types of pesticides, insecticides, herbicides, fungicides, and non-specific pesticides. A fixed-effect model with the Mantel–Haenszel method was used for analysis. The random-effect model of the DerSiomonian and Laird method was also used. The heterogeneity of selected studies was confirmed using the Cochran Q and I^2 tests. The heterogeneity was categorized into three criteria: low heterogeneity ($I^2 < 25\%$); moderate heterogeneity (I^2 25–50%); substantial heterogeneity ($I^2 > 50\%$). Funnel plots were tested to identify the publication bias of the selected studies. OR was plotted in the horizontal axis of the funnel plot, and standard error on the vertical axis. Two-tailed statistical tests at p-value < 0.05 were used. The data were analyzed using the STATA software package (Stata Corp. 2019. Stata Statistical Software: Release 16. College Station, TX, USA: Stata Corp LLC.).

3. Results

3.1. Association between Exposure to Insecticides and RA Development

Five studies were eligible for inclusion in the quantitative synthesis [6,17,18,20,21]: one study was a cohort study, two were case-control studies, and two were cross-sectional studies. Three studies were conducted in the USA ($n = 3$), with the others being conducted in Norway ($n = 1$) and Greece ($n = 1$). Of the five studies, two studies found an association between exposure to insecticides and RA, but three studies found no association. The study by Meyer et al. [6] found an association of increased risk of RA with exposure to fonofos (aOR = 1.7, 95% CI = 1.22–2.37) and carbaryl (aOR = 1.51, 95% CI = 1.03–2.23). The study by Koureas et al. [21] also found an association of increased risk of RA with exposure to organophosphates (aOR = 6.47, 95% CI = 1.00–45.43) and guanidines (aOR = 16.18, 95% CI = 1.58–165.97) (Table 1).

A total of 52,896 participants were included in the meta-analysis, and exposure to insecticides was found to be significantly associated with an increased risk of RA (aOR = 1.20, 95% CI = 1.12–1.28, p-value = 0.905 for heterogeneity $I^2 = 0\%$) (Figure 2).

Table 1. The association between exposure to insecticides and RA development.

Authors (Years)/Country	Study Design	Gender	Sample Size	Name of Chemicals	aOR (95% CI)	Confounding Variables
De Roos et al. (2005)/USA [17]	case-control	Female	810	Insecticides	1.2 (0.8–1.7)	Birth date, and state
				Carbamates	1.2 (0.8–1.7)	
				Organochlorines	1.1 (0.6–2.0)	
				Organophosphates	1.2 (0.8–1.8)	
				Carbaryl	1.2 (0.8–1.8)	
				Chlordane	0.5 (0.1–1.6)	
				Chlorpyrifos	0.8 (0.4–2.1)	
				Coumaphos	0.8 (0.2–3.4)	
				DDT	1.0 (0.4–2.2)	
				DDVP	1.4 (0.5–3.9)	
				Diazinon	0.9 (0.5–1.7)	
				Lindane	1.8 (0.6–5.0)	
				Malathion	1.3 (0.8–2.0)	
				Permethrin	1.0 (0.4–2.3)	
				Phorate	0.9 (0.2–4.3)	
				Terbufos	1.0 (0.3–3.4)	
				Toxaphene	2.3 (0.4–12.9)	
Lee et al. (2007)/Norway [18]	Cross-sectional	Both genders	1721	Organochlorines	3.5 (0.9–14.0)	Age, race, income status, BMI, and cigarette smoking
Parks et al. (2016)/USA [20]	Cohort	Female	23,841	Carbaryl	1.1 (0.85–1.4)	Age, state, and smoking pack-years
				Chlordane	0.99 (0.57–1.7)	
				DDT	1.5 (0.89–2.4)	
				Diazinon	1.2 (0.83–1.7)	
				Malathion	1.1 (0.80–1.4)	
				Permethrin	1.5 (0.83–2.7)	
				Dichlorvos	1.1 (0.56–2.4)	
Meyer et al. (2017)/USA [6]	case-control	Male	26,354	Aldrin	1.30 (0.82–2.05)	Age, state of enrollment, pack-years smoking, and education level
				Chlordane	1.32 (0.88–1.98)	
				DDT	115 (0.75–1.75)	
				Dieldrin	1.63 (0.77–3.43)	
				Heptachlor	0.88 (0.49–1.55)	
				Lindane	0.96 (0.58–1.59)	
				Toxaphene	1.44 (0.90–2.29)	
				Chlorpyrifos	1.30 (0.99–1.70)	
				Coumaphos	0.70 (0.40–1.23)	
				Diazinon	1.16 (0.77–1.75)	
				Dichlorvos	1.40 (0.91–2.14)	
				Fonofos	1.70 (1.22–2.37)	
				Malathion	1.05 (0.73–1.53)	
				Parathion	0.85 (0.45–1.60)	
				Phorate	1.14 (0.76–1.70)	
				Terbufos	1.24 (0.93–1.66)	
				Aldicarb	1.08 (0.58–2.01)	
				Carbaryl	1.51 (1.03–2.23)	
				Carbofuran	1.08 (0.80–1.46)	
				Permethrin [a]	1.17 (0.79–1.73)	
				Permethrin [b]	1.05 (0.68–1.62)	
Koureas et al. (2017)/Greece [21]	Cross-sectional	Male	170	Insecticides	2.82 (0.41–19.54)	Age, smoker, alcohol consumption, and use of a tractor on a farm
				Organophosphates	6.47 (1.00–45.43)	
				Pyrethroids	5.65 (0.39–81.82)	
				Guanidines	16.18 (1.58–165.97)	

[a] Used on crops; [b] used on poultry and livestock; aOR, adjusted odds ratio; 95% CI, 95% confidence interval; DDT, dichlorodiphenyltrichloroethane; DDVP, 2,2-dichlorovinyl dimethyl phosphate.

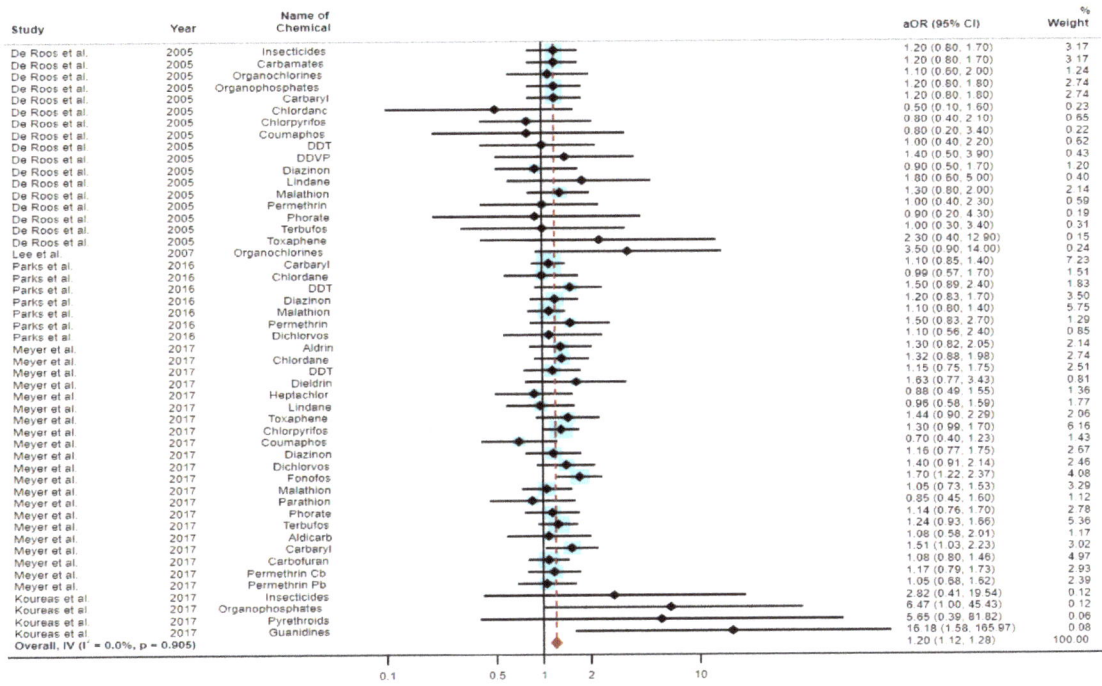

Figure 2. The association between exposure to insecticides and RA development [6,17,18,20,21]. aOR, adjusted odds ratio; 95% CI, 95% confidence interval.

3.2. Association between Exposure to Herbicides and RA Development

Four studies were eligible for inclusion in the quantitative synthesis [6,17,20,21]: one study was a cohort study, two were case-control studies, and one was a cross-sectional study. Three studies were conducted in the USA ($n = 3$), and one was conducted in Greece ($n = 1$). Of the four studies, only one study found an association between exposure to herbicides and RA, but three studies found no association. The study by Meyer et al. [6] found an association of increased risk of RA with exposure to chlorimuron ethyl (aOR = 1.45, 95% CI = 1.01–2.07) and EPTC (aOR = 0.62, 95% CI = 0.4–0.96). However, the study by De Roos et al. [17] found a negative association between RA and exposure to phenoxyacetic acids (aOR = 0.5, 95% CI = 0.3–0.9) and 2,4-D (aOR = 0.5, 95% CI = 0.3–0.9) (Table 2).

A total of 51,175 participants were included in the meta-analysis, and the results found that exposure to herbicides was not significantly associated with an increased risk of RA (aOR = 0.98, 95% CI = 0.89–1.08, p-value = 0.027 for heterogeneity $I^2 = 34.1\%$) (Figure 3).

3.3. Association between Exposure to Fungicides and RA Development

Four studies were eligible for inclusion in the quantitative synthesis [6,17,20,21]: one study was a cohort study, two were case-control studies, and one was a cross-sectional study. Three studies were conducted in the USA ($n = 3$), and one was conducted in Greece ($n = 1$). Of the four studies, only one study found an association between exposure to fungicides and RA, but three studies found no association. The study by Parks et al. [20] found an association of increased risk of RA with exposure to maneb/mancozeb (aOR = 2.0, 95% CI = 1.1–3.9) (Table 3).

Table 2. The association between exposure to herbicides and RA development.

Authors (Years)/Country	Study Design	Gender	Sample Size	Name of Chemicals	aOR (95% CI)	Confounding Variables
De Roos et al. (2005)/USA [17]	case-control	Female	810	Herbicides Phenoxyacetic acids Triazines 2,4-D Alachlor Atrazine Cyanazine Glyphosate Imazethapyr Metolachlor	1.1 (0.8–1.6) 0.5 (0.3–0.9) 0.5 (0.2–1.3) 0.5 (0.3–0.9) 0.5 (0.1–1.6) 0.5 (0.2–1.6) 0.8 (0.2–3.4) 1.2 (0.8–1.8) 1.5 (0.5–4.1) 0.4 (0.1–1.7)	Birth date and state
Parks et al. (2016)/USA [20]	Cohort	Female	23,841	2,4-D Atrazine Glyphosate Imazethapyr Trifluralin Dicamba	0.75 (0.51–1.1) 0.65 (0.32–1.3) 1.2 (0.95–1.6) 1.1 (0.55–2.3) 0.57 (0.28–1.1) 0.68 (0.32–1.5)	Age, state, and pack-years smoking
Meyer et al. (2017)/USA [6]	case-control	Male	26,354	2,4-D 2,4,5-T 2,4,5-TP Alachlor Atrazine Butylate Chlorimuron ethyl Cyanazine Dicamba EPTC Glyphosate Imazethapyr Metolachlor Metribuzin Paraquat Pendimethalin Trifluralin	1.16 (0.83–1.64) 1.11 (0.72–1.71) 1.00 (0.46–2.15) 1.26 (0.95–1.68) 1.29 (0.94–1.79) 1.04 (0.70–1.54) 1.45 (1.01–2.07) 0.96 (0.69–1.31) 0.90 (0.65–1.25) 0.62 (0.40–0.96) 0.90 (0.65–1.24) 1.32 (0.94–1.86) 0.90 (0.67–1.20) 1.08 (0.73–1.59) 0.92 (0.57–1.49) 0.98 (0.69–1.40) 1.23 (0.92–1.66)	Age, state of enrollment, pack-years smoking, and education level
Koureas et al. (2017)/Greece [21]	Cross-sectional	Male	170	Herbicides Paraquat	3.51 (0.45–27.20) 0.69 (0.09–5.03)	Age, smoker, alcohol consumption, and use of a tractor on a farm

aOR, adjusted odds ratio; 95% CI, 95% confidence interval; 2,4-D, 2,4-dichlorophenoxyacetic acid; 2,4,5-T, 2,4,5-trichlorophenoxyacetic acid; 2,4,5-TP, 2,4,5-trichlorophenoxy propionic acid; EPTC, S-ethyl-N, N-dipropylthiocarbamate.

A total of 51,175 participants were included in the analysis, and the results found that exposure to fungicides was not significantly associated with an increased risk of RA (aOR = 1.04, 95% CI = 0.86–1.27, p-value = 0.130 for heterogeneity I^2 = 33.5%) (Figure 4).

3.4. Association between Exposure to Non-Specific Pesticides and RA Development

Four studies were eligible for inclusion in the quantitative synthesis [20,22–24]: two studies were cohort studies, and two were case-control studies. Three studies were conducted in the USA (n = 3), and one was conducted in Sweden (n = 1).

Out of the four articles, two studies found an association between exposure to non-specific pesticides and RA, but two studies found no association. The study by Parks et al. [24] found an association with non-specific pesticides (aOR = 1.8, 95% CI = 1.1–2.9). Similarly, the study by Gold et al. [23] also found an association with non-specific pesticides (aOR = 1.14, 95% CI = 1.08–1.2) (Table 4).

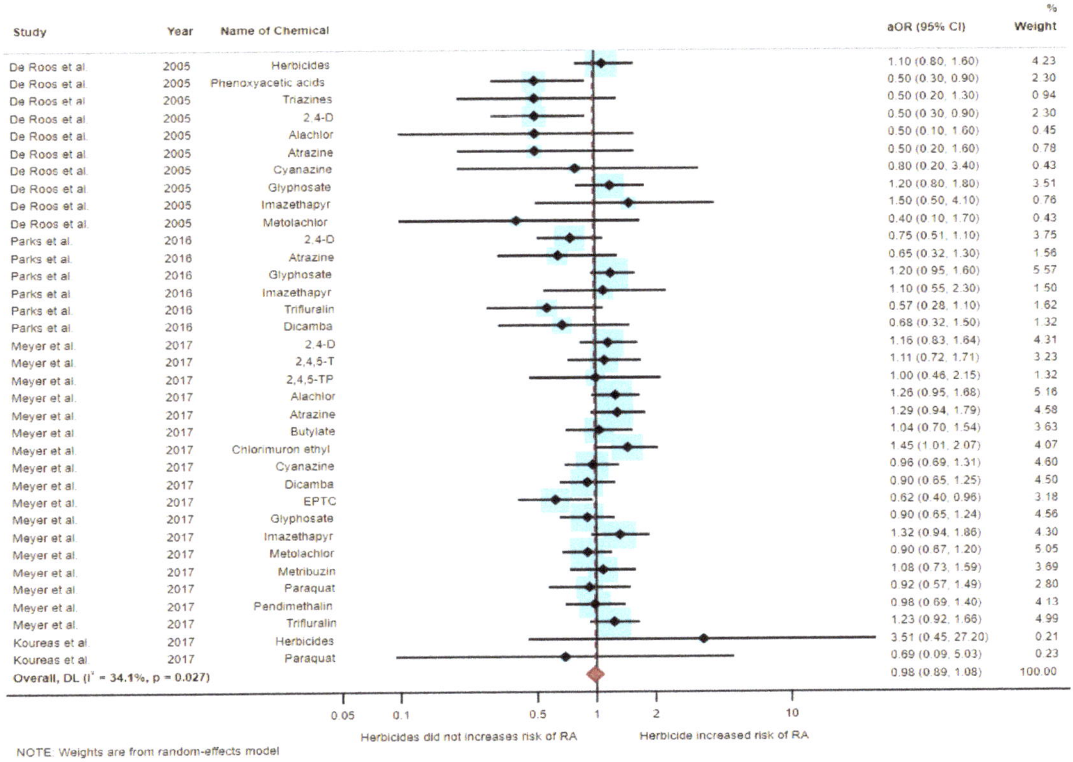
Study
Year
Name of Chemical
aOR (95% CI)
% Weight
De Roos et al. 2005 Herbicides 1.10 (0.80, 1.60) 4.23
De Roos et al. 2005 Phenoxyacetic acids 0.50 (0.30, 0.90) 2.30
De Roos et al. 2005 Triazines 0.50 (0.20, 1.30) 0.94
De Roos et al. 2005 2,4-D 0.50 (0.30, 0.90) 2.30
De Roos et al. 2005 Alachlor 0.50 (0.10, 1.60) 0.45
De Roos et al. 2005 Atrazine 0.50 (0.20, 1.60) 0.78
De Roos et al. 2005 Cyanazine 0.80 (0.20, 3.40) 0.43
De Roos et al. 2005 Glyphosate 1.20 (0.80, 1.80) 3.51
De Roos et al. 2005 Imazethapyr 1.50 (0.50, 4.10) 0.76
De Roos et al. 2005 Metolachlor 0.40 (0.10, 1.70) 0.43
Parks et al. 2016 2,4-D 0.75 (0.51, 1.10) 3.75
Parks et al. 2016 Atrazine 0.65 (0.32, 1.30) 1.56
Parks et al. 2016 Glyphosate 1.20 (0.95, 1.60) 5.57
Parks et al. 2016 Imazethapyr 1.10 (0.55, 2.30) 1.50
Parks et al. 2016 Trifluralin 0.57 (0.28, 1.10) 1.62
Parks et al. 2016 Dicamba 0.68 (0.32, 1.50) 1.32
Meyer et al. 2017 2,4-D 1.16 (0.83, 1.64) 4.31
Meyer et al. 2017 2,4,5-T 1.11 (0.72, 1.71) 3.23
Meyer et al. 2017 2,4,5-TP 1.00 (0.46, 2.15) 1.32
Meyer et al. 2017 Alachlor 1.26 (0.95, 1.68) 5.16
Meyer et al. 2017 Atrazine 1.29 (0.94, 1.79) 4.58
Meyer et al. 2017 Butylate 1.04 (0.70, 1.54) 3.63
Meyer et al. 2017 Chlorimuron ethyl 1.45 (1.01, 2.07) 4.07
Meyer et al. 2017 Cyanazine 0.96 (0.69, 1.31) 4.60
Meyer et al. 2017 Dicamba 0.90 (0.65, 1.25) 4.50
Meyer et al. 2017 EPTC 0.62 (0.40, 0.96) 3.18
Meyer et al. 2017 Glyphosate 0.90 (0.65, 1.24) 4.56
Meyer et al. 2017 Imazethapyr 1.32 (0.94, 1.86) 4.30
Meyer et al. 2017 Metolachlor 0.90 (0.67, 1.20) 5.05
Meyer et al. 2017 Metribuzin 1.08 (0.73, 1.59) 3.69
Meyer et al. 2017 Paraquat 0.92 (0.57, 1.49) 2.80
Meyer et al. 2017 Pendimethalin 0.98 (0.69, 1.40) 4.13
Meyer et al. 2017 Trifluralin 1.23 (0.92, 1.66) 4.99
Koureas et al. 2017 Herbicides 3.51 (0.45, 27.20) 0.21
Koureas et al. 2017 Paraquat 0.69 (0.09, 5.03) 0.23
Overall, DL (I² = 34.1%, p = 0.027) 0.98 (0.89, 1.08) 100.00
0.05
0.1
0.5
1
2
10
Herbicides did not increases risk of RA
Herbicide increased risk of RA
NOTE: Weights are from random-effects model

Figure 3. The association between exposure to herbicides and RA development [6,17,20,21]. aOR, adjusted odds ratio; 95% CI, 95% confidence interval.

Table 3. The association between exposure to fungicides and RA development.

Authors (Years)/Country	Study Design	Gender	Sample Size	Name of Chemicals	aOR (95% CI)	Confounding Variables
De Roos et al. (2005)/USA [17]	case-control	Female	810	Fungicides Maneb Thiocarbamates	0.5 (0.2–1.6) 0.8 (0.2–3.0) 0.4 (0.1–1.4)	Birth date and state
Parks et al. (2016)/USA [20]	Cohort	Female	23,841	Captan Maneb/Mancozeb	0.75 (0.31–1.8) 2.0 (1.1–3.9)	Age, state, and pack-years smoking
Meyer et al. (2017)/USA [6]	case-control	Male	26,354	Benomyl Captan Chlorothalonil Maneb Metalaxyl	0.64 (0.32–1.31) 0.90 (0.57–1.43) 1.27 (0.81–2.01) 0.97 (0.53–1.78) 1.20 (0.77–1.88)	Age, state of enrollment, pack-years smoking, and education level
Koureas et al. (2017)/Greece [21]	Cross-sectional	Male	170	Fungicides	5.85 (0.82–42.04)	Age, smoker, alcohol consumption, and use of a tractor on a farm

aOR, adjusted odds ratio; 95% CI, 95% confidence interval.

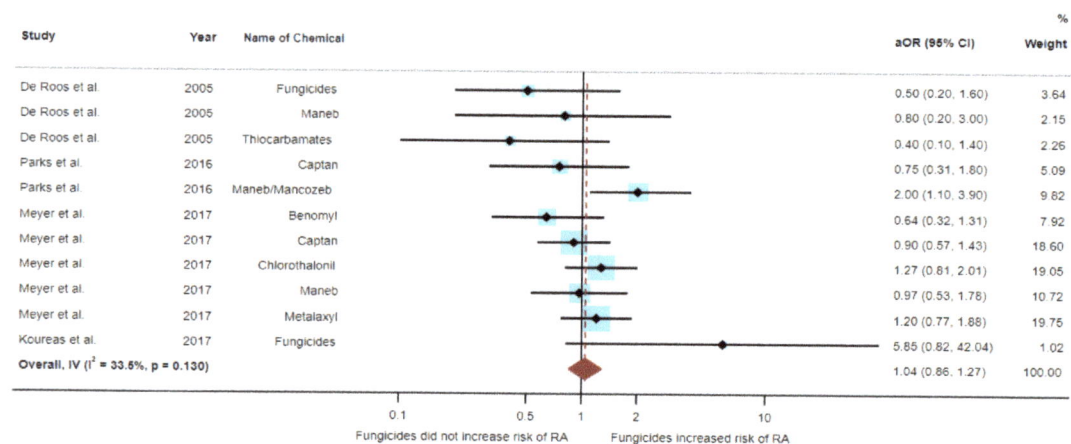

Figure 4. The association between exposure to fungicides and RA development [6,17,20,21]. aOR, adjusted odds ratio; 95% CI, 95% confidence interval.

Table 4. The association between exposure to non-specific pesticides and RA development.

Authors (Years)/ Country	Study Design	Gender	Sample Size	Adjusted OR (95% CI)	Confounding Variables
Parks et al. (2016)/USA [20]	Cohort	Female	23,841	1.3 (0.9–2.0)	Age, state, and pack-years smoking
Olsson et al. (2000)/Sweden [22]	case-control	Male	350	1.2 (0.4–4.1)	Age, smoking, and occupation
Gold et al. (2007)/USA [23]	case-control	Both genders	296,362	1.14 (1.08–1.20)	Age, sex, race, region, and socioeconomic status
Parks et al. (2017)/USA [24]	Cohort	Female	49,343	1.8 (1.1–2.9)	Age, race, education level, packyears of smoking, and childhood socioeconomic status

aOR, adjusted odds ratio; 95% CI, 95% confidence interval.

A total of 369,896 participants were included in the meta-analysis, and the results showed that exposure to non-specific pesticides was significantly associated with an increased risk of RA (aOR = 1.15, 95% CI = 1.09–1.21, p-value = 0.289 for heterogeneity I^2 = 20.1%) (Figure 5).

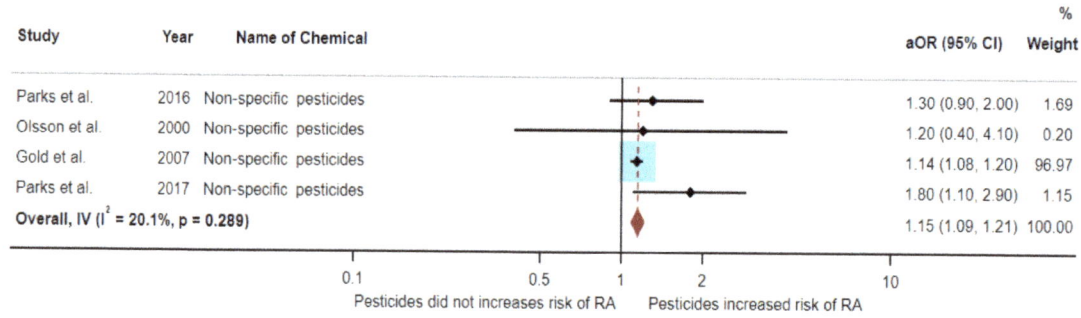

Figure 5. The association between exposure to non-specific pesticides and RA development [20,22–24]. aOR, adjusted odds ratio; 95% CI, 95% confidence interval.

3.5. Funnel Plots

Figure 6 presents the funnel plots of the subgroups of the studies, including insecticides, herbicides, fungicides, and non-specific pesticides. The results indicate that all funnel plots are asymmetrical, which may be a result of several factors, for example, the magnitude of the effect may vary with the study size and location bias.

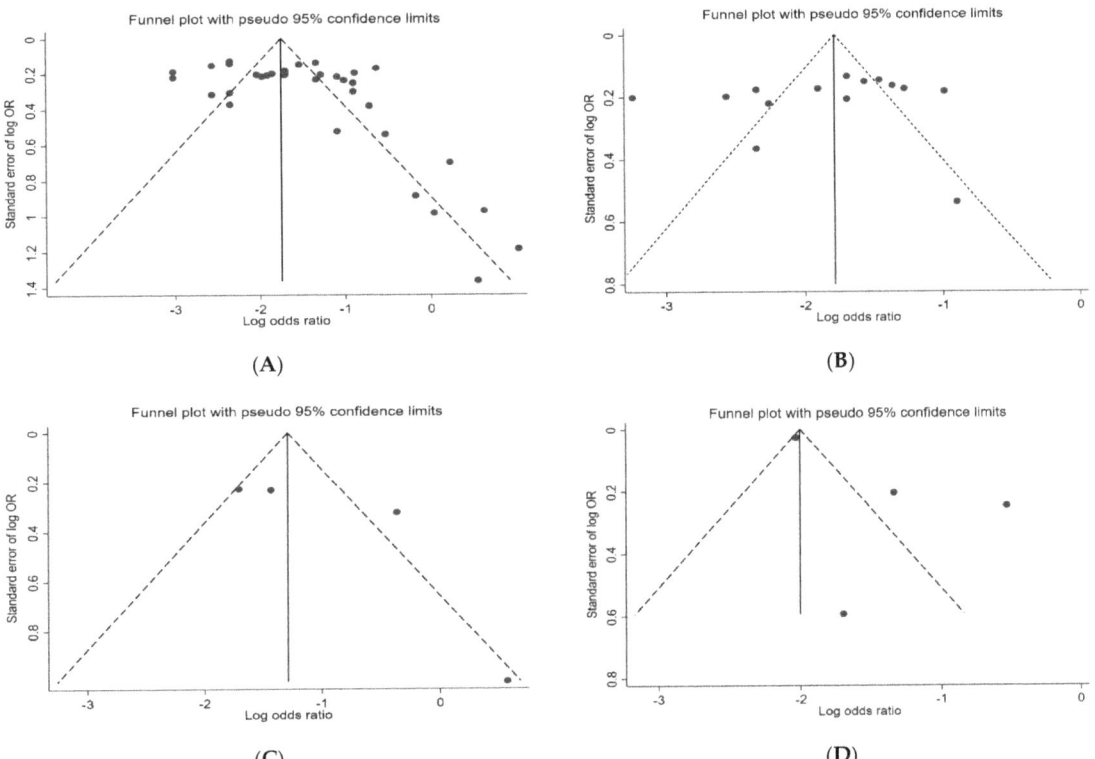

Figure 6. Funnel plots. (**A**) Insecticides; (**B**) herbicides; (**C**) fungicides; (**D**) non-specific pesticides.

4. Discussion

The studies currently available provided evidence that exposure to insecticides contributed to increased risk of RA (aOR = 1.20, 95% CI = 1.12–1.28). In addition, the specific insecticides that found a significant association were fonofos, cabaryl, and guanidines. Fonophos belongs to the organophosphate group, carbaryl is a carbamate, and guanidine a neonicotinoid. Importantly, the studies that found the association of exposure to insecticides with an increased risk of RA was found in insecticide applicators [6,21]. Therefore, this evidence provides considerable information that occupational exposure to insecticides is a possible risk factor for the development of RA.

RA is an illness of the immune system that causes joint inflammation [25]. Genetics and environmental factors are the two main divisions of risk factors for RA. Environmental risk factors are intriguing because they have the potential to affect a variety of physiological systems, including the immune system [26]. Pesticides have been found to be a major environmental risk factor. Several studies have revealed that pesticide exposure can harm the immune system and contribute to the onset of RA [6,20,21,23,26].

Direct immunotoxicity is the main mechanism associated with the impact of pesticide poisoning on the immune system [27]. Inhibition of acetylcholinesterase (AChE) by organophosphates and carbamates can result in inhibition of cholinergic signaling in lymphocytes. Exposure to high levels of insecticides can lead to accumulation of the neurotransmitter acetylcholine and overstimulation of cholinergic receptors. As a result, interleukin-2 (IL-2) is produced by T cells and B cells, resulting in stimulation of the inflammatory response in macrophages, which increases the risk of inflammatory disease [7,27,28]. However, exposure to low levels of insecticides for long periods may lead to a reduction in cholinergic receptors, which could lead to chronic disease or cancer [27].

T cells are lymphocytes that play an important role in immunity. Previously available studies have shown that insecticides had a negative effect on the viability and function of T cells by inducing apoptosis in different ways [29]. A previous study found that exposure to carbamates can induce apoptosis in human Jurkat T cells [29]. An investigation in an animal model also suggested that the intrinsic apoptotic pathway was stimulated due to the increase in the levels of caspase 3 and cytochrome C released from the mitochondria [30]. Carbamates also affect lymphocyte-specific kinases, resulting in an inhibitory effect on T cell and IL-2 production [29,31]. Several studies also suggested that chlorpyrifos and dimethyl 2,2-dichlorovinyl phosphate can inhibit cytotoxic T lymphocyte activity and decrease the T cell population [29,32,33]. With regard to B cells, pesticides can also inhibit B cell proliferation, leading to lower levels of B cells and reduced antibody production [29]. Some environmental chemicals can trigger an immunological response specific to antigens, which can cause polyclonal B cells to produce antibodies against themselves in some individuals, an autoimmune response [34]. Insecticides can also inhibit the development of M1 macrophages and increase M2 macrophage polarization, which leads to immunotoxicity in humans [27–29,35]. In addition, inhibition of the transcription levels of pro-inflammatory cytokines, which are related to oxidative stress, might be caused by insecticides. This results in increasing ROS and DNA damage, as well as the induction of apoptosis [36,37].

Although the studies currently available provided evidence that exposure to insecticides contributes to an increased risk of RA, there were some limitations in the study reviews. Firstly, some studies assessed the association between exposure to pesticides and RA by using cross-sectional studies; therefore, these studies were unable to describe the relationships between cause and effect. Secondly, most studies were conducted in the USA; therefore, the evidence cannot be directly generalized to other populations. Thirdly, the number of eligible studies was rather small; therefore, the interpretation of the evidence should be more careful. Fourthly, the eligible studies included for meta-analysis were both occupational and environmental exposure; therefore, the interpretation of the evidence should be concerned. Fifthly, most studies assessed the exposure to pesticides by using interviews or self-reporting procedures that may not quantitatively indicate the level of exposure and therefore may not be able to be directly correlated with the development of RA. Sixthly, exposure to multiple pesticides might result in the development of RA. Previous studies stated that co-exposure to pesticides affects toxicity in humans and may lead to chronic illness [38,39]. Therefore, further studies should be concerned on this point. Finally, there were several confounding factors contributing to RA. Therefore, in future studies, the confounding factors need to be considered, including age, race, genetics, income status, body mass index, resident area, occupation, education level, cigarette smoking and alcohol consumption, and exposure to other environmental chemicals.

5. Conclusions

There is some evidence to suggest that exposure to insecticides (especially fonofos, carbaryl, and guanidines) contributes to an increased risk of RA, while exposure to herbicides and fungicides has no impact on the development of RA. However, the evidence is limited because of a small number of studies. Therefore, further studies regarding the effect of pesticides on the development of RA need to be warranted. A continuous approach needs to be adopted to systematic review and meta-analysis of the evidence to ensure current updating of the knowledge pertinent to the effects of pesticides on RA development.

Supplementary Materials: The following supporting information can be downloaded at https://www.mdpi.com/article/10.3390/toxics10050207/s1, Table S1. Quality assessment of selected articles in accordance with the National Heart, Lung, and Blood Institute (NHLBI) Guidelines for reporting observational cohort and cross-sectional studies; Table S2. Quality assessment of selected articles in accordance with the National Heart, Lung, and Blood Institute (NHLBI) Guidelines for reporting case-control studies.

Author Contributions: Conceptualization, R.S., J.C. and W.S.; methodology, R.S., J.C. and W.S.; software, W.S.; validation, R.S., J.C. and W.S..; formal analysis, R.S., J.C. and W.S.; investigation, R.S., J.C. and W.S.; resources, R.S., J.C. and W.S.; data curation, R.S.; writing—original draft preparation, J.C. and R.S.; writing—review and editing, R.S.; visualization, R.S.; supervision, R.S.; project administration, R.S. All authors have read and agreed to the published version of the manuscript.

Funding: This research received no external funding.

Institutional Review Board Statement: The study was conducted in accordance with the Declaration of Helsinki and approved by the Research Ethics Committee, Faculty of Medicine, Chiang Mi University, Thailand (protocol code: EXEMPTION8712/2564, 17 December 2021).

Informed Consent Statement: Not applicable.

Data Availability Statement: Not applicable.

Acknowledgments: We thank the Research Administration Section, Faculty of Medicine, Chiang Mai University, for providing support.

Conflicts of Interest: The authors declare no conflict of interest.

References

1. Almutairi, K.; Nossent, J.; Preen, D.; Keen, H.; Inderjeeth, C. The global prevalence of rheumatoid arthritis: A meta-analysis based on a systematic review. *Rheumatol. Int.* **2021**, *41*, 863–877. [CrossRef]
2. Choy, E. Understanding the dynamics: Pathways involved in the pathogenesis of rheumatoid arthritis. *Rheumatology* **2012**, *51*, 3–11. [CrossRef] [PubMed]
3. Derksen, V.F.A.M.; Huizinga, T.W.J.; van der Woude, D. The role of autoantibodies in the pathophysiology of rheumatoid arthritis. *Semin. Immunopathol.* **2017**, *39*, 437–446. [CrossRef] [PubMed]
4. Tanaka, Y. Rheumatoid arthritis. *Inflamm. Regen.* **2020**, *40*, 20. [CrossRef] [PubMed]
5. George, G.; Shyni, G.L.; Raghu, K.G. Current and novel therapeutic targets in the treatment of rheumatoid arthritis. *Inflammopharmacology* **2020**, *28*, 1457–1476. [CrossRef]
6. Meyer, A.; Sandler, D.P.; Freeman, L.E.B.; Hofmann, J.N.; Parks, C.G. Pesticide exposure and risk of rheumatoid arthritis among licensed male pesticide applicators in the Agricultural Health Study. *Environ. Health Perspect.* **2017**, *125*, 077010. [CrossRef] [PubMed]
7. Corsini, E.; Sokooti, M.; Galli, C.L.; Moretto, A.; Colosio, C. Pesticide induced immunotoxicity in humans: A comprehensive review of the existing evidence. *Toxicology* **2013**, *307*, 123–135. [CrossRef]
8. Klak, A.; Raciborski, F.; Samel-Kowalik, P. Social implications of rheumatic diseases. *Reumatologia* **2016**, *54*, 73–78. [CrossRef]
9. Hsieh, P.; Wu, O.; Geue, C.; McIntosh, E.; McInnes, I.B.; Siebert, S. Economic burden of rheumatoid arthritis: A systematic review of literature in biologic era. *Ann. Rheum. Dis.* **2020**, *79*, 771–777. [CrossRef]
10. Boedeker, W.; Watts, M.; Clausing, P.; Marquez, E. The global distribution of acute unintentional pesticide poisoning: Estimations based on a systematic review. *BMC Public Health* **2020**, *20*, 1875. [CrossRef]
11. Akashe, M.M.; Pawade, U.C.; Nikam, A.V. Classification of pesticides: A review. *Int. J. Res. Ayurveda Pharm.* **2018**, *9*, 144–150. [CrossRef]
12. Damalas, C.A.; Koutroubas, S.D. Farmers' exposure to pesticides: Toxicity types and ways of prevention. *Toxics* **2016**, *4*, 1. [CrossRef] [PubMed]
13. Damalas, C.A.; Eleftherohorinos, I.G. Pesticide exposure, safety issues, and risk assessment indicators. *Int. J. Environ. Res. Public Health* **2011**, *8*, 1402–1419. [CrossRef]
14. Gangemi, S.; Miozzi, E.; Teodoro, M.; Briguglio, G.; De Luca, A.; Alibrando, C.; Polito, I.; Libra, M. Occupational exposure to pesticides as a possible risk factor for the development of chronic diseases in humans (Review). *Mol. Med. Rep.* **2016**, *14*, 4475–4488. [CrossRef] [PubMed]
15. Blair, A.; Ritz, B.; Wesseling, C.; Freeman, L.B. Pesticides and human health. *Occup. Environ. Med.* **2015**, *72*, 81–82. [CrossRef] [PubMed]
16. Chittrakul, J.; Sapbamrer, R.; Sirikul, W. Insecticide exposure and risk of asthmatic symptoms: A systematic review and meta-Analysis. *Toxics* **2021**, *9*, 228. [CrossRef]

17. De Roos, A.J.; Cooper, G.S.; Alavanja, M.C.; Sandler, D.P. Rheumatoid arthritis among women in the Agricultural Health Study: Risk associated with farming activities and exposures. *Ann. Epidemiol.* **2005**, *15*, 762–770. [CrossRef]
18. Lee, D.H.; Steffes, M.; Jacobs, D.R. Positive associations of serum concentration of polychlorinated biphenyls or organochlorine pesticides with self-reported arthritis, especially rheumatoid type, in women. *Environ. Health Perspect.* **2007**, *115*, 883–888. [CrossRef]
19. Guidelines for Reporting Observational Cohort and Cross-Sectional Studies. Available online: https://www.nhlbi.nih.gov/health-topics/study-quality-assessment-tools (accessed on 25 December 2021).
20. Parks, C.G.; Hoppin, J.A.; De Roos, A.J.; Costenbader, K.H.; Alavanja, M.C.; Sandler, D.P. Rheumatoid arthritis in Agricultural Health Study spouses: Associations with pesticides and other farm exposures. *Environ. Health Perspect.* **2016**, *124*, 1728–1734. [CrossRef]
21. Koureas, M.; Rachiotis, G.; Tsakalof, A.; Hadjichristodoulou, C. Increased frequency of rheumatoid arthritis and allergic rhinitis among pesticide sprayers and associations with pesticide use. *Int. J. Environ. Res. Public Health* **2017**, *14*, 865. [CrossRef]
22. Olsson, A.R.; Skogh, T.; Wingren, G. Occupational determinants for rheumatoid arthritis. *Scand. J. Work. Environ. Health* **2000**, *26*, 243–249. [CrossRef] [PubMed]
23. Gold, L.S.; Ward, M.H.; Dosemeci, M.; De Roos, A.J. Systemic autoimmune disease mortality and occupational exposures. *Arthritis Rheum.* **2007**, *56*, 3189–3201. [CrossRef] [PubMed]
24. Parks, C.G.; Aloisio, A.A.; Sandler, D.P. Childhood residential and agricultural pesticide exposures in relation to adult-onset rheumatoid arthritis in women. *Am. J. Epidemiol.* **2017**, *187*, 214–223. [CrossRef] [PubMed]
25. Guo, Q.; Wang, Y.; Xu, D.; Nossent, J.; Pavlos, N.J.; Xu, J. Rheumatoid arthritis: Pathological mechanisms and modern pharmacologic therapies. *Bone Res.* **2018**, *6*, 15. [CrossRef]
26. Domina, P. Review of toxins associated with autoimmune diseases. *ScienceOpen* **2021**, 1–7. [CrossRef]
27. Mokarizadeh, A.; Faryabi, M.R.; Rezvanfar, M.A.; Abdollahi, M. A comprehensive review of pesticides and the immune dysregulation: Mechanisms, evidence and consequences. *Toxicol. Mech. Methods* **2015**, *25*, 258–278. [CrossRef]
28. Dhouib, I.; Jallouli, M.; Annabi, A.; Marzouki, S.; Gharbi, N.; Elfazaa, S.; Lasram, M.M. From immunotoxicity to carcinogenicity: The effects of carbamate pesticides on the immune system. *Environ. Sci. Pollut. Res. Int.* **2016**, *23*, 9448–9458. [CrossRef]
29. Lee, G.H.; Choi, K.C. Adverse effects of pesticides on the functions of immune system. *Comp. Biochem. Physiol. C Toxicol. Pharmacol.* **2020**, *235*, 108789. [CrossRef]
30. Goldstein, J.C.; Waterhouse, N.J.; Juin, P.; Evan, G.I.; Green, D.R. The coordinate release of cytochrome c during apoptosis is rapid, complete and kinetically invariant. *Nat. Cell Biol.* **2000**, *2*, 156–2162. [CrossRef]
31. Martin, M.W.; Newcomb, J.; Nunes, J.J.; McGowan, D.C.; Armistead, D.M.; Boucher, C.; Buchanan, J.L.; Buckner, W.; Chai, L.; Elbaum, D.; et al. Novel 2-aminopyrimidine carbamates as potent and orally active inhibitors of Lck: Synthesis, SAR, and in vivo anti-inflammatory activity. *J. Med. Chem.* **2006**, *49*, 4981–4991. [CrossRef]
32. Li, Q.; Hirata, Y.; Piao, S.; Minami, M. The by-products generated during sarin synthesis in the Tokyo sarin disaster induced inhibition of natural killer and cytotoxic T lymphocyte activity. *Toxicology* **2000**, *146*, 209–220. [CrossRef]
33. Li, Q.; Nakadai, A.; Takeda, K.; Kawada, T. Dimethyl 2,2-dichlorovinyl phosphate (DDVP) markedly inhibits activities of natural killer cells, cytotoxic T lymphocytes and lymphokine-activated killer cells via the Fas-ligand/Fas pathway in perforin-knockout (PKO) mice. *Toxicology* **2004**, *204*, 41–50. [CrossRef] [PubMed]
34. Hess, E.V. Environmental chemicals and autoimmune disease: Cause and effect. *Toxicology* **2002**, *181*, 65–70. [CrossRef]
35. Khan, M.F.; Wang, H. Environmental exposures and autoimmune diseases: Contribution of gut microbiome. *Front. Immunol.* **2020**, *10*, 3094. [CrossRef]
36. Salem, I.B.; Boussabbeh, M.; Bacha, H. Dichlorvos-induced toxicity in HCT116 cells: Involvement of oxidative stress and apoptosis. *Pestic. Biochem. Physiol.* **2015**, *119*, 62–66. [CrossRef]
37. Sule, R.O.; Condon, L.; Gomes, A.V. A Common feature of pesticides: Oxidative stress-the role of oxidative stress in pesticide-induced toxicity. *Oxid. Med. Cell. Longev.* **2022**, *2022*, 5563759. [CrossRef] [PubMed]
38. Bossou, Y.M.; Cote, J.; Mantha, M.; Haddad, S.; Achard, S.; Bouchard, M. Impact of pesticide coexposure: An experimental study with binary mixtures of lambda-cyhalothrin (LCT) and captan and its impact on the toxicokinetics of LCT biomarkers of exposure. *Arch. Toxicol.* **2020**, *94*, 3045–3058. [CrossRef] [PubMed]
39. Timchalk, C.; Poet, T.S.; Hinman, M.N.; Busby, A.L.; Kousba, A.A. Pharmacokinetic and pharmacodynamic interaction for a binary mixture of chlorpyrifos and diazinon in the rat. *Toxicol. Appl. Pharmacol.* **2005**, *205*, 31–42. [CrossRef]

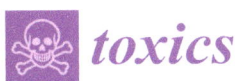

Article

The NOAEL Equivalent of Environmental Cadmium Exposure Associated with GFR Reduction and Chronic Kidney Disease

Soisungwan Satarug [1,*], Aleksandra Buha Đorđević [2], Supabhorn Yimthiang [3], David A. Vesey [1,4] and Glenda C. Gobe [1,5,6]

1. Kidney Disease Research Collaborative, Translational Research Institute, Brisbane 4102, Australia
2. Department of Toxicology "Akademik Danilo Soldatović", University of Belgrade-Faculty of Pharmacy, 11000 Belgrade, Serbia
3. Occupational Health and Safety, School of Public Health, Walailak University, Nakhon Si Thammarat 80160, Thailand
4. Department of Nephrology, Princess Alexandra Hospital, Brisbane 4102, Australia
5. School of Biomedical Sciences, The University of Queensland, Brisbane 4072, Australia
6. NHMRC Centre of Research Excellence for CKD QLD, UQ Health Sciences, Royal Brisbane and Women's Hospital, Brisbane 4029, Australia
* Correspondence: sj.satarug@yahoo.com.au

Abstract: Cadmium (Cd) is a highly toxic metal pollutant present in virtually all food types. Health guidance values were established to safeguard against excessive dietary Cd exposure. The derivation of such health guidance figures has been shifted from the no-observed-adverse-effect level (NOAEL) to the lower 95% confidence bound of the benchmark dose (BMD), termed BMDL. Here, we used the PROAST software to calculate the BMDL figures for Cd excretion (E_{Cd}) associated with a reduction in the estimated glomerular filtration rate (eGFR), and an increased prevalence of chronic kidney disease (CKD), defined as eGFR $\leq$ 60 mL/min/1.73 m^2. Data were from 1189 Thai subjects (493 males and 696 females) mean age of 43.2 years. The overall percentages of smokers, hypertension and CKD were 33.6%, 29.4% and 6.2%, respectively. The overall mean E_{Cd} normalized to the excretion of creatinine (E_{cr}) as E_{Cd}/E_{cr} was 0.64 µg/g creatinine. E_{Cd}/E_{cr}, age and body mass index (BMI) were independently associated with increased prevalence odds ratios (POR) for CKD. BMI figures $\geq$24 kg/m^2 were associated with an increase in POR for CKD by 2.81-fold ($p = 0.028$). E_{Cd}/E_{cr} values of 0.38–2.49 µg/g creatinine were associated with an increase in POR for CKD risk by 6.2-fold ($p = 0.001$). The NOAEL equivalent figures of E_{Cd}/E_{cr} based on eGFR reduction in males, females and all subjects were 0.839, 0.849 and 0.828 µg/g creatinine, respectively. The BMDL/BMDU values of E_{Cd}/E_{cr} associated with a 10% increase in CKD prevalence were 2.77/5.06 µg/g creatinine. These data indicate that Cd-induced eGFR reduction occurs at relatively low body burdens and that the population health risk associated with E_{Cd}/E_{cr} of 2.77–5.06 µg/g creatinine was not negligible.

Keywords: benchmark dose; BMDL; BMDU; cadmium; creatinine clearance; chronic kidney disease; eGFR; NOAEL; urine cadmium

1. Introduction

Environmental exposure to cadmium (Cd) is inevitable for most people because the metal is present in almost all food types [1–3]. The realization in the 1940s that the condition referred to as "itai-itai" disease was due to the consumption of rice heavily contaminated with Cd brought into focus the real threat to health posed by this metal [4,5]. Itai-itai disease is the most severe form of human Cd poisoning, characterized by severe damage to the kidneys and bones, resulting in multiple bone fractures due to osteoporosis and osteomalacia [4,5]. The pathologic symptoms of the itai-itai disease have been replicated in Cd-treated cynomolgus monkeys [6].

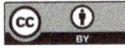

To safeguard against excessive dietary Cd exposure, health guidance such as a tolerable intake level of Cd was established [7]. The Joint FAO/WHO Expert Committee on Food Additives and Contaminants (JECFA) considered the kidney to be the critical target of Cd toxicity [8]. By definition, the provisional tolerable weekly intake (PTWI) for a chemical with no known biological function is an estimate of the amount that can be ingested weekly over a lifetime without appreciable health risk. Subsequently, the PTWI for Cd was amended to a tolerable monthly intake (TMI) of 25 µg per kg body weight per month, equivalent to 0.83 µg per kg body weight per day [8]. This tolerable intake level for Cd was derived from a risk assessment model that assumed an increase in excretion of β_2-microglobulin (β_2M) ($E_{\beta 2M}$) above 300 µg/g creatinine as the point of departure (POD) [8]. However, we have shown that such an increase in $E_{\beta 2M}$ reflected tubular dysfunction and nephron loss, evident from a reduction in estimated glomerular filtration rate (eGFR) to 60 mL/min/1.73 m^2 or below [9,10]. In effect, a tolerable intake level of Cd derived from the $E_{\beta 2M}$-based POD is not sufficiently low to be without an impact on human health.

Current evidence suggests that sufficient tubular injury disables glomerular filtration and leads to nephron atrophy and a decrease in GFR [11–13]. Accordingly, we argue that a reduction in eGFR due to Cd nephropathy could serve as the POD from which health guidance values should be derived. Owing to some shortcomings of the no-observed-adverse-effect level (NOAEL), the benchmark dose (BMD) has been used as the POD [7,14–16]. The BMD is a dose level, derived from an estimated dose–response curve, associated with a specified change in response, termed benchmark response (BMR) which can be set at 1%, 5%, or 10% as required [14–16].

The present study had two major aims. The first aim was to characterize a reduction in eGFR and risk factors of chronic kidney disease (CKD) in a sufficiently large group of people with a wide range of environmental Cd exposure. The risk factors considered included age, body mass index (BMI), smoking, hypertension, and Cd exposure measured as excretion of Cd (E_{Cd}). The second aim was to compute the lower 95% confidence bound of BMD (BMDL) and the BMD upper confidence limit (BMDU) of E_{Cd} associated with eGFR reduction and an increase in the prevalence of CKD.

2. Materials and Methods

2.1. Participants

To represent a large group of subjects with a wide range of environmental Cd exposure levels suitable for the dose–response analysis and health risk calculation, we assembled archived data from 1189 persons who participated in large population-based studies undertaken in a Cd contamination area in the Mae Sot District, Tak Province ($n = 537$), and low exposure locations in Bangkok and Nakhon–Si–Thammarat Province ($n = 652$). The Institutional Ethical Committees of Chulalongkorn University, Chiang Mai University and the Mae Sot Hospital approved the study protocol for the Mae Sot and Bangkok groups. The Office of the Human Research Ethics Committee of Walailak University in Thailand approved the study protocol for the Nakhon Si Thammarat group [17,18].

All participants gave informed consent prior to participation. They had lived at their current addresses for at least 30 years. Exclusion criteria were pregnancy, breastfeeding, a history of metalwork, and a hospital record or physician's diagnosis of advanced chronic disease. Because occupational exposure was an exclusion criterion, we presumed that all participants had acquired Cd from the environment. Diabetes was defined as fasting plasma glucose levels $\geq$ 126 mg/dL or a physician's prescription of anti-diabetic medications. Hypertension was defined as systolic blood pressure $\geq$ 140 mmHg, diastolic blood pressure $\geq$ 90 mmHg, a physician's diagnosis, or prescription of anti-hypertensive medications.

2.2. Collection and Analysis of Biological Specimens

Simultaneous blood and urine sampling are required to normalize E_{Cd}, to C_{cr}. Accordingly, second-morning urine samples were collected after an overnight fast, and whole blood samples were obtained within 3 hours after the urine sampling. Aliquots of urine, whole blood and plasma were stored at −20 °C or −80 °C for later analysis. The assay for urine and plasma concentrations of creatinine ($[cr]_u$ and $[cr]_p$) was based on the Jaffe reaction.

For the Bangkok group, urine concentration of Cd ($[Cd]_u$) was determined by inductively-coupled plasma mass spectrometry (ICP/MS, Agilent 7500, Agilent Technologies, Santa Clara, CA, USA). Multi-element standards (EM Science, EM Industries, Inc., Newark, NJ, USA) were used to calibrate the Cd analyses. Quality assurance and control were conducted with simultaneous analyses of samples of the reference urine Lyphochek® (Bio-Rad, Gladesville, New South Wales, Australia), which contained low- and high-range Cd levels. A coefficient of variation value of 2.5% was obtained for Cd in the reference urine. The low limit of detection (LOD) of urine Cd was 0.05 µg/L. The urine samples containing Cd below the LOD were assigned as the LOD divided by the square root of 2 [19].

For the Nakhon–Si–Thammarat group, $[Cd]_u$ was determined with the GBC System 5000 Graphite Furnace Atomic Absorption Spectrophotometer (AAS) (GBC Scientific Equipment, Hampshire, IL, USA). Instrumental metal analysis was calibrated with multi-element standards (Merck KGaA, Darmstadt, Germany). Reference urine metal control levels 1, 2, and 3 (Lyphocheck, Bio-Rad, Hercules, CA, USA) were used for quality control, analytical accuracy, and precision assurance. The analytical accuracy of metal detection was checked by an external quality assessment every 3 years. The LOD of urine Cd was 0.1 µg/L. When $[Cd]_u$ was below its detection limit, the Cd concentration assigned was the detection limit divided by the square root of 2 [19].

For the Mae Sot group, $[Cd]_u$ was determined with AAS (Shimadzu Model AA-6300, Kyoto, Japan). Urine standard reference material No. 2670 (National Institute of Standards, Washington, DC, USA) was used for quality assurance and control purposes. The LOD of Cd quantitation, defined as 3 times the standard deviation of blank measurements was 0.06 µg/L. None of the urine samples from this group contained $[Cd]_u$ below the detection limit.

2.3. Estimated Glomerular Filtration Rates (eGFR)

The GFR is the product of nephron number and mean single nephron GFR, and in theory, the GFR is indicative of nephron function [20–22]. In practice, the GFR is estimated from established chronic kidney disease-epidemiology collaboration (CKD-EPI) equations and is reported as eGFR [21].

Male eGFR = 141 × [plasma creatinine/0.9]^Y × 0.993^{age}, where Y = −0.411 if $[cr]_p \leq$ 0.9 mg/dL, Y = −1.209 if $[cr]_p >$ 0.9 mg/dL. Female eGFR = 144 × [plasma creatinine/0.7]^Y × 0.993^{age}, where Y = −0.329 if $[cr]_p \leq$ 0.7 mg/dL, Y = −1.209 if $[cr]_p >$ 0.7 mg/dL. For dichotomous comparisons, CKD was defined as eGFR $\leq$ 60 mL/min/1.73 m². CKD stages 1, 2, 3a, 3b, 4, and 5 corresponded to eGFR of 90–119, 60–89, 45–59, 30–44, 15–29, and <15 mL/min/1.73 m², respectively.

2.4. Normalization of E_{Cd} to E_{cr} and C_{cr}

E_x was normalized to E_{cr} as $[x]_u/[cr]_u$, where x = Cd; $[x]_u$ = urine concentration of x (mass/volume); and $[cr]_u$ = urine creatinine concentration (mg/dL). The ratio $[x]_u/[cr]_u$ was expressed in µg/g of creatinine.

E_x was normalized to C_{cr} as $E_x/C_{cr} = [x]_u[cr]_p/[cr]_u$, where x = Cd; $[x]_u$ = urine concentration of x (mass/volume); $[cr]_p$ = plasma creatinine concentration (mg/dL); and $[cr]_u$ = urine creatinine concentration (mg/dL). E_x/C_{cr} was expressed as the excretion of x per volume of filtrate [23].

2.5. Benchmark Dose Computation and Benchmark Dose–Response (BMR) Setting

We used the web-based PROAST software version 70.1 (https://proastweb.rivm.nl accessed on 13 October 2022) to compute the BMD figures for E_{Cd}/E_{cr} and E_{Cd}/C_{cr} associated with glomerular dysfunction. A specific effect size termed the benchmark response (BMR) was set at 5% for a continuous eGFR reduction endpoint and at 10%

for a quantal endpoint where eGFR $\leq$ 60 mL/min/1.73 m^2. For a continuous endpoint, BMD values were computed from fitting datasets to four dose–response models, including inverse exponential, natural logarithmic, exponential, and Hill models. For a quantal endpoint, BMD values were calculated from fitting datasets to seven dose–response models that included two-stage, logarithmic logistic, Weibull, logarithmic probability, gamma, exponential and Hill models. The BMD 95% confidence intervals of E_{Cd}/E_{cr} and E_{Cd}/C_{cr} were from model averaging using bootstrap with 200 repeats.

The BMDL and BMDU corresponded to the lower bound and upper bound of the 95% confidence interval (CI) of BMD. The wider the BMDL-BMDU difference, the higher the statistical uncertainty in the dataset [23–26]. BMDL/BMDU figures of E_{Cd} for the glomerular endpoint were calculated for males, females and all subjects.

2.6. Statistical Analysis

Data were analyzed with IBM SPSS Statistics 21 (IBM Inc., New York, NY, USA). The one-sample Kolmogorov–Smirnov test was used to identify departures of continuous variables from a normal distribution, and a logarithmic transformation was applied to variables that showed rightward skewing before they were subjected to parametric statistical analysis. The Mann–Whitney U-test was used to compare mean differences between the two groups. The Chi-square test was used to determine differences in percentage and prevalence data. The multivariable logistic regression analysis was used to determine the Prevalence Odds Ratio (POR) for CKD in relation to six independent variables; age, BMI, gender, smoking, hypertension and Cd exposure measures as E_{Cd}. We employed two models in each logistic regression analysis: model 1 incorporated $\log_2(E_{Cd}/Ecr)$ or three E_{Cd}/E_{cr} groups; model 2 incorporated $\log_2(E_{Cd}/C_{cr})$ or three E_{Cd}/C_{cr} groups. All other independent variables in models 1 and 2 were identical. For all tests, p-values $\leq$ 0.05 for two-tailed tests were assumed to indicate statistical significance.

3. Results

3.1. Characterization of Cadmium Exposure by Sex and Smoking

Table 1 provides demographic data of participants (493 males and 696 females) stratified by sex and smoking status.

The overall mean age of participants was 43.2 years, and the overall percentages of current smokers plus those who had stopped smoking for less than 10 years, hypertension and low eGFR were 33.6%, 29.4% and 6.2%, respectively. The overall mean [Cd]$_u$ and mean E_{Cd}/E_{cr} were 0.94 µg/L and 0.64 µg/g creatinine, while the overall mean $E_{Cd}/C_{cr} \times 100$ was 1.02 µg/L filtrate.

Smoking was higher among males (57.4%) than females (16.4%). In both sexes, % of smokers and non-smokers with hypertension did not differ. However, % of low eGFR among smokers was 3.7- and 3.8-fold higher than non-smokers in female and male groups, respectively. For the female group only, the mean BMI was 6 % lower in smokers than non-smokers (p = 0.004).

For the male group, the mean [Cd]$_u$ in smokers was 5.4-fold higher than nonsmokers (1.73 vs. 0.32 µg/L, p < 0.001). Mean E_{Cd}/E_{cr} and mean E_{Cd}/C_{cr} in smokers were 2.9- and 4.1-fold higher than in nonsmokers, respectively.

For the female group, the mean [Cd]$_u$ in smokers was 6.4-fold higher than nonsmokers (4.84 vs. 0.75 µg/L, p < 0.001). Mean E_{Cd}/E_{cr} and mean E_{Cd}/C_{cr} in smokers were 3.2-and 6-fold higher than in nonsmokers, respectively.

Table 1. Characteristics of participants stratified by sex and smoking status.

Parameters	All subjects n 1189 (33.6% Smokers)	Males, n 493 (57.4% Smokers)		Females, n 696 (16.8% Smokers)	
		Nonsmokers n 210	Smokers n 283	Nonsmokers n 579	Smokers n 117
Age, years	43.2 ± 14.0	35.9 ± 13.0	45.0 ± 14.8 ***	42.6 ± 12.9	54.2 ± 10.1 ###
Hypertension (%)	29.4	26.5	27.2	30.8	33.3
BMI, kg/m²	23.0 ± 3.9	22.4 ± 3.0	22.3 ± 3.4	23.8 ± 4.0	22.4 ± 4.6 #
BMI groups (%)					
12–18	10.5	9.2	12.2 *	7.4	21.4
19–23	47.1	56.9	57.2 **	41.6	36.8 ###
≥24	42.4	34.0	30.6	51.0	41.9 ###
eGFR [a], mL/min/1.73 m²	93.7 ± 20	96.6 ± 17.6	91.9 ± 22.1	95.9 ± 19.3	81.8 ± 22.0 ###
eGFR ≤ 60 mL/min/1.73 m² (%)	6.2	2.4	8.8 **	4.3	16.2 ###
eGFR, mL/min/1.73 m² (%) [b]					
>120	7.8	9.0	5.7	9.7	1.7 ###
90–120	53.8	61.0	56.5	54.1	33.3 ###
60–89	32.8	27.6	29.7 *	32.8	49.6 ###
30–59	5.0	1.9	7.1 **	3.3	13.7
15–29	0.6	0.5	1.1	0.2	1.7
Plasma creatinine, mg/dL	0.88 ± 0.24	1.00 ± 0.21	1.00 ± 0.27	0.76 ± 0.16	0.82 ± 0.27 ##
Urine creatinine, mg/dL	104.4 ± 73.5	81.1 ± 78	107.0 ± 75.6 ***	67.9 ± 68.9	79.8 ± 64.8
Urine Cd, µg/L	0.94 ± 9.69	0.32 ± 5.96	1.73 ± 15.9 ***	0.75 ± 6.46	4.84 ± 6.38 ###
Normalized to E_{cr} as E_x/E_{cr} [c] E_{Cd}/E_{cr}, µg/g creatinine	0.64 ± 6.12	0.32 ± 3.29	0.94 ± 8.85 ***	0.57 ± 4.62	1.83 ± 7.27 ###
Normalized to C_{cr} as E_x/C_{cr} [d] E_{Cd}/C_{cr} × 100, µg/L filtrate	1.02 ± 8.19	0.39 ± 4.75	1.61 ± 12.61 ***	0.83 ± 5.27	5.00 ± 9.36 ###

n, number of subjects; BMI, body mass index; eGFR, estimated glomerular filtration rate; E_x, excretion of x; cr, creatinine; C_{cr}, clearance of creatinine. [a] eGFR determined with Chronic Kidney Disease Epidemiology Collaboration (CKD–EPI) equations [20]; [b] eGFR of 90–119, 60–89, 45–59, 30–44, 15–29, and <15 mL/min/1.73 m² corresponded to CKD stages 1, 2, 3a, 3b, 4, and 5, respectively. [c] $E_x/E_{cr} = [x]_u/[cr]_u$; [d] $E_x/C_{cr} = [x]_u[cr]_p/[cr]_u$, where x = Cd [23]. Data for age, eGFR and BMI are arithmetic means ± standard deviation (SD). Data for all other continuous variables are geometric means ± SD. Data for BMI are from 951 subjects; data for hypertension are from 917 subjects; data for all other variables are from 1189 subjects. For each test, $p ≤ 0.05$ identifies statistical significance, determined by Chi-Square test and Mann–Whitney U test for % differences and mean differences, respectively. Compared with non-smoking males * $p = 0.029$–0.042, ** $p = 0.001$–0.006, *** $p ≤ 0.001$. Compared with non-smoking females, # $p = 0.004$, ## $p = 0.001$, ### $p ≤ 0.001$.

3.2. Characterization of CKD Risk factors

Table 2 provides the results of a logistic regression analysis where E_{Cd}/E_{cr} and E_{Cd}/C_{cr} were continuous variables, while age and BMI were categorical variables.

An independent effect on the POR for CKD was observed for E_{Cd}/E_{cr}, BMI and age (Table 2). Sex, smoking and hypertension were not associated with the POR for CKD. Doubling of E_{Cd}/E_{cr} was associated with an increase in POR for CKD by 1.47-fold ($p < 0.001$). BMI figures ≥ 24 kg/m² were associated with 2.81-fold increase in POR for CKD ($p = 0.028$). Compared with those aged 16–45 years, the POR values for CKD were 14-, 28- and 141-fold higher in those aged 46–55, 56–65, and 66–87 years, respectively.

In an equivalent analysis of the C_{cr}-normalized datasets, E_{Cd}/C_{cr}, BMI and age were independently associated with increased POR for CKD. Sex, smoking and hypertension were not associated with the POR for CKD. Doubling of E_{Cd}/C_{cr} was associated with an increase in POR for CKD by 1.96-fold ($p < 0.001$). BMI figures ≥ 24 kg/m² were associated with a 3.12-fold increase in POR for CKD ($p = 0.022$). Compared with those aged 16–45 years, the POR values for CKD were 10-, 35- and 199-fold higher in those aged 46–55, 56–65, and 66–87 years, respectively.

Table 2. Increment in risk of chronic kidney disease in relation to age, BMI and cadmium exposure.

Independent Variables/ Factors	Number of Subjects	β Coefficients (SE)	POR	95% CI Lower	95% CI Upper	p
			[a] CKD			
Model 1						
$Log_2[(E_{Cd}/E_{cr}) \times 10^3]$, µg/g creatinine	917	0.385 (0.072)	1.470	1.276	1.692	<0.001
Hypertension	276	0.490 (0.312)	1.632	0.885	3.008	0.117
Gender (female)	562	0.028 (0.340)	1.029	0.528	2.002	0.934
Smoking	335	0.209 (0.337)	1.232	0.637	2.383	0.536
BMI, kg/m²						
12–18	99	Referent				
19–23	431	0.057 (0.426)	1.058	0.459	2.439	0.894
≥24	387	1.033 (0/470)	2.810	1.118	7.064	0.028
Age, years						
16–45	392	Referent				
46–55	348	2.655 (1.036)	14.23	1.867	108.4	0.010
56–65	100	3.340 (1.059)	28.21	3.538	224.9	0.002
66–87	77	4.950 (1.055)	141.2	17.87	1116	<0.001
Model 2						
$Log_2[(E_{Cd}/C_{cr}) \times 10^5]$, µg/L filtrate	917	0.674 (0.107)	1.962	1.589	2.422	<0.001
Hypertension	276	0.551 (0.326)	1.735	0.916	3.287	0.091
Gender (female)	562	−0.174 (0.366)	0.840	0.410	1.719	0.633
Smoking	335	−0.058 (0.351)	0.944	0.474	1.879	0.869
BMI, kg/m²						
12–18	99	Referent				
19–23	431	0.103 (0.457)	1.109	0.452	2.717	0.822
≥24	387	1.147 (0.500)	3.150	1.181	8.400	0.022
Age, years						
16–45	392	Referent				
46–55	348	2.298 (1.036)	9.951	1.305	75.88	0.027
56–65	100	3.543 (1.062)	34.57	4.312	277.2	0.001
66–87	77	5.292 (1.066)	198.6	24.59	1605	<0.001

POR, Prevalence Odds Ratio; S.E., standard error of mean; CI, confidence interval. [a] CKD was defined as estimated glomerular filtration rate (eGFR) ≤ 60 mL/min/1.73 m². Coding; female = 1, male = 2, hypertensive = 1, normotensive = 2, smoker = 1, non-smoker = 2. Data were generated from logistic regression analyses relating POR for CKD to six independent variables, listed in the first column. For all tests, p-values < 0.05 indicate statistical significance. $Log_2[(E_{Cd}/E_{cr}) \times 10^3]$ was incorporated into model 1; $log_2[(E_{Cd}/C_{cr}) \times 10^5]$ was incorporated into model 2. Other independent variables in models 1 and 2 were identical. β coefficients indicate an effect size of each independent variable on POR for CKD.

3.3. Cadmium Excretion in Relation to the Risk of CKD

Table 3 provides the results of a logistic regression analysis where age and BMI were continuous variables, while E_{Cd}/E_{cr} was a categorical variable in model 1, and E_{Cd}/C_{cr} was categorical in model 2.

Table 3. Dose–response relationship between cadmium excretion and the risk of chronic kidney disease.

Independent Variables/ Factors	Number of Subjects	β Coefficients (SE)	POR	95% CI Lower	95% CI Upper	p
Model 1						
Age, years	917	0.126 (0.016)	1.135	1.100	1.170	<0.001
BMI, kg/m^2	917	0.082 (0.038)	1.086	1.009	1.169	0.028
Gender (female)	562	0.124 (0.337)	1.132	0.585	2.190	0.713
Hypertension	276	0.304 (0.310)	1.355	0.738	2.486	0.327
Smoking	335	0.173 (0.345)	1.189	0.605	2.338	0.615
E_{Cd}/E_{cr}, µg/g creatinine						
≤0.37	358	Referent				
0.38–2.49	333	1.819 (0.565)	6.164	2.035	18.67	0.001
≥2.5	226	2.362 (0.557)	10.61	3.562	31.60	<0.001
Model 2						
Age, years	917	0.141 (0.016)	1.152	1.116	1.189	<0.001
BMI, kg/m2	917	0.099 (0.039)	1.104	1.023	1.191	0.011
Gender (female)	562	0.191 (0.356)	1.211	.602	2.434	0.591
Hypertension	276	0.240 (0.314)	1.271	0.687	2.353	0.445
Smoking	335	−0.033 (0.359)	0.968	0.479	1.956	0.927
E_{Cd}/C_{cr}, ng/L filtrate						
≤9.9	346	Referent				
10–49.9	326	1.470 (0.642)	4.350	1.237	15.30	0.022
≥50	245	3.036 (0.637)	20.82	5.979	72.52	<0.001

POR, Prevalence Odds Ratio; S.E., standard error of mean; CI, confidence interval. [a] CKD was defined as estimated glomerular filtration rate (eGFR) ≤ 60 mL/min/1.73 m^2. Coding; female = 1, male = 2, hypertensive = 1, normotensive = 2, smoker = 1, non-smoker = 2. Data were generated from logistic regression analyses relating POR for CKD to six independent variables listed in the first column. For all tests, p-values < 0.05 indicate statistical significance. Three E_{Cd}/E_{cr} categories were incorporated into model 1; three E_{Cd}/C_{cr} × 100 categories were incorporated into model 2. Other independent variables in models 1 and 2 were identical. β coefficients indicate an effect size of each independent variable on POR for CKD.

Age and BMI were independently associated with increased POR for CKD in both models 1 and 2. Compared with E_{Cd}/E_{cr} ≤ 0.37 µg/g creatinine (model 1), the POR for CKD was increased by 6.2- and 10.6-fold in those with E_{Cd}/E_{cr} values of 0.38–2.49 and ≥2.5 µg/g creatinine, respectively. Compared with E_{Cd}/C_{cr} ≤ 9.9 ng/L filtrates (model 2), the POR for CKD was increased by 4.4- and 20.8-fold in those with E_{Cd}/C_{cr} values of 10–49.9 and ≥50 ng/L filtrate, respectively.

3.4. BMDL/BMDU Figures of E_{Cd} Associated with Reduced Glomerular Function
3.4.1. E_{cr}-Normalized Dataset

As data in Figures 1 and 2 indicate, the differences between BMDL and BMDU figures of E_{Cd}/E_{cr} were small for both continuous and quantal endpoints. The BMDL-BMDU figures of E_{Cd}/E_{cr} calculated from Cd-dose and eGFR response models were higher in females than males.

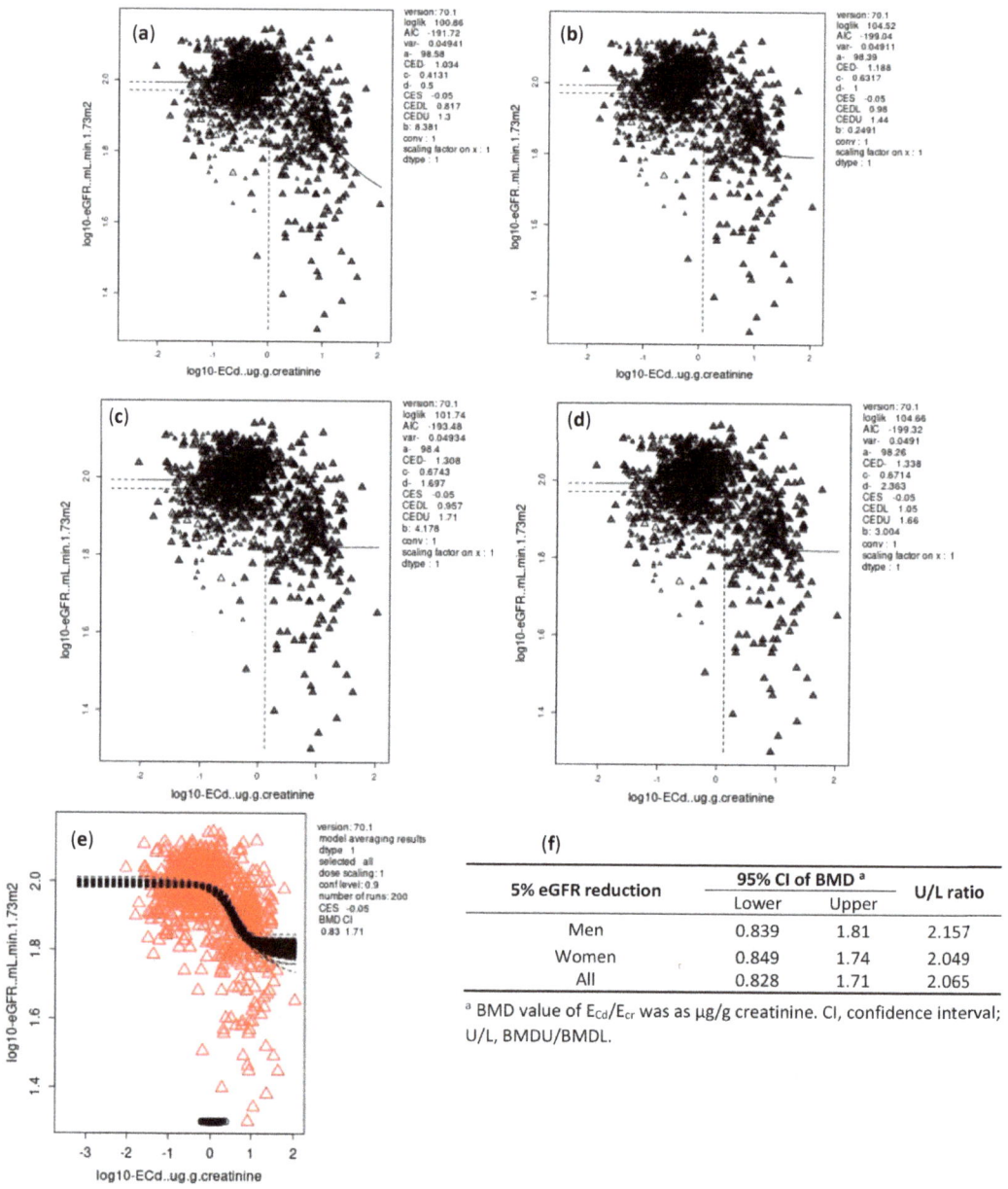

Figure 1. BMD estimates of E_{Cd}/E_{cr} from eGFR reduction endpoint with BMR at 5%. E_{Cd}/E_{cr} and eGFR data were fitted to an inverse exponential model (**a**), a natural logarithmic model (**b**), an exponential model (**c**), and Hill model (**d**). Bootstrap curves were based on model averaging of E_{Cd}/E_{cr} BMD estimates for all subjects (**e**). Outputs of all fitted models as BMDL and BMDU estimates of E_{Cd}/E_{cr} associated with a 5 % reduction in eGFR (**f**).

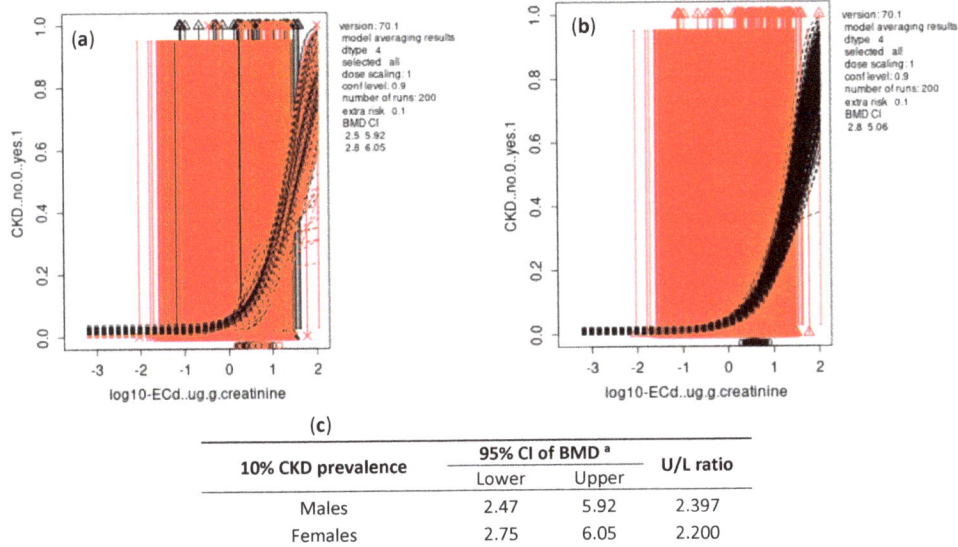

Figure 2. BMD estimates of E_{Cd}/E_{cr} from quantal eGFR endpoint with BMR at 10%. Bootstrap curves were based on model averaging 95% confidence intervals of BMD of E_{Cd}/E_{cr} in males and females (**a**) and in all subjects (**b**). Outputs of all fitted models as BMDL and BMDU estimates of E_{Cd}/E_{cr} associated with a 10% increase in prevalence of CKD (**c**).

For all subjects, the BMDL/BMDU of E_{Cd}/E_{cr} for continuous and quantal endpoints were 0.828/1.71 and 2.77/5.06 μg/g creatinine, respectively.

3.4.2. C_{cr}-Normalized Dataset

As data in Figures 3 and 4 indicate, the differences between BMDL and BMDU figures of E_{Cd}/C_{cr} were small for both continuous and quantal endpoints. The BMDL-BMDU figures of E_{Cd}/E_{cr} calculated by Cd-dose and eGFR response models in males and females were nearly identical.

For all subjects, the BMDL/BMDU of E_{Cd}/C_{cr} for continuous and quantal endpoints were 10.4/24 and 56.1/83.1 ng/L filtrate, respectively.

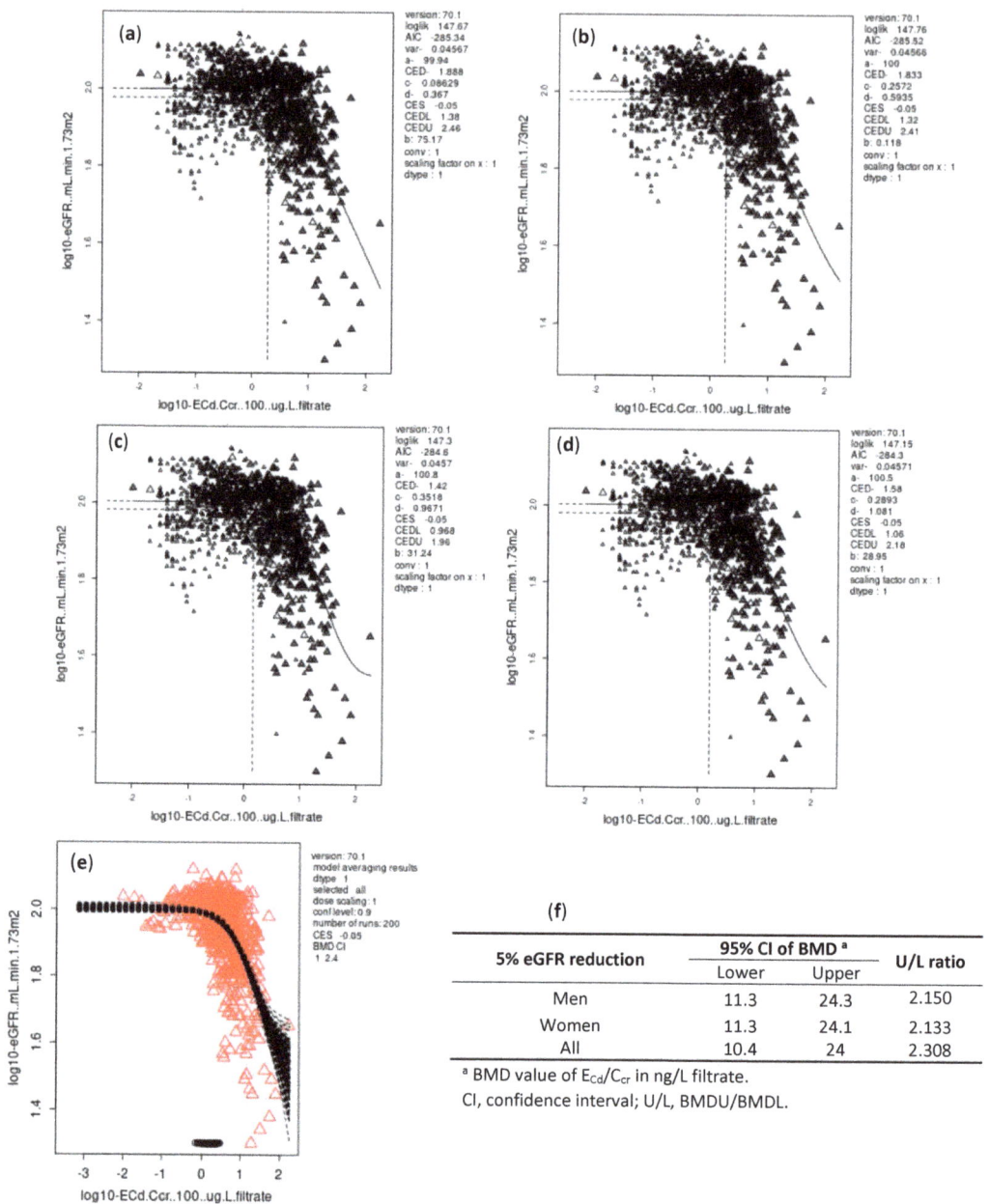

Figure 3. BMD estimates of E_{Cd}/C_{cr} from eGFR reduction endpoint with BMR at 5%. E_{Cd}/C_{cr} and eGFR data were fitted to an inverse exponential model (**a**), a natural logarithmic model (**b**), an exponential model (**c**), and Hill model (**d**). Bootstrap curves were based on model averaging of E_{Cd}/C_{cr} BMD estimates for all subjects (**e**). Outputs of all fitted models as BMDL and BMDU estimates of E_{Cd}/C_{cr} associated with a 5% reduction in eGFR (**f**).

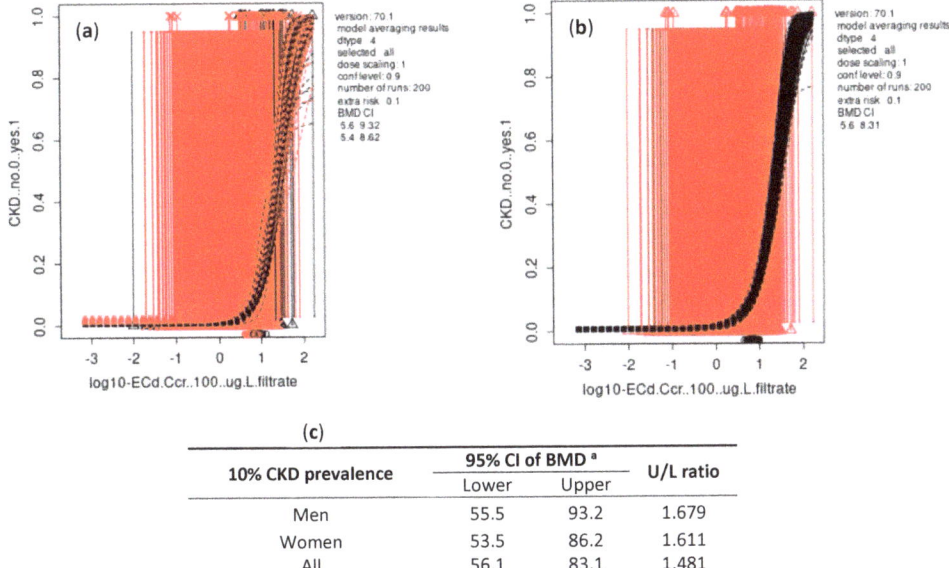

10% CKD prevalence	95% CI of BMD [a]		U/L ratio
	Lower	Upper	
Men	55.5	93.2	1.679
Women	53.5	86.2	1.611
All	56.1	83.1	1.481

[a] BMD value of E_{Cd}/C_{cr} in ng/L filtrate.
CI, confidence interval; U/L, BMDU/BMDL.

Figure 4. BMD estimates of E_{Cd}/C_{cr} from quantal eGFR endpoint with BMR at 10%. Bootstrap curves were based on model averaging 95% confidence intervals of BMD of E_{Cd}/C_{cr} in males and females (**a**) and in all subjects (**b**). Outputs of all fitted models as BMDL and BMDU estimates of E_{Cd}/E_{cr} associated with a 10% increase in the prevalence of CKD (**c**).

4. Discussion

In a dose–response analysis of a large dataset from apparently healthy participants (mean age 48.3 years), older age and higher BMI were independently associated with higher risks of CKD, based on the low eGFR criterion (Table 2). These findings are consistent with the literature reports of age, overweight and obesity as common CKD risk factors [27–30]. In addition to these two risk factors, we have found the measure of long-term exposure to Cd (E_{Cd}/E_{cr}) to be another independent risk factor of CKD (Table 3). An association between low environmental Cd exposure and a decrease in eGFR to levels commensurate with CKD has been observed in population-based studies in the U.S. [31–34], Taiwan [35] and Korea [36–38].

In this study, the risk of CKD was increased by 6.2- and 10.6-fold, when $E_{Cd}/E_{cr} \leq 0.37$ μg/g creatinine rose to 0.38–2.49 and ≥ 2.5 μg/g creatinine, respectively. These Cd-dose dependent increases in the risk of CKD were strengthened by the results obtained from the C_{cr}-normalized dataset where the risk of CKD was increased by 4.4- and 20.8-fold, comparing $E_{Cd}/C_{cr} \leq 9.9$ ng/L filtrates with E_{Cd}/C_{cr} of 10–49.9 and ≥ 50 ng/L filtrate, respectively. This confirmation is noteworthy because normalizing E_{Cd} to E_{cr} can cause a wide dispersion of dataset due to the interindividual differences in E_{cr} such as muscle mass which is unrelated to neither Cd exposure nor nephron function [11,12].

Because of such increased variance in datasets introduced by E_{cr}-normalization, the effect of chronic exposure to low-dose Cd on eGFR was not realized. For example, a systematic review and meta-analysis of pooled data from 28 studies reported that the risk of proteinuria was increased by 1.35-fold when comparing the highest vs. lowest category of Cd dose metrics, but an increase in the risk of low eGFR was statistically insignificant (p = 0.10) [39]. An erroneous conclusion that chronic Cd exposure was not associated with a progressive eGFR reduction was also made in another systematic review [40].

A significant relationship was seen between E_{Cd} and a decrease in eGFR with adjustment for covariates (Table 3). We subsequently applied the BMD method to our E_{cr}- and C_{cr}-normalized datasets to identify E_{Cd}/E_{cr} and E_{Cd}/C_{cr} values below which an adverse effect of Cd on eGFR can be discerned. The BMDL/BMDU figures of E_{Cd}/E_{cr}, estimated from the eGFR reduction endpoint were 0.839/1.81, 0.849/1.74 and 0.828/1.71 µg/g creatinine in males, females and all subjects, respectively (Figure 1). The corresponding BMDL/BMDU figures of E_{Cd}/C_{cr} were 11.3/24.3, 11.3/24.1 and 10.4/24 ng/L filtrate in males, females and all subjects, respectively (Figure 3).

The BMD values of Cd exposure levels calculated from toxic tubular cell injury and reduced tubular reabsorption of the filtered protein β₂M can be found in numerous studies [41,42]. In contrast, a report of BMDL/BMDU of Cd exposure levels associated with eGFR reduction could only be found in a study of 790 Swedish women, aged 53–64 years, where the reported BMDL values for the glomerular endpoint were 0.7–1.2 µg/g creatinine [43]. These BMD values were slightly lower than those calculated for females in the present study (0.849/1.74 µg/g creatinine). The differences may be attributable to lower E_{cr} in Thai women than in Swedish women. Nevertheless, all these BMD values were lower than E_{Cd}/E_{cr} of 5.24 µg/g creatinine, which suggested to be a threshold level for the nephrotoxicity of Cd when $E_{β2M}/E_{cr} > 300$ was used as the POD [8].

In our quantal eGFR endpoint analysis (Figure 2), the BMDL/BMDU values of E_{Cd} associated with a 10% increase in CKD prevalence were 2.77/5.06 µg/g creatinine (56.1/83.1 ng/L filtrate). These data suggested that population CKD prevalence was likely to be smaller than 10% at $E_{Cd}/E_{cr} < 2.77$ µg/g creatinine (<56.1 ng/L filtrates). Thus, the population health risk associated with $E_{Cd}/E_{cr} < 2.77$ µg/g creatinine could not be discerned. The impact of Cd exposure on GFR has long been underestimated due to the common practice of normalizing E_{Cd} to E_{cr}. The comparability of guidelines between populations could be improved by the universal acceptance of a consistent normalization of E_{Cd} to Ccr that eliminates the effect of muscle mass on E_{cr}, thereby giving a more accurate assessment of the severity of Cd nephropathy [10].

A tolerable intake level of 0.28 µg/kg body weight per day was derived in a risk calculation using pooled data from Chinese population studies [44]. This consumption level, equivalent to 16.8 µg/day for a 60 kg person, was derived from an $E_{β2M}/E_{cr}$ endpoint where the BMDL value of E_{Cd}/E_{cr} for such an endpoint was 3.07 µg/g creatinine. This BMDL estimate was 3.7-fold higher than the BMDL of 0.828 µg/g creatinine derived in the present study. In another Chinese population study, dietary Cd intake estimates at 23.2, 29.6, and 36.9 µg/d were associated with 1.73-, 2.93- and 4.05-fold increments in the prevalence of CKD, compared with the 16.7 µg/d intake level [45]. A diet high in rice, pork, and vegetables was associated with a 4.56-fold increase in the prevalence of CKD [45].

The European Food Safety Authority (EFSA) also used the β₂M endpoint. However, the EFSA included an uncertainty factor (safety margin), and an intake of 0.36 µg/kg body weight per day for 50 years as an acceptable Cd ingestion level or a reference dose (RfD) [46]. The EFSA designated E_{Cd}/E_{cr} of 1 µg/g creatinine as the toxicity threshold level for an adverse effect on kidneys. This Cd excretion of 1 µg/g creatinine is 17 % higher than our NOAEL equivalent of Cd excretion of 0.828 µg/g creatinine.

The Cd toxicity threshold level, RfD and an acceptable consumption level derived from the β₂M excretion above ≥300 µg/ g creatinine do not appear to be without an appreciable health risk. In theory, health-risk assessment should be based on the most sensitive endpoint with consideration given to subpopulations with increased susceptibility to Cd toxicity such as children.

In the present study, the body burden of Cd, measured as E_{Cd}/E_{cr}, was increased by 3-fold in men and women who smoked cigarettes (Table 1). These results are expected, given that the tobacco plant accumulates high levels of Cd in its leaves, and the volatile metallic Cd and oxide (CdO) generated from cigarette burning are more bioavailable than Cd that enters the body through the gut [47,48].

The diet is the main Cd exposure source for non-smoking and non-occupationally-exposed populations. In a temporal trend analysis of environmental Cd exposure in the U.S., the mean urinary Cd fell by 29% in men (0.58 vs. 0.41 µg/g creatinine, $p < 0.001$) over 18 years (NHANES 1988–2006), but not in women (0.71 vs. 0.63 µg/g creatinine, $p = 0.66$) [49]. Such a reduction in Cd exposure among men was attributable to a decrease in smoking prevalence [50]. In contrast, total diet studies in Australia [51], France [52], Spain [53] and the Netherlands [2] reported that dietary Cd exposure levels among young children exceeded the current health guidance values. These data are concerning for the reasons below.

CKD is a progressive syndrome with high morbidity and mortality and affects 8% to 16% of the world's population [27–30]. An upward trend of its incidence continues, while an adverse effect of Cd on eGFR and the risk of CKD have increasingly been reported. Higher Cd excretion was associated with lower eGFR in studies from Guatemala [54] and Myanmar [55]. The effect of Cd exposure on eGFR observed in children is particularly concerning. In a prospective cohort study of Bangladeshi preschool children, an inverse relationship between urinary Cd excretion and kidney volume was seen in children at 5 years of age. This was in addition to a decrease in eGFR [56]. Urinary Cd levels were inversely associated with eGFR, especially in girls. In another prospective cohort study of Mexican children, the reported mean for Cd intake at the baseline was 4.4 µg/d, which rose to 8.1 µg/d after nine years, when such Cd intake levels showed a marginally inverse association with eGFR [57].

5. Conclusions

Environmental exposure to Cd, old age, and elevated BMI are independent risk factors for reduced eGFR. For the first time, the BMDL/BMDU figures of Cd excretion levels associated with a decrease in eGFR have been computed for men and women. The narrow BMDL-BMDU differences indicate the high degree of statistical certainty in these derived NOAEL equivalent figures. The BMDL/BMDU estimates of the Cd excretion associated with a decrease in eGFR in all subjects are 0.828/1.71 µg/g creatinine. The BMDL/BMDU estimates of Cd excretion associated with a 10% increase in the prevalence of CKD are 2.77/5.06 µg/g creatinine. These NOAEL equivalents indicate a decrease in eGFR due to Cd nephropathy occurs at the body burdens lower than those associated with Cd excretion of 5.24 µg/g creatinine and an increase in β_2M excretion above 300 µg/g creatinine. The established nephrotoxicity threshold level for Cd is outdated and is not protective of human health. Human health risk assessment should be based on current scientific research data.

Author Contributions: Conceptualization, S.S.; methodology, S.S., S.Y. and A.B.Đ.; formal analysis, S.S. and A.B.Đ.; investigation, S.S. and S.Y.; resources, G.C.G. and D.A.V.; writing—original draft preparation, S.S.; writing—review and editing, G.C.G. and D.A.V.; project administration, S.S. and S.Y. All authors have read and agreed to the published version of the manuscript.

Funding: This research received no external funding.

Institutional Review Board Statement: This study analyzed archived data taken from published reports [17,18]. Ethical review and approval were not applicable.

Informed Consent Statement: All participants took part in the study after giving informed consent.

Data Availability Statement: All data are contained within this article.

Acknowledgments: This work was supported with resources from the Kidney Disease Research Collaborative, Translational Research Institute and the Department of Nephrology, Princess Alexandra Hospital. It was also supported by the resources of the Department of Toxicology "Akademik Danilo Soldatović", University of Belgrade-Faculty of Pharmacy, Serbia.

Conflicts of Interest: The authors have declared no potential conflict of interest.

References

1. Satarug, S.; Vesey, D.A.; Gobe, G.C. Current health risk assessment practice for dietary cadmium: Data from different countries. *Food Chem. Toxicol.* **2017**, *106*, 430–445. [CrossRef] [PubMed]
2. Boon, P.E.; Pustjens, A.M.; Te Biesebeek, J.D.; Brust, G.M.H.; Castenmiller, J.J.M. Dietary intake and risk assessment of elements for 1- and 2-year-old children in the Netherlands. *Food Chem. Toxicol.* **2022**, *161*, 112810. [CrossRef] [PubMed]
3. Fechner, C.; Hackethal, C.; Höpfner, T.; Dietrich, J.; Bloch, D.; Lindtner, O.; Sarvan, I. Results of the BfR MEAL Study: In Germany, mercury is mostly contained in fish and seafood while cadmium, lead, and nickel are present in a broad spectrum of foods. *Food Chem. X* **2022**, *14*, 100326. [CrossRef] [PubMed]
4. Aoshima, K. Epidemiology of renal tubular dysfunction in the inhabitants of a cadmium-polluted area in the Jinzu River basin in Toyama Prefecture. *Tohoku J. Exp. Med.* **1987**, *152*, 151–172. [CrossRef]
5. Horiguchi, H.; Aoshima, K.; Oguma, E.; Sasaki, S.; Miyamoto, K.; Hosoi, Y.; Katoh, T.; Kayama, F. Latest status of cadmium accumulation and its effects on kidneys, bone, and erythropoiesis in inhabitants of the formerly cadmium-polluted Jinzu River Basin in Toyama, Japan, after restoration of rice paddies. *Int. Arch. Occup. Environ. Health* **2010**, *83*, 953–970. [CrossRef] [PubMed]
6. Kurata, Y.; Katsuta, O.; Doi, T.; Kawasuso, T.; Hiratsuka, H.; Tsuchitani, M.; Umemura, T. Chronic cadmium treatment induces tubular nephropathy and osteomalacic osteopenia in ovariectomized cynomolgus monkeys. *Vet. Pathol.* **2014**, *51*, 919–931. [CrossRef] [PubMed]
7. Wong, C.; Roberts, S.M.; Saab, I.N. Review of regulatory reference values and background levels for heavy metals in the human diet. *Regul. Toxicol. Pharmacol.* **2022**, *130*, 105122. [CrossRef] [PubMed]
8. JECFA. Summary and Conclusions. In Proceedings of the Joint FAO/WHO Expert Committee on Food Additives and Contaminants, Seventy-Third Meeting, Geneva, Switzerland, 8–17 June 2010; JECFA/73/SC. Food and Agriculture Organization of the United Nations/World Health Organization: Geneva, Switzerland, 2011. Available online: https://apps.who.int/iris/handle/10665/44521 (accessed on 21 September 2022).
9. Satarug, S.; Vesey, D.A.; Nishijo, M.; Ruangyuttikarn, W.; Gobe, G.C. The inverse association of glomerular function and urinary β2-MG excretion and its implications for cadmium health risk assessment. *Environ. Res.* **2019**, *173*, 40–47. [CrossRef]
10. Satarug, S.; Vesey, D.A.; Gobe, G.C. Dose-response analysis of the tubular and glomerular effects of chronic exposure to environmental cadmium. *Int. J. Environ. Res. Public Health* **2022**, *19*, 10572. [CrossRef]
11. Satarug, S.; Vesey, D.A.; Ruangyuttikarn, W.; Nishijo, M.; Gobe, G.C.; Phelps, K.R. The source and pathophysiologic significance of excreted cadmium. *Toxics* **2019**, *7*, 55. [CrossRef]
12. Satarug, S.; Vesey, D.A.; Nishijo, M.; Ruangyuttikarn, W.; Gobe, G.C.; Phelps, K.R. The effect of cadmium on GFR is clarified by normalization of excretion rates to creatinine clearance. *Int. J. Mol. Sci.* **2021**, *22*, 1762. [CrossRef]
13. Schnaper, H.W. The tubulointerstitial pathophysiology of progressive kidney disease. *Adv. Chronic Kidney Dis.* **2017**, *24*, 107–116. [CrossRef]
14. Sand, S.; Victorin, K.; Filipsson, A.F. The current state of knowledge on the use of the benchmark dose concept in risk assessment. *J. Appl. Toxicol.* **2008**, *28*, 405–421. [CrossRef] [PubMed]
15. EFSA Scientific Committee. Update: Use of the benchmark dose approach in risk assessment. *EFSA J.* **2017**, *15*, 4658.
16. Moffett, D.B.; Mumtaz, M.M.; Sullivan, D.W., Jr.; Whittaker, M.H. Chapter 13, General Considerations of Dose-Effect and Dose-Response Relationships. In *Handbook on the Toxicology of Metals*, 5th ed.; Volume I: General Considerations; Nordberg, G., Costa, M., Eds.; Academic Press: Cambridge, MA, USA, 2022; pp. 299–317.
17. Satarug, S.; Swaddiwudhipong, W.; Ruangyuttikarn, W.; Nishijo, M.; Ruiz, P. Modeling cadmium exposures in low- and high-exposure areas in Thailand. *Environ. Health Perspect.* **2013**, *121*, 531–536. [CrossRef] [PubMed]
18. Yimthiang, S.; Pouyfung, P.; Khamphaya, T.; Kuraeiad, S.; Wongrith, P.; Vesey, D.A.; Gobe, G.C.; Satarug, S. Effects of environmental exposure to cadmium and lead on the risks of diabetes and kidney dysfunction. *Int. J. Environ. Res. Public Health* **2022**, *19*, 2259. [CrossRef] [PubMed]
19. Denic, A.; Elsherbiny, H.; Rule, A.D. In-vivo techniques for determining nephron number. *Curr. Opin. Nephrol. Hypertens.* **2019**, *28*, 545–551. [CrossRef] [PubMed]
20. Levey, A.S.; Becker, C.; Inker, L.A. Glomerular filtration rate and albuminuria for detection and staging of acute and chronic kidney disease in adults: A systematic review. *JAMA* **2015**, *313*, 837–846. [CrossRef]
21. Soveri, I.; Berg, U.B.; Björk, J.; Elinder, C.G.; Grubb, A.; Mejare, I.; Sterner, G.; Bäck, S.E.; SBU GFR Review Group. Measuring GFR: A systematic review. *Am. J. Kidney Dis.* **2014**, *64*, 411–424. [CrossRef]
22. White, C.A.; Allen, C.M.; Akbari, A.; Collier, C.P.; Holland, D.C.; Day, A.G.; Knoll, G.A. Comparison of the new and traditional CKD-EPI GFR estimation equations with urinary inulin clearance: A study of equation performance. *Clin. Chim. Acta* **2019**, *488*, 189–195. [CrossRef]
23. Phelps, K.R.; Gosmanova, E.O. A generic method for analysis of plasma concentrations. *Clin. Nephrol.* **2020**, *94*, 43–49. [CrossRef] [PubMed]
24. Slob, W.; Moerbeek, M.; Rauniomaa, E.; Piersma, A.H. A statistical evaluation of toxicity study designs for the estimation of the benchmark dose in continuous endpoints. *Toxicol. Sci.* **2005**, *84*, 167–185. [CrossRef] [PubMed]
25. Slob, W.; Setzer, R.W. 2014. Shape and steepness of toxicological dose-response relationships of continuous endpoints. *Crit. Rev. Toxicol.* **2014**, *44*, 270–297. [CrossRef] [PubMed]

26. Zhu, Y.; Wang, T.; Jelsovsky, J.Z. Bootstrap estimation of benchmark doses and confidence limits with clustered quantal data. *Risk Anal.* **2007**, *27*, 447–465. [CrossRef] [PubMed]
27. Nichols, G.A.; Déruaz-Luyet, A.; Brodovicz, K.G.; Kimes, T.M.; Rosales, A.G.; Hauske, S.J. Kidney disease progression and all-cause mortality across estimated glomerular filtration rate and albuminuria categories among patients with vs. without type 2 diabetes. *BMC Nephrol.* **2020**, *21*, 167.
28. George, C.; Mogueo, A.; Okpechi, I.; Echouffo-Tcheugui, J.B.; Kengne, A.P. Chronic kidney disease in low-income to middle-income countries: *Case Increased Screening*. *BMJ Glob Health.* **2017**, *2*, e000256. [CrossRef]
29. George, C.; Echouffo-Tcheugui, J.B.; Jaar, B.G.; Okpechi, I.G.; Kengne, A.P. The need for screening, early diagnosis, and prediction of chronic kidney disease in people with diabetes in low- and middle-income countries-a review of the current literature. *BMC Med.* **2022**, *20*, 247. [CrossRef] [PubMed]
30. Kalantar-Zadeh, K.; Jafar, T.H.; Nitsch, D.; Neuen, B.L.; Perkovic, V. Chronic kidney disease. *Lancet* **2021**, *398*, 786–802. [CrossRef]
31. Ferraro, P.M.; Costanzi, S.; Naticchia, A.; Sturniolo, A.; Gambaro, G. Low level exposure to cadmium increases the risk of chronic kidney disease: Analysis of the NHANES 1999–2006. *BMC Public Health* **2010**, *10*, 304. [CrossRef] [PubMed]
32. Navas-Acien, A.; Tellez-Plaza, M.; Guallar, E.; Muntner, P.; Silbergeld, E.; Jaar, B.; Weaver, V. Blood cadmium and lead and chronic kidney disease in US adults: A joint analysis. *Am. J. Epidemiol.* **2009**, *170*, 1156–1164. [CrossRef]
33. Lin, Y.S.; Ho, W.C.; Caffrey, J.L.; Sonawane, B. Low serum zinc is associated with elevated risk of cadmium nephrotoxicity. *Environ. Res.* **2014**, *134*, 33–38. [CrossRef] [PubMed]
34. Madrigal, J.M.; Ricardo, A.C.; Persky, V.; Turyk, M. Associations between blood cadmium concentration and kidney function in the U.S. population: Impact of sex, diabetes and hypertension. *Environ. Res.* **2018**, *169*, 180–188. [CrossRef] [PubMed]
35. Tsai, K.F.; Hsu, P.C.; Lee, C.T.; Kung, C.T.; Chang, Y.C.; Fu, L.M.; Ou, Y.C.; Lan, K.C.; Yen, T.H.; Lee, W.C. Association between enzyme-linked immunosorbent assay-measured kidney injury markers and urinary cadmium levels in chronic kidney disease. *J. Clin. Med.* **2021**, *11*, 156. [CrossRef] [PubMed]
36. Myong, J.-P.; Kim, H.-R.; Baker, D.; Choi, B. Blood cadmium and moderate-to-severe glomerular dysfunction in Korean adults: Analysis of KNHANES 2005–2008 data. *Int. Arch. Occup. Environ. Health* **2012**, *85*, 885–893. [CrossRef]
37. Chung, S.; Chung, J.H.; Kim, S.J.; Koh, E.S.; Yoon, H.E.; Park, C.W.; Chang, Y.S.; Shin, S.J. Blood lead and cadmium levels and renal function in Korean adults. *Clin. Exp. Nephrol.* **2014**, *18*, 726–734. [CrossRef]
38. Park, Y.; Lee, S.J. Association of blood heavy metal levels and renal function in Korean adults. *Int. J. Environ. Res. Public Health* **2022**, *19*, 6646. [CrossRef]
39. Jalili, C.; Kazemi, M.; Cheng, H.; Mohammadi, H.; Babaei, A.; Taheri, E.; Moradi, S. Associations between exposure to heavy metals and the risk of chronic kidney disease: A systematic review and meta-analysis. *Crit. Rev. Toxicol.* **2021**, *51*, 165–182. [CrossRef]
40. Byber, K.; Lison, D.; Verougstraete, V.; Dressel, H.; Hotz, P. Cadmium or cadmium compounds and chronic kidney disease in workers and the general population: A systematic review. *Crit. Rev. Toxicol.* **2016**, *46*, 191–240. [CrossRef]
41. Liu, C.; Li, Y.; Zhu, C.; Dong, Z.; Zhang, K.; Zhao, Y.; Xu, Y. Benchmark dose for cadmium exposure and elevated N-acetyl-β-D-glucosaminidase: A meta-analysis. *Environ. Sci. Pollut. Res. Int.* **2016**, *23*, 20528–20538. [CrossRef]
42. Pócsi, I.; Dockrell, M.E.; Price, R.G. Nephrotoxic biomarkers with specific indications for metallic pollutants: Implications for environmental health. *Biomark. Insights* **2022**, *17*, 11772719221111882. [CrossRef]
43. Suwazono, Y.; Sand, S.; Vahter, M.; Filipsson, A.F.; Skerfving, S.; Lidfeldt, J.; Akesson, A. Benchmark dose for cadmium-induced renal effects in humans. *Environ. Health Perspect.* **2006**, *114*, 1072–1076. [CrossRef] [PubMed]
44. Qing, Y.; Yang, J.; Zhu, Y.; Li, Y.; Zheng, W.; Wu, M.; He, G. Dose-response evaluation of urinary cadmium and kidney injury biomarkers in Chinese residents and dietary limit standards. *Environ. Health* **2021**, *20*, 75. [CrossRef] [PubMed]
45. Shi, Z.; Taylor, A.W.; Riley, M.; Byles, J.; Liu, J.; Noakes, M. Association between dietary patterns, cadmium intake and chronic kidney disease among adults. *Clin. Nutr.* **2018**, *37*, 276–284. [CrossRef] [PubMed]
46. EFSA. European Food Safety Agency, Statement on tolerable weekly intake for cadmium. *EFSA J.* **2011**, *9*, 1975.
47. Repić, A.; Bulat, P.; Antonijević, B.; Antunović, M.; Džudović, J.; Buha, A.; Bulat, Z. The influence of smoking habits on cadmium and lead blood levels in the Serbian adult people. *Environ. Sci. Pollut. Res. Int.* **2020**, *27*, 751–760. [CrossRef]
48. Pappas, R.S.; Fresquez, M.R.; Watson, C.H. Cigarette smoke cadmium breakthrough from traditional filters: Implications for exposure. *J. Anal. Toxicol.* **2015**, *39*, 45–51. [CrossRef]
49. Ferraro, P.M.; Sturniolo, A.; Naticchia, A.; D'Alonzo, S.; Gambaro, G. Temporal trend of cadmium exposure in the United States population suggests gender specificities. *Intern. Med. J.* **2012**, *42*, 691–697. [CrossRef]
50. Tellez-Plaza, M.; Navas-Acien, A.; Caldwell, K.L.; Menke, A.; Muntner, P.; Guallar, E. Reduction in cadmium exposure in the United States population, 1988–2008: The contribution of declining smoking rates. *Environ. Health Perspect.* **2012**, *120*, 204–209. [CrossRef]
51. Callan, A.; Hinwood, A.; Devine, A. Metals in commonly eaten groceries in Western Australia: A market basket survey and dietary assessment. *Food Addit. Contam. A* **2014**, *31*, 1968–1981. [CrossRef]
52. Arnich, N.; Sirot, V.; Riviere, G.; Jean, J.; Noel, L.; Guerin, T.; Leblanc, J.-C. Dietary exposure to trace elements and health risk assessment in the 2nd French Total Diet Study. *Food Chem. Toxicol.* **2012**, *50*, 2432–2449. [CrossRef]

53. González, N.; Calderón, J.; Rúbies, A.; Timoner, I.; Castell, V.; Domingo, J.L.; Nadal, M. Dietary intake of arsenic, cadmium, mercury and lead by the population of Catalonia, Spain: Analysis of the temporal trend. *Food Chem. Toxicol.* **2019**, *132*, 110721. [CrossRef] [PubMed]
54. Butler-Dawson, J.; James, K.A.; Krisher, L.; Jaramillo, D.; Dally, M.; Neumann, N.; Pilloni, D.; Cruz, A.; Asensio, C.; Johnson, R.J.; et al. Environmental metal exposures and kidney function of Guatemalan sugarcane workers. *J. Expo. Sci. Environ. Epidemiol.* **2022**, *32*, 461–471. [CrossRef] [PubMed]
55. Win-Thu, M.; Myint-Thein, O.; Win-Shwe, T.-T.; Mar, O. Environmental cadmium exposure induces kidney tubular and glomerular dysfunction in the Myanmar adults. *J. Toxicol. Sci.* **2021**, *46*, 319–328. [CrossRef] [PubMed]
56. Skröder, H.; Hawkesworth, S.; Kippler, M.; El Arifeen, S.; Wagatsuma, Y.; Moore, S.E.; Vahter, M. Kidney function and blood pressure in preschool-aged children exposed to cadmium and arsenic-potential alleviation by selenium. *Environ. Res.* **2015**, *140*, 205–213. [CrossRef] [PubMed]
57. Rodríguez-López, E.; Tamayo-Ortiz, M.; Ariza, A.C.; Ortiz-Panozo, E.; Deierlein, A.L.; Pantic, I.; Tolentino, M.C.; Estrada-Gutiérrez, G.; Parra-Hernández, S.; Espejel-Núñez, A.; et al. Early-life dietary cadmium exposure and kidney function in 9-year-old children from the PROGRESS cohort. *Toxics* **2020**, *8*, 83. [CrossRef]

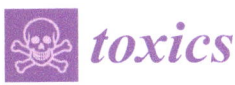

Review

Cadmium: A Focus on the Brown Crab (*Cancer pagurus*) Industry and Potential Human Health Risks

Ronan Lordan [1,2,3,4,*] and Ioannis Zabetakis [1,2,3]

1 Department of Biological Sciences, University of Limerick, V94 T9PX Limerick, Ireland
2 Health Research Institute, University of Limerick, V94 T9PX Limerick, Ireland
3 Bernal Institute, University of Limerick, V94 T9PX Limerick, Ireland
4 Institute for Translational Medicine and Therapeutics, Perelman School of Medicine, University of Pennsylvania, Philadelphia, PA 19104, USA
* Correspondence: ronan.lordan@pennmedicine.upenn.edu

Abstract: Cadmium is a major health risk globally and is usually associated with pollution and anthropogenic activity. The presence of cadmium in food is monitored to ensure that the health and safety of consumers are maintained. Cadmium is ubiquitous in the Asian and Western diets, with the highest levels present in grains, leafy greens, and shellfish. As part of their natural lifecycle of moulting and shell renewal, all crustaceans—including the brown crab (*Cancer pagurus*)—bioaccumulate cadmium from their environment in their hepatopancreas. The brown crab is an important species to the crab-fishing industries of many European countries, including Ireland. However, the industry has come under scrutiny in Europe due to the presence of cadmium in the brown crab meat intended for live export to Asia. This review explores evidence regarding the effects of cadmium consumption on human health, with a focus on the brown crab. Differences in cadmium surveillance have given rise to issues in the crab industry, with economic consequences for multiple countries. Currently, evidence suggests that brown crab consumption is safe for humans in moderation, but individuals who consume diets characterised by high levels of cadmium from multiple food groups should be mindful of their dietary choices.

Keywords: cadmium; crab; crustaceans; heavy metal toxicity; nutrition; pollution; biomagnification; biomonitoring

Citation: Lordan, R.; Zabetakis, I. Cadmium: A Focus on the Brown Crab (*Cancer pagurus*) Industry and Potential Human Health Risks. *Toxics* **2022**, *10*, 591. https://doi.org/10.3390/toxics10100591

Academic Editors: Virgínia Cruz Fernandes, Diogo Pestana and Soisungwan Satarug

Received: 5 September 2022
Accepted: 1 October 2022
Published: 6 October 2022

Publisher's Note: MDPI stays neutral with regard to jurisdictional claims in published maps and institutional affiliations.

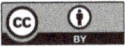

Copyright: © 2022 by the authors. Licensee MDPI, Basel, Switzerland. This article is an open access article distributed under the terms and conditions of the Creative Commons Attribution (CC BY) license (https://creativecommons.org/licenses/by/4.0/).

1. Introduction

Cadmium is a major health risk globally and is associated with pollution and anthropogenic activity. Consequently, cadmium levels in foods are monitored to ensure the health and safety of consumers [1]. Some foods are more likely to contain cadmium than others. These foods include rice, potatoes, leafy greens such as spinach, and various seafoods such as crustaceans (e.g., lobster, prawns, and crab) [2,3]. Crab fishing is an important industry around the world, including in Ireland and Northern Europe, where the brown crab (*Cancer pagurus*) (Figure 1) is the main species traded. The brown crab is of considerable value to the European economy, contributing to the income of the communities around the coastlines of trading nations such as Ireland [4,5]. The brown crab is caught off the Irish, Atlantic, and Mediterranean shores and occasionally found inshore in countries such as Norway using baited traps called pots or creels, which can be set individually or in strings [6].

The crab-fishing industry in general has come under scrutiny for cadmium levels present in the meat of frozen products and live exports to Asia [7–9]. Cadmium and other heavy metals bioaccumulate in the hepatopancreas of crustaceans, including the brown crab, due to this organ's detoxifying function [10–14]. Cadmium may also be present transiently in low concentrations in the haemolymph [15].

Strict regulations exist in some Asian countries, such as the People's Republic of China (PRC) and Hong Kong, where regulatory authorities require testing of cadmium levels of the combined white and brown meat of all crabs imported from abroad [16]. Ensuring the health of consumers is of critical importance; hence, the strict regulation of food products. However, the methods employed to sample and monitor cadmium levels in the crab industry generally appear to vary [17], as discussed in this review. In the European Union, cadmium limits are prescribed for the white crab meat intended for consumption (0.5 mg/kg) [18–20], whereas the same limits are applied to the total of the white and brown crab meat in the PRC and Hong Kong (0.5 mg/kg) [9,17,21]. These discrepancies have caused considerable tension between these trading nations [7]. However, cadmium is an issue for all crab-producing nations, but not all nations have the same issues with exports to Asian countries; therefore, it is possible that the "political climate between trading countries" may play a role [9], with preferences evident for some countries over others [22].

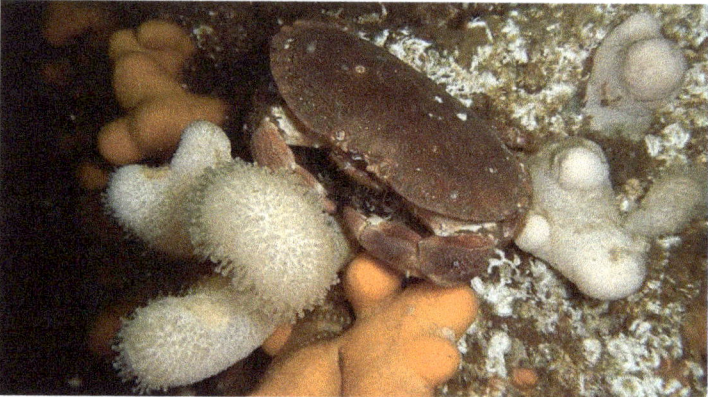

Figure 1. The brown crab (*Cancer pagurus*). Reproduced with permission from [23], licensed under CC BY 2.0.

Chronic consumption of cadmium due to a cumulative dietary intake from cadmium-exposed foods is dangerous and carries a serious risk of toxicity [24]. Although cadmium toxicity is extremely rare in modern times [25], monitoring cadmium levels in various foods is nevertheless a critical safety net to maintain health.

Brown crab is mostly treated as a delicacy and, thus, is consumed in low amounts in most countries. However, there are countries that are exceptions, including South Korea [26], Portugal [27], and Norway [28], where regular consumption is common among some of their populations. For the consumption of any species of crab, factors such as the age of the crab, the part of the crab consumed, and the origin of the crab may contribute to the ingestion of cadmium over time [29–31]. Consuming the white meat of the crab from the appendages, claws, and legs, and avoiding the cephalothorax that contains the gonadal tissue and hepatopancreas (known as the brown meat or tomalley), can be considered low-risk, as cadmium is mostly concentrated in the latter tissues [27]. While the brown meat is edible and enjoyed around the world due to its distinctive flavour, as a precaution, some health authorities and those in the scientific domain advise against its regular consumption from crab [9,32,33] and other crustaceans [34]. In 2009, a scientific opinion was published followed by an information note in 2011 by the European Commission, who recommended that member states should advise consumers about the consumption of brown crab meat due to the higher levels of cadmium in the cephalothorax [35]. However, as discussed in this review, a person's diet as a whole must be taken into consideration when attempting to determine their intake of cadmium. Thus, we consider the consumption of crab in relation to various dietary patterns, the monitoring of cadmium in crabs, and human studies of brown crab consumption.

2. Brown Crab (*Cancer pagurus*)

The brown crab is a long-lived, benthic, carnivorous, nocturnal predator species that resides on the seafloor, commonly found at depths of 6–100 m, but they are generally found between 6 and 40 m, where smaller crabs can be seen closer to the intertidal zone. The male brown crab is easily identified by its large, black-tipped claws and its "pie-crust" edged carapace (Figure 1), while the female brown crab has a domed and rounded carapace, which offers greater meat yield. However, the most reliable and common method used for sex determination is to inspect the shape of their tail, where the male abdomen is relatively narrow, while that of the females is wider [36–38]. Brown crabs largely consume molluscs and other decapod species. They achieve a carapace width of up to 270 mm in males and 250 mm in females, although there is regional variation and there have been reports of larger males reaching 300 mm. They are 5 years old when they reach minimum landing size, but they can live to 25–30 years, with some living to almost 100 years old. Brown crab can moult (the process of ecdysis) several times per year when young but less often as they become larger in size, even up to once every 4 years [4,31,37,39,40]. This can make it difficult to determine the age of a crab. After moulting, mating occurs generally from July to September when the female carapace is soft. The male transfers spermatozoa to the female, who stores the spermatozoa in a specialised organ (the spermatheca) by forming a plug, pending internal fertilisation, which usually occurs 1–14 months post-mating. The female spawns the fertilised eggs onto the pleopods and carries them over winter into the hatching season from spring to summer. During this time, the (berried) females generally remain in pits dug into the sediment or under rocks, where they mostly refrain from movement or feeding. Notably, females can spawn and inseminate the eggs without any need for mating up to several times, due to the presence of sperm plugs that can keep the spermatozoa viable for up to 3 years. Hatching can occur at any time in this period depending on numerous environmental conditions, including water temperatures and latitude. As many as 1–4 million eggs may hatch from one female brown crab, indicating their high fecundity. Because crabs are known to be migratory due to mating patterns, the hatchlings may be found over a vast distance [4,37,39,41–43], although the distribution and density of brown crabs are affected by many factors—not only fecundity or migration. For example, water temperature and access to food are additional important factors, and there tends to be greater population density inshore [37]. The biology of brown crabs is important to consider in order to understand their distribution and their availability for human consumption. The geographic distribution of brown crabs in Europe is presented in Figure 2.

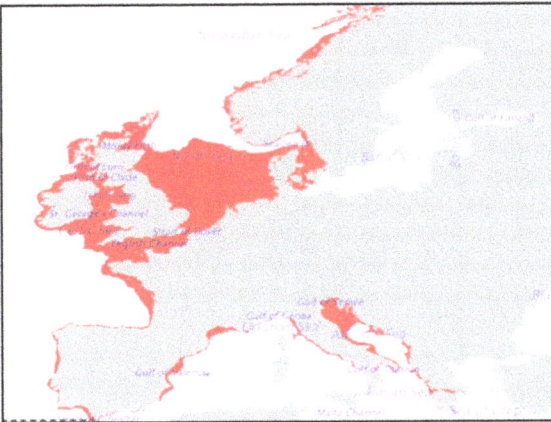

Figure 2. A diagram of the geographic distribution of brown crabs in Europe. Reproduced with permission from the European Market Observatory for Fisheries and Aquaculture Products [9].

3. The Importance of the Brown Crab Fishing Industry and the Challenge of Cadmium: Ireland as an Example of a Crab-Trading Nation

The seafood industry is significant to the Irish economy and contributes to a vibrant export trade with European and Asian countries, especially the PRC. The brown crab, or "portán dearg", is the heaviest Irish crab and is landed by most major and some minor fishing ports in the country. The brown crab is a non-quota species and can be legally caught by vessels operating with a polyvalent or potting license [44]. Globally, the brown crab is a seafood species with increasing value, totalling a catch greater than 50,000 tonnes per year [45]. Exports of crustaceans and molluscs to the PRC from Ireland in 2018 increased by 68%, accounting for a total of 12,700 tonnes of seafood and growing the market to almost EUR 46 million [46]. Ireland has become one of the top three producers of brown crab products in Europe [47]. In 2018, landings of Irish brown crab reached 5500 tonnes, representing EUR 1 million in domestic sales and EUR 60 million in exports. Additionally, the price of Irish brown crab that year increased by 58% due to considerable demand from the Asian market, making brown crab the third most valuable export species that year. This increase in exports and price is of particular value to small-scale inshore fishermen in coastal communities around Ireland [48], although it should be noted that the Irish market was affected by the coronavirus disease 2019 (COVID-19) pandemic, with lower exports reported in 2020. The Irish brown crab exports reached a total of 2878 tonnes in 2020, representing a decrease of 47% compared with 2019, recording an exports value decrease of 27% for the same period [9].

Chinese food import authorities have always been concerned regarding the levels of cadmium in all crustacean species originating from multiple countries, as they may exceed their limits of 0.5 mg/kg [9,49,50]. Ireland is not the only nation affected, as there are also reports of similar issues in Britain, Spain, France, Norway, Portugal, the Netherlands (mitten crab), the United States (Dungeness crab), and even Taiwan for various crab species exported to the PRC [8,9,49,51–53]. The main European countries exporting brown crab to the PRC have traditionally been the United Kingdom, Ireland, and France [6]. Initially, those countries used the basic health certificates (HCs) approved by their individual regulatory bodies, which were relatively non-specific regarding heavy metal testing but guaranteed that seafood was not contaminated by pollutants [9,54].

Over the past decade, the supply of brown crab from the main European exporting countries has been rejected due to cadmium for a period one or more years, and with high-level negotiations ongoing including delegations from the PRC visiting the exporting countries [55–57]. In all cases, more specific testing and health certificate (HC) formats have been agreed, which has restored some level of export of brown crab to the PRC. In Ireland, the Sea Fisheries Protection Authority (SFPA) is responsible for the issuance of Irish HCs and operates a monitoring plan whereby samples are collected and tested in a state laboratory [9,58]; however, difficulties still persist, particularly around the export of live crabs under these systems.

Questions have been raised in relation to whether the strict limits of cadmium intake in seafood might be misguided. Indeed, in the PRC there has been public consultation to raise the permitted level of cadmium in brown crab from 0.5 mg/kg to 3.0 mg/kg, but an update on this consultation has not been released yet. It is undeniable that cadmium does indeed accumulate in humans due to dietary exposure and that this does have deleterious effects on health, as discussed later in the review. However, one must consider the entirety of the dietary intake of cadmium from various sources before limits of cadmium in a specific food are imposed for specific populations. Equally, the frequency of consumption of a particular food product that is naturally high in cadmium must also be considered when determining dietary guidance on cadmium-containing products. This concept is discussed further in Section 5.

4. Cadmium Accumulation and Monitoring in Crabs and Crustaceans

The Industrial Revolution over the last two centuries has led to anthropogenic-derived pollution that ultimately has negatively affected various global biomes and ecosystems. While cadmium is ubiquitous in the environment at very low levels, industrial and technological advancement has occurred at the expense of the environment, with an increased release of cadmium (Cd^{2+}) into the environment. Cadmium is an element that can accumulate in the food chain, with potential human and ecosystem risks [59,60]. Cadmium can bioaccumulate in various marine organisms, but most prominently within crustaceans such as lobsters, crabs, crayfish, and prawns. The elemental composition of crabs has mainly been studied in crabs from the Norwegian and Scottish coasts and the English Channel [31]. See Table 1 for an overview of cadmium measurements in brown crabs. As mentioned above, crabs and other crustaceans accumulate metals mostly via diet, with some negligible amounts coming from their environment [61–63].

Table 1. An overview of cadmium concentrations in brown crab (*Cancer pagurus*) expressed as mg/kg ww.

Crab Meat Type (State)	Location	Estimated Cadmium Levels (mg/kg)		Detection Method	Reference
		Mean ± SD			
		Spring Caught	Summer Caught		
White meat (raw)	Portugal	0.07 ± 0.06	0.01 ± 0.01	FAAS	[14]
White meat (steamed)	Portugal	0.24 ± 0.38	0.10 ± 0.14		
White meat (boiled)	Portugal	0.05 ± 0.05	0.10 ± 0.16		
Brown meat (raw)	Portugal	8.4 ± 8.3	8.1 ± 14.2		
Brown meat (steamed)	Portugal	7.6 ± 5.2	11 ± 13		
Brown meat (boiled)	Portugal	5.6 ± 5.6	5.0 ± 8.2		
		Mean ± SD			
White claw meat (raw)	Northern Norway	0.024 ± 0.012		ICP-MS	[30]
White claw meat (raw)	Southern Norway	0.007 ± 0.005			
Brown meat (raw)	Northern Norway	1.15 ± 0.76			
Brown meat (raw)	Southern Norway	0.21 ± 0.14			
White claw meat (boiled)	Northern Norway	0.30 ± 0.29			
White claw meat (boiled)	Southern Norway	0.065 ± 0.075			
Brown meat (boiled)	Northern Norway	0.45 ± 0.26			
Brown meat (boiled)	Southern Norway	0.16 ± 0.12			
		Yearly median concentration range between 2016 and 2017			
Brown meat (raw)	Mausund, Norway	2.11–4.37		ICP-MS	[33]
		Estimated mean			
White meat (raw)	English Channel	0.10		FAAS	[13]
Brown meat (raw)	English Channel	15–18			
White meat (raw)	Scottish coast	0.10			
Brown meat (raw)	Scottish coast	20–30			
		Mean/range			
White meat (raw)	Birsay, Scotland	-/0.08–0.27		FAAS	[64]
Brown meat (raw)	Birsay, Scotland	7.30/1.12–49.4			
White meat (raw)	Norwegian coast	0.62/0.002–4.5		ICP-MS	[33,65]
Brown meat (raw)	Norwegian coast	8.7/0.24–43.0			
White meat (raw)	Senja, Norway	0.53/0.03–3.2		ICP-MS	[33,66]
Brown meat (raw)	Senja, Norway	9.3/1.6–29.0			
White meat (raw)	Kvaløya, Norway	0.25/0.06–0.74			
Brown meat (raw)	Kvaløya, Norway	30.0/7.3–58.0			

Several methods have been employed over the years to detect cadmium in biological samples. The most effective method to date that is commonly used is inductively coupled plasma mass spectrometry (ICP-MS), where cadmium can be detected at levels as low as 0.003 µg/L [67,68]. Indeed, most food and environment surveillance agencies use ICP-MS or similar methods to monitor cadmium in crabs [17,69]. However, alternative methods are available and have been used to measure cadmium in crabs, as shown in Table 1. For example, atomic absorption spectroscopy (AAS) is another effective analytical tool used to measure cadmium in biological materials [68]. Graphite furnace atomic absorption spectroscopy (GFAAS) was previously a common method used for the detection of cadmium in foods, with a sample detection limit of 0.4 µg/L [70]. However, other methods of cadmium detection exist that are not commonly used today for seafood analysis. For instance, radiochemical neutron activation analysis (RNAA) is a method that has been used to detect cadmium burden in humans, but its detection limits are not preferential [68]. Other methods include differential pulse ASV [71] and the calorimetric dithizone method [68].

Various factors affect cadmium accumulation in crab species. In *Carcinus maenas* (shore crab), factors such as ovarian maturation, moulting stage, condition (e.g., water content of the crab), tissue hydration, sex, and size all affect cadmium bioaccumulation [62,63,72–74]. In brown crabs specifically, there is evidence that cadmium levels differ due to location and cooking (which increases cadmium in claw meat while reducing the concentration in the inner meat), and there is a correlation between crab size and levels of cadmium in the hepatopancreas [30,75], which implies that cadmium accumulates as the crab ages. However, season, moulting, and gonad maturation have limited effects on cadmium concentrations in brown crabs [31]. Although no account has been provided regarding the age of the crabs sampled and the correlation between age and cadmium levels, this is likely because crustaceans are very difficult to age due to the process of moulting their exoskeleton throughout their life and their indeterminate growth [76]. Processing conditions are also an important consideration. Frozen crab that has been defrosted may leech cadmium with the haemolymph, which may be lost during the cooking process. Indeed, claws taken from frozen crab before thawing had lower cadmium levels than claws taken from the carapace after thawing, indicating that there can be redistribution of cadmium in the crab. This may indicate biases when assessing cadmium levels in crabs that have been processed [30]. Studies have also linked cadmium levels to seasons, where lower levels have been detected in the summer months [63,72], potentially due to the shorter biological half-life of cadmium as the temperature increases during summer [63]. However, the effect of season was inconclusive in another study [31].

The tissue hydration and water content of the crab have significant effects on the levels of cadmium measured in the crab—particularly when considering that a lot of trade involves live transport of crabs. This has significant implications for obtaining accurate measurements of cadmium in crabs, as once taken from its environment the animal will begin to lose water content. For live export, it is important that the crabs are in a suitable environment as they are osmoconformers and, therefore, are reliant on their external environment to maintain body fluid osmolarity [77]. The longer the crab is out of the water before testing and consumption, the more likely the cadmium is to concentrate. However, it should be noted that only some water loss in the interior organs can be tolerated before the crab dies and is no longer suitable for human consumption. Indeed, feeding is also an important consideration for export, as the hepatopancreas and the reproductive tissue may fill the crab's entire body or may dwindle during periods of poor feeding [78]. These changes in biological condition can, in turn, affect the overall relative levels of cadmium in laboratory samples during testing. Therefore, there are potentially discrepancies in testing for cadmium, as various laboratories will have different schedules for testing and follow different butchering, sample preparation, and testing protocols, and crab samples may be in storage for a considerable amount of time prior to testing. This is an important consideration for the transport of live crabs that are often traded from European countries such as Ireland and Scotland to Asian regions such as the PRC and Hong Kong, where crabs may have to wait at ports to be tested [17,21]. However, it should be noted that Wiech, Frantzen, Duinker, Rasinger, and Maage [31] did not note an association between condition and cadmium levels.

The rates of uptake of cadmium in crustaceans appear to increase according to metal concentration, but are also determined by various other factors, including the uptake rates of other metals, such as zinc [79]. Indeed, it seems that even acute exposure to cadmium can result in an increase in its accumulation [80]. This implies that even a localised increase in cadmium levels in an area supporting the habitat of crabs could affect the levels of cadmium in the crabs, even over a short period of time. This is particularly concerning considering the long biological half-life of cadmium in the kidneys (10–30 years) [81]. Heavy industry can contribute to the geospatial occurrence of cadmium in fishing grounds, particularly around the mouths of some large European rivers [82]. Certainly, there is evidence of geospatial cadmium accumulation in crabs, as demonstrated by the higher cadmium levels in brown crabs in the north of Norway versus the south [31].

It is important to note that the crabs themselves may not always be unscathed by acute exposure. A study by Zhu et al. [83] determined that cadmium exposure induced the expression of stress-related genes and histological alterations in the gills and hepatopancreas of mud crabs (*Scylla paramamosain*). However, this was a laboratory experiment with cadmium levels ranging from 0 to 60 mg/L. Therefore, it is important to determine how relevant these experiments are to real-world situations. For instance, the study neglected to include another arm to examine the length of time required for the crab tissues to heal or return to homeostasis and to measure the internal cadmium uptake in relation to the pathology observed; however, in any case, their findings are a cause for concern. Another study found that 24 h of acute exposure to cadmium in Chinese mitten crabs (*Eriocheir japonica sinensis*) led to transcriptomic differences in the expression of genes relating to the immune and antioxidant defence functions of the crab [84]. These are not the only studies to investigate cadmium toxicity in crabs, as there is concern that cadmium may affect their reproductive capacity [85]. Likewise, a study in other crustaceans—crayfish (*Procambarus clarkii*)—indicated that cadmium may alter their gut histology and the function of their gut microbiota [86,87]. However, some species of crab may adopt mechanisms to mitigate cadmium toxicity. One study showed that the hepatopancreas of freshwater crabs (*Sinopotamon henanense*) altered the expression of a considerable amount of miRNAs in response to acute and subchronic cadmium exposure, which is thought to be an adaptive mechanism to prevent oxidative stress [88].

Considering that there may be histological and transcriptomic changes specific to cadmium exposure, there is the potential to develop rapid diagnostics to determine whether crabs have been exposed to cadmium. Although speculative, lateral flow tests akin to pregnancy tests in their operation could be designed for the detection of stress proteins related to cadmium exposure using haemolymph or another biological fluid. Such a test could be conducted on live crabs at sea, allowing for the release of the crab should an issue be detected. Further research is required to determine whether there are unique signatures in brown crabs that correlate with exposure to cadmium and could be leveraged to improve the industry. An alternative approach to mitigate cadmium levels in crabs is to alter the cooking process. One study has suggested that temperature and ultrasound could be used to reduce cadmium levels in crabs during the cooking process [89]. Such technology could be optimised to reduce cadmium levels in pre-packaged products such as cooked canned crab. Indeed, developing novel testing capacities or processing steps to reduce cadmium levels in crab products is necessary to save time and money and protect consumer health. Another potential way to reduce the risk of capturing cadmium-laden crabs is to carry out biomonitoring of other crabs or, indeed, other flora and fauna for cadmium bioaccumulation or related effects. For example, one could monitor the spermatozoa of *Mytilus galloprovincialis* for conformational alterations of protamine-like proteins, which have been shown to change as a result of cadmium exposure, potentially acting as early sentinels for the health of the environment [90]. However, this approach may be limited to crabs that are present close to the intertidal zone and may not be relevant to crabs that migrate far from the habitats of *Mytilus galloprovincialis*.

In summary, the sampling and analysis of cadmium in crabs is important, and there can be significant health and economic consequences if not properly conducted; hence, the necessity for standardised sampling, butchery, and analysis of cadmium in brown crabs. However, standardisation of protocols and even limits of cadmium in crabs is not consistent or uniform worldwide, even between trading nations.

5. Cadmium and Human Health

5.1. Cadmium Exposure in Humans

Understanding all possible routes of human cadmium exposure is important to consider when assessing one's risk of excessive exposure. Cadmium exposure occurs through three possible routes: dermal, gastrointestinal, or pulmonary. Inhalation of cadmium by industrial workers or smokers is a significant exposure risk, but for the general population of non-smokers, exposure most commonly occurs via ingestion of contaminated foods or water [91]. Previously, it was suggested that atmospheric changes in cadmium levels due to increased pollution may affect blood cadmium levels. However, a recent study found that ingestion of dietary cadmium has a stronger impact on blood cadmium levels [92], likely due to the biomagnification of cadmium in dietary sources versus occasional acute exposure from atmospheric pollution. Therefore, it is important to consider dietary sources of cadmium, which may contain excessive cadmium, so that people and public health authorities can decide whether to mitigate excessive cadmium exposure risk by eliminating or reducing these food sources in the diet. Notably, cadmium is found ubiquitously in nature, and not all anthropogenic sources are the result of industrial emissions. For example, it has been documented that metal pollution can occur due to mining, aquaculture, wastewater treatment, crop farming, and animal breeding [93,94].

Diet is the most prevalent source of cadmium exposure in the general population, and it is also a source that can be mitigated to reduce cadmium exposure. It is estimated that daily dietary cadmium intake in unpolluted European areas can vary from 0.1 to 0.45 µg/kg bodyweight. However, in polluted areas, the total intake may be significantly more than the tolerable daily cadmium intake and reach several hundred µg/day [95,96]. This has major implications when considering the overall intake of cadmium from various foods, which tends to govern what limits are applied to the cadmium content of foods intended for human consumption. Lifestyle choices are certainly one of the biggest determinants of cadmium exposure. Smoking is a significant modifiable risk factor for cadmium exposure, as the tobacco plant accumulates cadmium from the soil into its leaves with great efficiency [97]. The United States national geometric mean blood cadmium level for non-smoking adults is 0.47 µg/L, whereas the mean of smokers is approximately thrice as high at 1.58 µg/L [98]. Smoking is estimated to at least double the body burden of cadmium exposure in one's lifetime. Cadmium oxide (CdO) is a highly bioavailable form of cadmium that is responsible for the high concentrations of cadmium in the blood, urine, and tissues of smokers compared with non-smokers [99,100].

Whether there are specific foods that one should avoid, or dietary alterations required to reduce a person's exposure to dietary cadmium is a topic of interest. The European Food Safety Authority (EFSA) noted that it is not the foods with the highest cadmium levels but, rather, the foods that are consumed in larger quantities most often that have the largest impact on dietary exposure to cadmium [1]. EFSA, using the food description and classification system FoodEx, determined that dietary cadmium exposure in European populations mainly originated from grains and grain-derived products (26.9%), vegetables and vegetable products (16.0%), and starchy roots and tubers (13.2%). In more detail, the following food categories contributed the most to dietary cadmium exposure across all age groups: potatoes (13.2%), bread and rolls (11.7%), fine bakery goods (5.1%), chocolate products (4.3%), leafy vegetables (3.9%), and molluscs (3.2%). However, it was noted that crustaceans were among a group of foods that exceeded 100 µg/kg, along with algal formulations, cocoa powder, offal, some seafood, mushrooms, and water molluscs [20]. Lifetime cadmium dietary exposure for Europeans is estimated to be approximately 2 µg/kg bodyweight/week (averaged for all age groups)—within the EFSA's tolerable weekly intake (TWI) of 2.5 µg/kg bodyweight/week.

In Ireland, weekly adult intake of cadmium has been estimated to be between 1.1 and 2.5 µg/kg bodyweight/week, which is between 44 and 62% of the EFSA's TWI [101]. These findings indicate that the majority of Irish people are not exposed to excess dietary cadmium levels. These findings are supported by the National Adult Nutrition Survey, which examined urinary cadmium excretion in the general population They and that 95% of participants had urinary cadmium levels below the 1 µg cadmium/g creatinine that the EFSA has deemed safe [102]. The main cadmium-contributing foods in the Irish diet were cereals (39%), vegetables (36%), and dairy (12%), where fish and shellfish only accounted for approximately 1% [101], likely due to the low consumption of fish and shellfish in Ireland.

In the United States, a recent study was conducted to determine the intake and sources of cadmium [103]. The average intake of dietary cadmium in the general population was 4.6 µg/day, or 0.54 µg/kg body weight/week—that is, approximately 22% of the tolerable weekly intake (TWI), which is considered to be 2.5 µg/kg body weight/week. However, certain demographics—such as elderly men, those who were well-educated and had a high income, and those with high adiposity—had higher levels of cadmium intake [103]. The food groups that contributed the most to the majority of the cadmium intake in the United States were cereals and bread (34%), leafy vegetables (20%), potatoes (11%), legumes and nuts (7%), and root vegetables (6%). Notably, the individual foods that contributed the most to the overall cadmium intake included lettuce (14%), spaghetti (8%), bread (7%), and potatoes (6%) (Figure 3A).

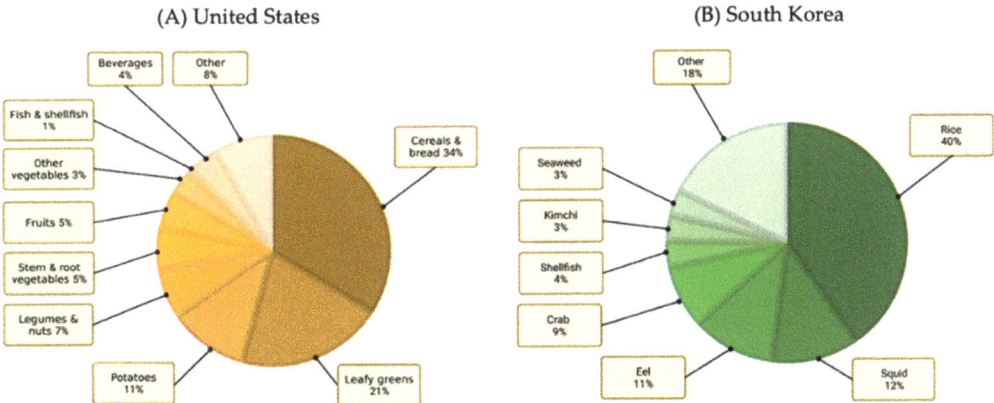

Figure 3. (**A**) The estimated contribution of major food components to cadmium intake as a percentage of total daily intake among a United States cohort of 12,523 aged 2 years and above in the NHANES 2007–2012 study, adapted from [103]. (**B**) The estimated percentage of the major food components contributing to daily cumulative cadmium intake in a South Korean cohort of 1245 people, adapted from [26].

Interestingly, but unsurprisingly, due to the many cultures that coexist in the United States, there were ethnic and cultural differences in cadmium intake due to differences in dietary preferences. Lettuce was a major cadmium source for Caucasian and Black populations, whereas tortillas were the main source for Hispanics, and rice was the top contributor to the Asian population. Notably, the trends of cadmium intake in the United States seem to be very similar overall to those in the European Union. This is also unsurprising because despite there being many culinary differences in the foods and cultures of the US and Europe, the prevailing dietary pattern in both regions is the so-called "Western

Diet" characterised by highly processed foods [104]. Amongst the Asian populations of the United States, smoking was the main exposure route for cadmium, followed by dietary exposure [105], which increases one's risk for many non-communicable diseases—including cardiovascular, renal, and pulmonary diseases [104,106]. It is notable that fish and shellfish comprise a low contribution of cadmium to the American diet, but fish consumption is traditionally low in the United States [107].

Looking further afield, there are similarities between the so-called Western countries and Asian countries such as the PRC and South Korea. The average total daily cadmium intake in healthy Koreans is estimated to be 20.8 µg/day [26]. Figure 3B shows the food groups that contribute the most cadmium to the diet in South Korea. Notably, the food groups recorded are starkly different to the food groups associated with higher cadmium exposure in Europe or the United States. In particular, they seem to be culturally relevant. For example, there are much higher levels of rice (40.3%), as was noted in Asian groups from the United States cohort [103], but also higher intake of seafood and specific foods associated with Korean cuisine, such as kimchi and seaweed. Indeed, crab in this case was shown to contribute 8.6% of the cumulative cadmium intake in this South Korean population.

Many parts of the PRC share similar food consumption patterns to South Korea and, thus, similar cadmium exposure [108]. In one study [108], freshwater crab and sea-caught crab samples obtained contained 0.101 ± 0.323 and 0.544 ± 1.203 mg/kg (mean $\pm$ standard deviation) cadmium, respectively, which were estimated to be consumed at 0.7 ± 7.3 and 0.8 ± 8.9 g/day by the general population. This contrasts with rice and wheat, which contain 0.062 ± 0.128 and 0.021 ± 0.026 mg/kg of cadmium and are consumed at 218 ± 174.5 and 145.4 ± 168 g/day (mean $\pm$ standard deviation), respectively. These data show that while it is true that crab contains higher concentrations of cadmium in mg/kg weight, its consumption levels are markedly different. A further examination of the specific food groups contributing dietary cadmium to the Chinese population is presented in Table 2. The interesting point of this research is that for the high-exposure subpopulation with cadmium exposure higher than the 95th percentile, rice was the largest contributor (58.6%), followed by shellfish (13.2%), and leafy vegetables (9.2%). This is a very small sub-fraction of the population that are exposed to such high levels of cadmium because of their dietary choices; it would be interesting to break down the subcategory of shellfish further to determine the impact that crab may have on the consumption of cadmium in this cohort. The study determined that the mean dietary cadmium exposure of the general Chinese population was 15.3 µg/kg body weight/month (30.6 µg/day for a 60 kg average body weight of adults). A similar study in Shanghai found that the average exposure to dietary and environmental cadmium was 167 µg/day (34% of the PTDI). Similarly, vegetables and rice were the main sources of dietary cadmium, and tobacco accounted for 25% of the total cadmium exposure from non-occupational sources [109]. Considering that almost 20% of agricultural soil in the PRC is contaminated with cadmium [110], it is likely that their dietary exposure to cadmium will only increase with their growing economy. Furthermore, the daily exposure to dietary cadmium in the Chinese population is significantly higher than that in either Europe or the United States.

The total diet study (TDS) is a food safety monitoring program that is conducted by various food agencies, including the United States Food and Drug Administration (FDA), the Food Standards of Australia and New Zealand (FSANZ), and the European Food Safety Agency (EFSA) [111]. These are "market basket surveys" that collection of various food samples from groceries and retailers for the quantitation of food additives, pesticide residues, contaminants, nutrients and, of course, heavy metals [112,113]. The TDS provides a realistic approach to gauge the relative contribution of each food group and specific item to estimate the total intake of cadmium in the diet. Foods that were consumed in large quantities at high frequency contributed the most to cadmium intake [111]. Currently, TDS data are available for a limited number of countries, including Australia, the United States, France, Spain, Sweden, Chile, Denmark, and Serbia [100]. Overall, data from TDS show that these countries' cadmium intake varies between 8 and 25 µg/day for the average consumer with staple foods (e.g., rice, wheat, and potatoes), which accounted for 40–60% of total dietary cadmium ingestion. Shellfish, crustaceans, molluscs, offal, and spinach were considered to be additional cadmium sources [100,111]. These types of studies are often thought to underestimate dietary cadmium, as they fail to demonstrate an association between estimated cadmium intake and the incidence of cancer and bone diseases [114–117].

Table 2. Data depicting the main contributors to dietary cadmium intake in (A) the general Chinese population and (B) the highly exposed Chinese population. Data adapted with permission from [108].

General Population (A)		High-Exposure Population (B) *	
Food Group	Percentage (%) Contribution of Dietary Cadmium Intake	Food Group	Percentage (%) Contribution of Dietary Cadmium Intake
Rice	55.8	Rice	58.6
Leafy vegetables	10.5	Leafy vegetables	9.2
Wheat flour	11.8	Wheat flour	2
Shellfish	4.8	Shellfish	13.2
Meat	2.6	Meat	2
Seaweed	2.4	Seaweed	6.4
Other vegetables	2.4	Other vegetables	1.4
Other cereals	2.1	Other cereals	0.9
Root and stalk vegetables	2.0	Root and stalk vegetables	1.7
Mushrooms	1.1	Mushrooms	1.5
Fish	1.1	Fish	1
Legumes	0.9	Legumes	0.6
Fruits	0.6	Fruits	0.4
Eggs	0.6	Eggs	0.2
Nuts	0.4	Nuts	0.4
Offal	0.4	Offal	0.2
Other	0.5	Other	0.3

* The highly exposed population was determined to be those within the 95th percentile of the mean dietary cadmium exposure of the general Chinese population.

Overall, these epidemiological and dietary studies demonstrate that dietary cadmium exposure is affected by many factors and that the main contributor of dietary cadmium in all instances around the world mostly originates from staple foods such as rice, wheat, and other grains. In Asian diets, seafood and shellfish were contributors to dietary cadmium intake, but this is not necessarily the main source in countries that consume Western diets. Overall, it seems that it is important to strike a balance and be cautious of foods that are potentially significant contributors of cadmium to the diet. Indeed, moderate consumption of shellfish should not significantly affect one's risk of illness from cadmium ingestion, but further research specific to crab consumption is required.

5.2. Cadmium Ingestion and Accumulation in Humans

Depending on the exact dose and nutritional composition of a food, the human gastrointestinal tract can take up 3–5% of ingested cadmium [20,118]. Various factors can affect cadmium uptake in humans, such as low intakes of calcium, vitamin D, zinc, and copper [91]. One possible mechanism of high cadmium resorption is related to the assumption that cadmium shares molecular homology with zinc and calcium; as a result, low levels of these minerals are compensated by higher cadmium resorption [119]. This observation was closely replicated in competitive resorption studies in rats against other polyvalent cations such as Cr^{3+}, Mg, Ni, Pb, and Sr [120]. Notably, a low zinc/iron status in individuals who subsist on diets characterised by high rice intake may cause high absorption of cadmium in contrast to other staple diets [121]. Other factors that affect cadmium uptake include gender, nutritional status, diet, and smoking status can also affect the bioavailability of cadmium in humans [68].

Indeed, various human studies show that cadmium intake can be increased by dietary fibre intake [96]. Animal experiments have shown that diets with high concentrations of protein and lipids can also increase net intestinal uptake of cadmium and that diets high in wheat bran may reduce cadmium intake [95]. The exact mechanisms of these effects on cadmium intake are yet to be fully elucidated. On the other hand, cadmium can bind to low-molecular-weight proteins rich in cysteine such as metallothionein, which may increase its bioavailability [122]. This has been demonstrated naturally in various marine organisms where cadmium seems to be bound to small, soluble cytoplasmic proteins, including in oysters, mussels, scallops [122], and green crab (*Carcinus maenas*) [62,63,123]. In rat studies, cadmium binds to amino acids and peptides in the intestinal tract [124], which undoubtedly has implications for its bioavailability. What these studies suggest is that these effects may be the result of a food matrix effect in a similar way to dairy products, where nutrients are more or less bioavailable depending on the food's structure and composition [125]. This implies that the foods or ingredients that we mix with foods containing high cadmium levels may affect the overall bioavailability of cadmium. Therefore, it may be possible to mitigate cadmium's bioavailability when preparing foods that may have higher levels of cadmium by altering the food matrix. However, research is very limited in this area, and further studies are required to confirm such associations.

Evidence from animal studies shows that marginal deficiencies in zinc, iron, and calcium can enhance the absorption, organ accumulation, and retention of dietary cadmium [121]. Moreover, marginal deficiencies can enhance cadmium absorption as much as 10-fold in diets containing low cadmium concentrations similar to those consumed by some human populations, indicating that people who are nutritionally marginal with respect to zinc, iron, and calcium are at higher risk of cadmium-related diseases than those who are nutritionally adequate [126–128]. Indeed, similar studies in humans show that an individual's iron levels may be a metabolic factor of concern in the resorption of cadmium. It has been demonstrated that a lack of iron leads to a 6% higher uptake of cadmium in individuals with normal iron levels [129]. A study of iron-deficient children in the United States found elevated blood cadmium levels [130]. This accounts for higher cadmium absorption in individuals with a habitual iron deficit (e.g., children or menstruating women) or people with anaemia [91]. It seems that these observations are the result of the expression of DCT-1 and MTP1—metal ion transporters in the gastrointestinal tract that act as a gate for cadmium resorption when low iron levels occur [131,132]. Overall, the evidence presented supports the notion that dietary components and trace element status can affect the fractional intestinal uptake of cadmium, as reviewed by Andersen et al. [95].

These findings hint at the possibility of ensuring that individuals who may be at high risk of exposure to cadmium have a healthy nutritional status. Those who may be deficient in some minerals may consider dietary alterations or dietary supplements to ameliorate mineral deficiencies.

5.3. Cadmium's Transport, Bioavailability, and Excretion in Humans

Cadmium is well-known for its toxicity to humans, as evidenced by decades of observational studies and research. Like many heavy metals, bioaccumulation of cadmium in mammals can differentially affect certain tissues, including bone, the liver, muscle, and the kidneys. Indeed, Cd^{2+} is dangerous in that it can substitute for Zn in enzyme structures. Likewise, calcium and cadmium have similar ionic radii (109 pm and 114 pm, respectively), meaning that cadmium can accumulate in the bone along with calcium [133].

Once taken up by the gastrointestinal tract and deposited into the bloodstream, cadmium binds to proteins such as albumin and metallothionein. From there, it is transported to the liver, where cadmium can induce the production of metallothionein. Following the necrosis and apoptosis of hepatocytes, cadmium–metallothionein (Cd–M) complexes form, which are washed from sinusoidal blood. Some cadmium then enters the enterohepatic cycle via secretion into the biliary tract in the form of cadmium–glutathione conjugates. Cadmium can then be enzymatically degraded to cadmium–cysteine complexes in the biliary tree, where it can re-enter the small intestine [91,134]. Cadmium accumulates in the renal tubular cells in the cortex of the kidneys via the transport of metallothionein. It resides there, where it can have a half-life of 10–30 years [135]. Lifelong exposure to and consumption of foods containing cadmium can lead to the accumulation of cadmium, and as it is very slowly excreted from the body, it causes irreversible tubular cell necrosis in the kidneys [91]. Unfortunately, the kidneys are the organs most susceptible to damage from cadmium accumulation [136], although chronic and prolonged exposure to cadmium can have devastating effects on various tissues of the human body and can even cause bone demineralisation [137]. When cadmium arrives at the kidneys in the form of Cd–M, it is filtered in the glomerulus and reabsorbed in the proximal convoluted tubules, where it tends to remain [91].

Cadmium concentrations can be measured in urine, hair, blood, nail, and saliva samples. Cadmium-induced kidney damage correlates with urinary cadmium excretion. Indeed, proteinuria characterised by the excretion of low-molecular-weight proteins such as retinol-binding protein or ß$_2$-microglobulin [138] is likely to occur with a 10% response rate when the concentration of cadmium in the cortex exceeds approximately 200 µg/g wet weight (200 ppm) [135]. Moreover, urinary cadmium has been used as a non-invasive detection method of the accumulation of cadmium in the kidneys, and as a marker of tubular dysfunction in industrial workers and those who have had low environmental exposure. This is due to the curvilinear relationship between urinary cadmium and cadmium accumulation in the kidneys [118,139]. This allows for the urinary cadmium value corresponding to the critical kidney cadmium level of 200 ppm to be estimated at 10 µg/g creatinine, which is estimated in concordance with the relationship between urinary cadmium and proteinuria [138,140,141]. These measurements are now well-established and, in populations with excessive exposure to cadmium, urinary cadmium is correlated with the renal cadmium levels or body burden. Worryingly, these levels remain elevated many years after cessation of exposure [142].

While measuring ß$_2$-microglobulin was previously thought to be the most reliable and accepted method of measuring cadmium burden and levels in humans, there are several other urinary biomarkers for the assessment of the renal effects of cadmium. A significant debate about the utility of these various biomarkers is ongoing [111]. These markers are outlined in Table 3 as per the publication of Satarug [111]. The associated renal biological effects are also enclosed in Table 3. These biomarkers are currently being used to assess the impacts of seafood and crab consumption on human health [143,144].

Table 3. Urinary biomarkers for the assessment of cadmium burden on the kidneys. Adapted from Satarug [111].

Biomarkers	Abnormal Values	Interpretations and Associations
NAG	>4 U/g creatinine	Tubular injury, mortality
Lysozyme	>4 mg/g creatinine	Tubular injury
Total protein	>100 mg/g creatinine	Glomerular dysfunction, CKD
Albumin	>30 mg/g creatinine	Glomerular dysfunction, CKD
ß$_2$MG	≥1000 µg/g creatinine	Irreversible tubular dysfunction
ß$_2$-MG	≥300 µg/g creatinine	Mild tubular dysfunction, rapid GFR decline
ß$_2$-MG	≥145 µg/g creatinine	Increased hypertension risk
α1-MG	≥400 µg/g creatinine	Mild tubular dysfunction
α1-MG	≥1500 µg/g creatinine	Irreversible tubular dysfunction
KIM-1	≥1.6 mg/g creatinine in men ≥2.4 mg/g creatinine in women	Kidney injury, urinary KIM-1 levels correlated with blood cadmium levels

Abbreviations: NAG = N-acetyl-β-D-glucosaminidinase; ß$_2$-MG = beta-2 microglobulin; α1-MG = α1-microglobulin; KIM-1 = kidney injury molecule-1; CKD = chronic kidney disease; GFR = glomerular filtration rate.

An interesting in vivo study assessed the bioavailability of cadmium from boiled crab hepatopancreas, inorganic cadmium, or dried wild mushroom fed to mice [145]. The study design included a control group of mice that received low levels of cadmium (<0.007 ppm) in their feed, which did not lead to detectable levels of cadmium over a 9-week exposure period. The authors used cadmium accumulation in the kidneys and liver as a measure of absorption. Notably, the bioavailability of cadmium from boiled crab hepatopancreas was lower than that of cadmium from mushroom or even inorganic cadmium. Cadmium in the crab hepatopancreas is mainly associated with denatured proteins with low solubility, whereas a large proportion of cadmium in dried mushroom is associated with soluble ligands. Therefore, there was an indication that the difference in cadmium speciation might account for the lower bioavailability of cadmium from crab than from mushroom. However, the authors commented that the difference in bioavailability was low, and that restricting intake was recommended if the products were high in cadmium. This may be evidence of cadmium speciation or, indeed, a food matrix effect. A similar study in which rats consumed a diet consisting of high crab intake (4 mg/kg organic-bound cadmium), a low-crab diet (0.2 mg/kg organic-bound cadmium), or a casein-based cadmium diet (4 mg/kg as cadmium chloride) for 6 months showed that cadmium intake from the high-crab diet was only half that of the diet consisting of cadmium chloride [146]. These findings also appear to indicate that there may be a food matrix effect at play. Other studies in humans have shown that cadmium is more bioaccessible from fish (84%) than from shellfish (73%) [147]. Worryingly, individuals who smoke cigarettes and have a high consumption of seafood can experience exacerbated adverse effects of cadmium exposure [147]. This is particularly dangerous for populations such as the PRC, where many of the people smoke frequently. There are still many questions regarding cadmium's bioavailability that require further investigation, particularly regarding the food matrix effect and how it may be leveraged to mitigate dietary cadmium intake.

Another point to note is that current health risk assessments relating to cadmium exposure in humans rely heavily on the evaluation of the toxicity to the kidneys alone. In 2010, the Joint Food and Agriculture Organisation (FAO) and World Health Organisation (WHO) Expert Committee on Food Additives and Contaminants (JECFA) deemed the kidneys to be a suitable target for evaluating cadmium toxicity, as measurements of $ß_2$-microglobulin could be used as a surrogate biomarker for the effects of dietary cadmium intake [148]. The JECFA established a tolerable monthly intake of 25 µg/kg/bodyweight per month, with a urinary cadmium excretion rate of 5.24 µg/g creatinine or 0.8 µg/kg/day as a nephrotoxicity threshold [148–150]. While the EFSA and JECFA share the same critical $ß_2$-microglobulin endpoint of 300 µg/g creatinine, the EFSA adopted a different cadmium excretion rate of 1 µg/g creatinine as the nephrotoxicity threshold, along with an uncertainty factor of 0.36 µg/kg bodyweight per day for 50 years as a benchmark dose [151]. While these values are important references to monitor to stay within safe levels of cadmium exposure, relying on one biomarker ($ß_2$-microglobulin) is insufficient. In 2019, Satarug et al. [152] showed that $ß_2$-microglobulin excretion levels as low as 100–299 µg/g creatinine were associated with a 4.7-fold increase in eGFR to $\leq$60 mL/min/1.73 m^2—a measurement consistent with chronic kidney disease. Therefore, a $ß_2$-microglobulin endpoint of 300 µg/g creatinine may not be a low enough threshold to detect early nephrotoxicity [149].

Considering the emerging evidence that many organ systems are affected by cadmium exposure, other toxicity endpoints may be informative for risk assessment. As reviewed by Satarug et al. [149], other biomarkers of chronic low-dose cadmium exposure may contribute to risk assessments. For example, reductions in estimated glomerular filtration rate (eGFR) and lower fecundity have been observed at cadmium excretion levels as low as 0.5 µg/g creatinine, with worsening outcomes noted in a dose-dependent manner [149]. In men, sperm cadmium levels are inversely associated with sperm motility [153,154] and appear to be associated with other measures of sperm quality, viability, and acrosome reactions [149]. In females, high blood cadmium levels have been associated with infertility [155]. High urinary cadmium levels (~0.70 µg/L) have been associated with ovarian reserve depletion and ovarian insufficiency, with serum follicle-stimulating hormone (FSH) levels $\geq$ 10 IU/L [156] and $\geq$25 IU/L [157], respectively. However, sampling and monitoring of reproductive health is intrusive and inconvenient; therefore, surrogate markers such as serum FSH or anti-Mullerian hormone (AMH) in females may be useful. Blood biomarkers are preferred because of the convenience of analysing a blood sample. Therefore, alternative approaches have been sought, including monitoring of epigenetic factors [158]. Preliminary research indicates that cadmium exposure induces epigenetic changes in micro ribonucleic acids (miRNAs) that may lead to the development of novel blood-borne biomarkers [159,160]. Collectively, these findings indicate that additional novel biomarkers of human cadmium exposure are necessary to determine one's risk of toxicity and disease, as opposed to the reliance on monitoring kidney function alone.

5.4. Cadmium Toxicity in Humans

Cadmium can affect important cellular functions such as cell differentiation, proliferation, and apoptosis, which is of concern considering that these processes overlap with the important processes of the generation of reactive oxygen species (ROS) and DNA repair mechanisms [81]. Cadmium at low concentrations even has the capacity to bind to mitochondria and can inhibit cellular oxidative phosphorylation and cellular respiration [161]. Cadmium exposure results in chromosomal aberrations, DNA strand breaks, sister chromatid exchange, and DNA–protein crosslinks. Cadmium can potentially cause mutations and chromosomal deletions [162]. Cadmium toxicity encompasses the depletion of reduced glutathione (GSH), binds sulfhydryl groups with proteins, and causes the enhanced production of ROS, resulting in oxidative stress, which may promote organ toxicity, apoptotic cell death, and carcinogenicity [81]. Cadmium can also inhibit the capacity of the natural antioxidant enzymes, such as catalase, manganese superoxide dismutase, and copper/zinc-dismutase [163]. Metallothionein is also involved in these processes and can act as a free-radical scavenger of hydroxyl and superoxide radicals [164]. Largely, the cells that contain metallothioneins are resilient to the effects of cadmium toxicity. However, it has been observed that cells that do not synthesise metallothioneins are sensitive to cadmium [81].

Cadmium has also been shown to be an endocrine disruptor. Cadmium may affect thyroid function, as demonstrated in both animal and human studies [165], where tissue damage in the thyroid led to hyperplasia and hypertrophy [166–168]. Moreover, cadmium has been linked with changes in hormone function [169,170], and there is suspicion that chronic cadmium exposure may lead to thyroid cancer, but further research is required [171]. Cadmium may also act as a metalloestrogen, as it can bind to the oestrogen receptor [172], which has led to a concern that chronic cadmium exposure may be associated with breast cancer [173–175]. There have also been links drawn between cadmium and the inhibition of progesterone synthesis, ovarian and reproductive tract morphological alterations, disruption to menstrual cycles, and issues with pregnancy and birth [176]. Likewise, cadmium may mimic some of the effects of androgens and may play a role in prostate cancer [177,178] and reduce male fertility by affecting spermatogenesis and motility [179].

The vast and various effects of cadmium exposure on the human body that have been explored in the previous sections lead to various clinical manifestations. As such, it is known that different forms of cadmium compounds lead to different clinical manifestations. However, the details of this require further investigation. While cadmium poisoning is very rare, it can happen. Itai-itai disease is the most severe form of chronic cadmium toxicity in humans, caused by the prolonged ingestion of cadmium. Areas severely polluted by cadmium, such as the Jinzu River Basin in Toyama, Japan, have high incidences of cadmium-related pathologies. In that example, the river was polluted with slag from a mine upstream. The cadmium-polluted water was subsequently used to irrigate crops and rice between the 1910s and 1960s. The water from this river was used as potable water and for cooking, bathing, etc. [25]. This was significant, as cadmium is a food-chain contaminant that has high rates of soil-to-plant transference [111] and, thus, a high risk of ingestion. Itai-itai disease is characterised by renal tubular disorder and renal osteomalacia [180]. Even if people did not get itai-itai disease in the Jinzu Basin, they were at serious risk of cancer [181]. Some of the main effects of cadmium on the human body are presented in Figure 4. Patients with cadmium toxicity require significant treatment, including gastrointestinal tract irrigation, supportive care, and chemical decontamination via traditional chelation therapy with novel chelating agents and nanoparticle-based antidotes [81].

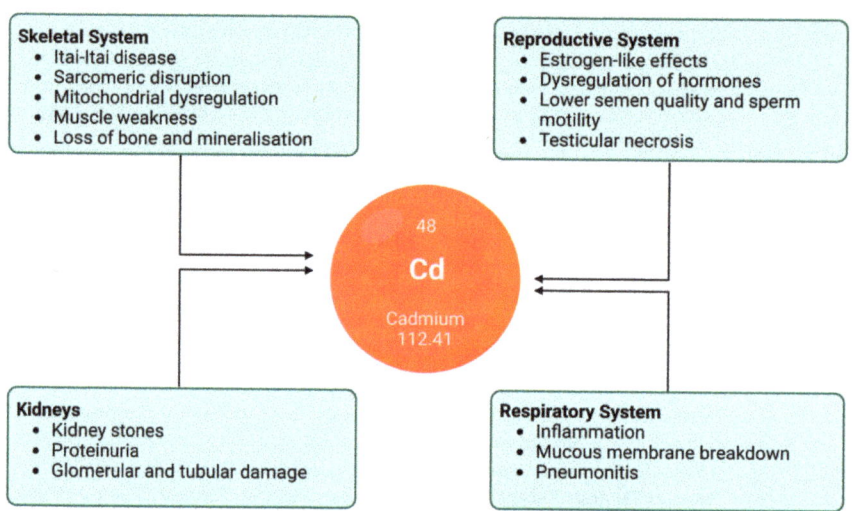

Figure 4. An illustration depicting the effects of chronic cadmium exposure on various human organs and systems. While not an exclusive list, this figure demonstrates the importance of mitigating excess cadmium ingestion.

6. Crab Consumption, Cadmium, and Human Health

There are limited studies that have investigated the effects of crab consumption on cadmium ingestion and human health. A recent study examined whether regular crab meat consumers exhibited increased levels of ß$_2$-microglobulin or cadmium in their urine compared to those who did not eat crab meat [143]. They determined that whole blood cadmium levels can be both a short- and long-term marker of cadmium intake. However, while it was expected that cadmium levels would be elevated in the crab meat consumers, the study showed that crab meat consumers did not show increased levels of urinary cadmium and, consistent with this, showed no changes in cadmium-induced kidney toxicity markers. Consequently, the authors concluded that compared to consumers who reported very little crab meat consumption, healthy middle-aged consumers who regularly consumed brown crab meat products (an average of 447 g/week) for an average of 16 years showed no changes in long-term cadmium exposure or kidney toxicity. A study of French seafood consumers demonstrated that the mean dietary ingestion of cadmium was 2.4 ± 3.3 mg/kg bodyweight/week. The authors also determined that the mean urinary cadmium level was 0.65 ± 0.45 mg/g creatinine, and was significantly higher in women than in men. This is particularly interesting, as sexual dimorphism was observed in populations of Japan who suffered itai-itai disease, where women generally had a more severe prognosis [100].

In the United States, the Long Island Study of Seafood Consumption, conducted in New York, examined the relationship between seafood intake and blood cadmium levels in 252 people who were avid seafood consumers [182]. After the researchers adjusted for age, BMI, sex, smoking status, and other factors, a linear regression model was employed. They determined that there was no association with regular seafood intake ($\beta = -0.01; p = 0.11$) but did identify an association between salmon intake in cups/week (ln transformed)

(β = 0.20; p = 0.001) and blood cadmium levels. The study determined that only salmon was meaningfully associated with blood cadmium levels and that seafood was most likely not a significant source of cadmium exposure. They suggested that as the cadmium levels in salmon are not higher than those in many other seafood species, the association with salmon intake was likely due to higher consumption of salmon within this cohort. A similar study—the Norwegian Fish and Game study—assessed cadmium concentrations in spot urine and blood samples and conducted a food frequency questionnaire (FFQ) with 179 volunteers. The median urinary cadmium level was 0.16 µg/L when corrected for creatinine, and the median (5th to 95th percentile) blood cadmium level was 0.45 µg/L. According to the FFQ, 24% of individuals designated as high cadmium consumers and 8% of the controls (i.e., those with lower levels of cadmium in the diet) had intakes above the TWI. Notably, there was an association between high cadmium levels and seafood consumption, which was thought to be partially driven by crab consumption [183]. This may be unsurprising, as both white and brown crab meat is consumed in Norway and is a contributor of cadmium to the diets of Norwegian seafood consumers [28].

Considering these collective findings and some of the mechanisms of cadmium's bioavailability discussed in this review, it is likely that while it is necessary to monitor cadmium levels in foods, these levels may not directly translate to 1:1 absorption from the bioavailable cadmium pool. It is likely that the food matrix also plays a considerable role in cadmium's bioavailability. As discussed previously, the preparation of crab may also play a significant role in the cadmium levels of crab for consumption [30]. Finally, it is likely that the health and nutritional status of the individual consuming the product, along with various other factors, contribute to whether a person is at risk of cadmium bioaccumulation and associated negative health effects.

7. Conclusions

Trace cadmium is naturally present in the food chain due to its ubiquitous presence in nature. Some food sources, including crustaceans such as the brown crab, naturally bioaccumulate cadmium and, therefore, are thought to pose a health risk. However, cadmium exposure from dietary sources may be mitigated by individuals and public health authorities by limiting exposure. As discussed in this review, evidence supports the notion that moderate consumption of brown crab is unlikely to pose a significant health risk when one's lifestyle and dietary choices offer little risk of excessive cadmium exposure. In particular, evidence supports the safe consumption of white crab meat due to its low cadmium levels and other beneficial health benefits, including its role as a source of protein and omega-3 fatty acids. On the other hand, the brown meat containing the hepatopancreas does have high levels of cadmium, but this is unlikely to pose a significant health threat if the brown meat is consumed in low amounts. However, regular consumption of the brown meat is not recommended until further dietary research deems frequent consumption safe. Finally, as discussed, there are discrepancies and various interpretations of adequate testing for cadmium in crab products in the industry. Furthermore, the sampling, butchery, and analysis of brown crab would appear to vary from region to region. Differences in legislation and interpretation of cadmium's risks have led to rifts in the export trade of live crabs between Europe and Asia, which have caused significant issues to trade for exporters such as Ireland and the United Kingdom. This review also raises questions regarding how legislation is put forward and what are the most reasonable assessments to make when considering individual and public health risks. Collective agreement on how to determine cadmium risk factors and the standardisation of crab monitoring are required to ensure a safe and equitable crab market internationally.

Author Contributions: Conceptualisation, R.L. and I.Z.; methodology, R.L.; software, R.L.; investigation, R.L.; writing—original draft preparation, R.L.; writing—review and editing, R.L. and I.Z.; visualisation, R.L.; project administration, R.L.; funding acquisition, R.L. and I.Z. All authors have read and agreed to the published version of the manuscript.

Funding: Bord Iascaigh Mhara and the European Maritime and Fisheries Fund (19/SRDP/002).

Acknowledgments: The authors would like to acknowledge the Department of Biological Sciences at the University of Limerick, Ireland, for their continued support. Funding was provided by Bord Iascaigh Mhara and the European Maritime and Fisheries Fund and was used to conduct a report on cadmium levels in Irish brown crab that has been referenced in this review. We would also like to thank members from multiple agencies who guided us in the right direction to seek information for this review, including the South Australian Research and Development Institute (SARDI), Australia; the Department of Agriculture, Water, and the Environment, Residues and Food Branch, Export Division, Queensland, Australia; the Ocean Frontier Institute, Dalhousie University, Nova Scotia, Canada; Canada Health, Ottawa, Canada; the Canadian Food Inspection Agency, Ottawa, Canada; the Department of Agriculture, Food, and the Marine, Dublin, Ireland; John Fagan, Bord Iascaigh Mhara, Dublin, Ireland; and Norah Parke, Killybegs Fishermen's Organisation, Donegal, Ireland.

Conflicts of Interest: Bord Iascaigh Mhara and the European Maritime and Fisheries Fund (19/SRDP/002) requested an independent review of cadmium and crab consumption. The authors are not affiliated with Bord Iascaigh Mhara and declare no other competing interest. The grant providers had no role in the literature collection, analyses, or interpretation of the data, in the writing of the manuscript, or in the decision to publish.

References

1. European Food Safety Authority. Cadmium dietary exposure in the European population. *EFSA J.* **2012**, *10*, 2551. [CrossRef]
2. Schaefer, H.R.; Dennis, S.; Fitzpatrick, S. Cadmium: Mitigation strategies to reduce dietary exposure. *J. Food Sci.* **2020**, *85*, 260–267. [CrossRef] [PubMed]
3. Bolam, T.; Bersuder, P.; Burden, R.; Shears, G.; Morris, S.; Warford, L.; Thomas, B.; Nelson, P. Cadmium levels in food containing crab brown meat: A brief survey from UK retailers. *J. Food Compos. Anal.* **2016**, *54*, 63–69. [CrossRef]
4. Tully, O.; Robinson, M.; O'Keeffe, E.; Cosgrove, R.; Doyle, O.; Lehane, B. The Brown Crab (*Cancer pagurus* L.) fishery: Analysis of the resource in 2004–2005. *Fish. Resour. Ser.* **2006**, *4*, 48.
5. Fahy, E.; Carroll, J.; Stokes, D. *The Inshore Pot Fishery for Brown Crab (Cancer pagurus) Landing into South East Ireland: Estimate of Yield and Assessment of Status*; 0578-7467; Marine Institute: Galway, Ireland, 2002.
6. European Market Observatory for Fisheries and Aquaculture Products. Species Analyses 2014–2018 Edition. Available online: https://www.eumofa.eu/documents/20178/136822/Species+analyses.pdf/26ae5573-7f6c-47e1-b928-7ec5941c8ac8?version=1.0 (accessed on 26 April 2022).
7. Seafood Source. Irish Brown Crab Exports to China Squeezed by New Testing Regime. Available online: https://www.seafoodsource.com/news/food-safety-health/irish-brown-crab-exports-to-china-squeezed-by-new-testing-regime (accessed on 11 April 2020).
8. Seafood Source. Scottish Live Crab Exporters Feel the Pinch of Chinese Cadmium Crackdown. Available online: https://www.seafoodsource.com/news/premium/food-safety-health/scottish-live-crab-exporters-feel-the-pinch-of-chinese-cadmium-crackdown (accessed on 11 April 2020).
9. European Market Observatory for Fisheries and Aquaculture Products. *Brown Crab: COVID-19 Impact of the Supply Chain*; European Market Observatory for Fisheries and Aquaculture Products: Luxembourg, 2021.
10. Centre for Environment F. & Aquaculture Sciences (CEFAS). Survey of Cadmium in Brown Meat from Crabs and Products Made with Brown Meat from Crabs. Available online: https://www.food.gov.uk/research/research-projects/survey-of-cadmium-in-brown-meat-from-crabs-and-products-made-with-brown-meat-from-crabs (accessed on 11 April 2022).
11. Angeletti, R.; Binato, G.; Guidotti, M.; Morelli, S.; Pastorelli, A.A.; Sagratella, E.; Ciardullo, S.; Stacchini, P. Cadmium bioaccumulation in Mediterranean spider crab (*Maya squinado*): Human consumption and health implications for exposure in Italian population. *Chemosphere* **2014**, *100*, 83–88. [CrossRef]
12. Chavez-Crooker, P.; Pozo, P.; Castro, H.; Dice, M.S.; Boutet, I.; Tanguy, A.; Moraga, D.; Ahearn, G.A. Cellular localization of calcium, heavy metals, and metallothionein in lobster (*Homarus americanus*) hepatopancreas. *Comp. Biochem. Physiol. Part C Toxicol. Pharmacol.* **2003**, *136*, 213–224. [CrossRef]
13. Barrento, S.; Marques, A.; Teixeira, B.; Carvalho, M.L.; Vaz-Pires, P.; Nunes, M.L. Accumulation of elements (S, As, Br, Sr, Cd, Hg, Pb) in two populations of *Cancer pagurus*: Ecological implications to human consumption. *Food Chem. Toxicol.* **2009**, *47*, 150–156. [CrossRef] [PubMed]
14. Maulvault, A.L.; Anacleto, P.; Lourenço, H.M.; Carvalho, M.L.; Nunes, M.L.; Marques, A. Nutritional quality and safety of cooked edible crab (*Cancer pagurus*). *Food Chem.* **2012**, *133*, 277–283. [CrossRef]
15. Martin, D.J.; Rainbow, P.S. The kinetics of zinc and cadmium in the haemolymph of the shore crab *Carcinus maenas* (L.). *Aquat. Toxicol.* **1998**, *40*, 203–231. [CrossRef]
16. Market Advisory Council. Testing for Cadmium Levels in Brown Crab Exported to People's Republic of China. Available online: https://marketac.eu/testing-for-cadmium-levels-in-brown-crab-exported-to-peoples-republic-of-china/ (accessed on 11 April 2022).

17. Lordan, R.; Zabetakis, I. Report: Cadmium Mitigation in Brown Crab. In *19/SRDP/002*; Bord Iascaigh Mhara: Dublin, Ireland, 2020.
18. European Commission. Commission Regulation (EU) No 488/2014 of 12 May 2014 Amending Regulation (EC) No 1881/2006 as Regards Maximum Levels of Cadmium in Foodstuffs. Available online: https://leap.unep.org/countries/eu/national-legislation/commission-regulation-eu-no-4882014-amending-regulation-ec-no (accessed on 17 August 2022).
19. European Commission. Commission Regulation (EC) No 1881/2006 of 19 December 2006 setting maximum levels for certain contaminants in foodstuffs. *Off. J. Eur. Union* **2006**, *364*, 5–24.
20. Authority, E.F.S. Cadmium in food-Scientific opinion of the Panel on Contaminants in the Food Chain. *EFSA J.* **2009**, *7*, 980. [CrossRef]
21. Guilbert, S. Brown Crab and the Triple Challenge of Cadmium, Covid, and Brexit. In *University of Exeter-Food System Impacts of COVID-19*; University of Exeter: Exeter, UK, 2021.
22. Seafood Source. Enhanced Food Safety Inspections Bite into Market for Chinese Demand for Irish, UK-Sourced Brown Crab. Available online: https://www.seafoodsource.com/news/premium/food-safety-health/enhanced-food-safety-inspections-bite-into-market-for-chinese-demand-for-irish-uk-sourced-brown-crab (accessed on 12 April 2022).
23. Milligan, G. Edible Crab (Cancer pagurus). 2014. Available online: https://commons.wikimedia.org/wiki/File:Edible_Crab_(Cancer_pagurus).jpg (accessed on 4 September 2022).
24. Bernhoft, R.A. Cadmium toxicity and treatment. *Sci. World J.* **2013**, *2013*, 394652. [CrossRef]
25. Aoshima, K. Itai-itai disease: Lessons from the investigations of environmental epidemiology conducted in the 1970's, with special reference to the studies of the Toyama Institute of Health. *Nihon Eiseigaku Zasshi. Jpn. J. Hyg.* **2017**, *72*, 149–158. [CrossRef]
26. Kim, H.; Lee, J.; Woo, H.D.; Kim, D.W.; Choi, I.J.; Kim, Y.-I.; Kim, J. Association between dietary cadmium intake and early gastric cancer risk in a Korean population: A case–control study. *Eur. J. Nutr.* **2019**, *58*, 3255–3266. [CrossRef] [PubMed]
27. Maulvault, A.L.; Cardoso, C.; Nunes, M.L.; Marques, A. Risk–benefit assessment of cooked seafood: Black scabbard fish (*Aphanopus carbo*) and edible crab (*Cancer pagurus*) as case studies. *Food Control* **2013**, *32*, 518–524. [CrossRef]
28. Knutsen, H.K.; Amlund, H.; Brantsæter, A.L.; Engeset, D.; Fæste, C.K.; Holene, E.; Ruus, A.; Lillegaard, I.; Eriksen, G.S.; Kvalem, H.E. Risk assessment of dietary Cadmium exposure in the Norwegian population. *Eur. J. Nutr. Food Saf.* **2015**, *8*, 157–161. [CrossRef]
29. Turoczy, N.J.; Mitchell, B.D.; Levings, A.H.; Rajendram, V.S. Cadmium, copper, mercury, and zinc concentrations in tissues of the King Crab (Pseudocarcinus gigas) from southeast Australian waters. *Environ. Int.* **2001**, *27*, 327–334. [CrossRef]
30. Wiech, M.; Vik, E.; Duinker, A.; Frantzen, S.; Bakke, S.; Maage, A. Effects of cooking and freezing practices on the distribution of cadmium in different tissues of the brown crab (*Cancer pagurus*). *Food Control* **2017**, *75*, 14–20. [CrossRef]
31. Wiech, M.; Frantzen, S.; Duinker, A.; Rasinger, J.D.; Maage, A. Cadmium in brown crab *Cancer pagurus*. Effects of location, season, cooking and multiple physiological factors and consequences for food safety. *Sci. Total Environ.* **2020**, *703*, 134922. [CrossRef] [PubMed]
32. New York State Department of Health. New York State Blue Crab Cooking & Eating Guide. Available online: https://www.health.ny.gov/publications/6502/index.htm (accessed on 20 August 2022).
33. Ervik, H.; Lierhagen, S.; Asimakopoulos, A.G. Elemental content of brown crab (*Cancer pagurus*)—Is it safe for human consumption? A recent case study from Mausund, Norway. *Sci. Total Environ.* **2020**, *716*, 135175. [CrossRef]
34. Seafood Source. FDA Warns Consumers to Avoid Eating Lobster Tomalley. Available online: https://www.seafoodsource.com/news/food-safety-health/fda-warns-consumers-to-avoid-eating-lobster-tomalley (accessed on 18 August 2022).
35. European Commission. Information Note: Consumption of Brown Crab Meat. Available online: https://food.ec.europa.eu/system/files/2016-10/cs_contaminants_catalogue_information_note_cons_brown_crab_en.pdf (accessed on 20 August 2022).
36. Coleman, M.; Rodrigues, E. Orkney brown crab (*Cancer pagurus*) tagging project. *Orkney Shellfish Res. Proj.* **2017**, *21*, 19.
37. Tonk, L.; Rozemeijer, M. *Ecology of the Brown Crab (Cancer pagurus): And Production Potential for Passive Fisheries in Dutch Offshore Wind Farms*; Wageningen Marine Research: Yerseke, The Netherlands, 2019.
38. Skajaa, K.; Fernö, A.; Løkkeborg, S.; Haugland, E.K. Basic movement pattern and chemo-oriented search towards baited pots in edible crab (*Cancer pagurus* L.). *Hydrobiologia* **1998**, *371*, 143–153. [CrossRef]
39. Edwards, E. *A Contribution to the Bionomics of the Edible Crab (Cancer pagurus L.) in English and Irish Waters*; National University of Ireland: Dublin, Ireland, 1971.
40. Neal, K.; Wilson, E. Edible Crab (*Cancer pagurus*). Available online: https://www.marlin.ac.uk/species/detail/1179 (accessed on 30 August 2022).
41. Öndes, F.; Emmerson, J.A.; Kaiser, M.J.; Murray, L.G.; Kennington, K. The catch characteristics and population structure of the brown crab (*Cancer pagurus*) fishery in the Isle of Man, Irish Sea. *J. Mar. Biol. Assoc. UK* **2019**, *99*, 119–133. [CrossRef]
42. Öndes, F.; Kaiser, M.J.; Murray, L.G.; Torres, G. Reproductive Ecology, Fecundity, and Elemental Composition of Eggs in Brown Crab *Cancer pagurus* in The Isle of Man. *J. Shellfish Res.* **2016**, *35*, 539–547. [CrossRef]
43. Anilkumar, G.; Sudha, K.; Anitha, E.; Subramoniam, T. Aspects of Sperm Metabolism in the Spermatheca of the Brachyuran Crab Metopograpsus Messor (Forskal). *J. Crustac. Biol.* **1996**, *16*, 310–314. [CrossRef]
44. Bord Bia. Irish Brown Carb. Available online: https://www.bordbia.ie/industry/news/food-alerts/irish-brown-crab-cancer-pagrus/ (accessed on 11 April 2022).
45. FAO Fisheries and Aquaculture Department. Species Fact Sheets: Cancer pagurus (Linnaeus, 1758). Available online: http://www.fao.org/fishery/species/2627/en (accessed on 20 April 2020).

46. Bord Bia. Irish Fish & Seafood: An Analysis of the Irish Fish and Seafood Sector. Available online: https://www.bordbia.ie/industry/sector-profiles/fish-seafood/ (accessed on 10 January 2020).
47. McDermott, A.; Whyte, P.; Brunton, N.; Lyng, J.; Bolton, D.J. Increasing the Yield of Irish Brown Crab (*Cancer pagurus*) during Processing without Adversely Affecting Shelf-Life. *Foods* **2018**, *7*, 99. [CrossRef] [PubMed]
48. Bord Iascaigh Mhara. *The Business of Seafood 2018: A Snapshot of Irelands Seafood Sector*; BIM: Dublin, Ireland, 2019.
49. The Irish Examiner. China Fears for Irish Crab Meat Exceeding Cadmium Limits. Available online: https://www.irishexaminer.com/farming/arid-20367120.html (accessed on 12 April 2022).
50. Johnson, P. Chinese Market for Crab and Salmon Suffers Sudden Decline. Available online: https://www.shetnews.co.uk/2020/02/05/chinese-market-for-crab-and-salmon-suffers-sudden-decline/ (accessed on 20 August 2020).
51. Seafood News. Live Dungeness Shipments to China Hampered by Rumors of Cadmium Contamination. Available online: https://www.seafoodnews.com/Story/1059810/Live-Dungeness-Shipments-to-China-Hampered-By-Rumors-of-Cadmium-Contamination (accessed on 12 April 2022).
52. South China Morning Post. Mainland Halt on Hairy Crab Exports Keeps Them off the Menu in Hong Kong, as Peak Season Nears. Available online: https://www.scmp.com/news/hong-kong/health-environment/article/2115619/mainland-halt-hairy-crab-exports-keeps-them-menu (accessed on 27 April 2020).
53. Hoogenboom, R.L.A.P.; Kotterman, M.J.J.; Hoek-van Nieuwenhuizen, M.; van der Lee, M.K.; Mennes, W.C.; Jeurissen, S.M.F.; van Leeuwen, S.P.J. Dioxins, PCBs and heavy metals in Chinese mitten crabs from Dutch rivers and lakes. *Chemosphere* **2015**, *123*, 1–8. [CrossRef]
54. CBI Ministry of Foreign Affairs. Entering the European Market for Crab. Available online: https://www.cbi.eu/market-information/fish-seafood/crab/market-entry (accessed on 1 September 2022).
55. BBC. Chinese Ban Imposed on 'Contaminated' Crabs. Available online: https://www.bbc.com/news/uk-wales-north-west-wales-34006259 (accessed on 22 March 2022).
56. The Times. Chinese Ban on Crabmeat Costs Millions. Available online: https://www.thetimes.co.uk/article/chinese-ban-on-crabmeat-costs-millions-krcj73thk (accessed on 1 January 2022).
57. Garret, A.; Lawler, I.; Ballesteros, M.; Marques, A.; Dean, C.; Schnabele, D. *SR681 Outlook for European Brown Crab: Understanding Brown Crab Production and Consumption in the UK, Republic of Ireland, France, Spain and Portugal*; Seafish: Edinburgh, UK, 2015.
58. SFPA. Certification of Fishery Products. Available online: https://www.sfpa.ie/What-We-Do/Trade-Market-Access-Support/Exports/Certification-of-Fishery-Products (accessed on 23 March 2022).
59. Mazzei, V.; Longo, G.; Brundo, M.V.; Sinatra, F.; Copat, C.; Oliveri Conti, G.; Ferrante, M. Bioaccumulation of cadmium and lead and its effects on hepatopancreas morphology in three terrestrial isopod crustacean species. *Ecotoxicol. Environ. Saf.* **2014**, *110*, 269–279. [CrossRef]
60. Signa, G.; Mazzola, A.; Tramati, C.D.; Vizzini, S. Diet and habitat use influence Hg and Cd transfer to fish and consequent biomagnification in a highly contaminated area: Augusta Bay (Mediterranean Sea). *Environ. Pollut.* **2017**, *230*, 394–404. [CrossRef] [PubMed]
61. Bjerregaard, P. Relationship between physiological condition and cadmium accumulation in *Carcinus maenas* (L.). *Comp. Biochem. Physiol. Part A Physiol.* **1991**, *99*, 75–83. [CrossRef]
62. Bondgaard, M.; Nørum, U.; Bjerregaard, P. Cadmium accumulation in the female shore crab *Carcinus maenas* during the moult cycle and ovarian maturation. *Mar. Biol.* **2000**, *137*, 995–1004. [CrossRef]
63. Bjerregaard, P.; Bjørn, L.; Nørum, U.; Pedersen, K.L. Cadmium in the shore crab *Carcinus maenas*: Seasonal variation in cadmium content and uptake and elimination of cadmium after administration via food. *Aquat. Toxicol.* **2005**, *72*, 5–15. [CrossRef]
64. Davies, I.; Topping, G.; Graham, W.; Falconer, C.; McIntosh, A.; Saward, D. Field and experimental studies on cadmium in the edible crab *Cancer pagurus*. *Mar. Biol.* **1981**, *64*, 291–297. [CrossRef]
65. Frantzen, A.; Duinker, A.; Måge, A. *Kadmiumanalyser i taskekrabbe fra Nordland Høsten/Vinteren 2013–2014*; Norway Report; National Institute of Nutrition and Seafood Research (NIFES): Bergen, Norway, 2015.
66. Frantzen, S.; Måge, A. *Fremmedstoffer i Villfisk Med Vekt På Kyst-Nære Farvann. Brosme, Lange og Bifangstarter. Gjelder Tall for Prøver Samlet Inn i 2013–2015*; NIFES: Bergen, Norway, 2016.
67. Espinosa Almendro, J.M.; Bosch Ojeda, C.; Garcia de Torres, A.; Cano Pavón, J.M. Determination of cadmium in biological samples by inductively coupled plasma atomic emission spectrometry after extraction with 1,5-bis(di-2-pyridylmethylene) thiocarbonohydrazide. *Analyst* **1992**, *117*, 1749–1751. [CrossRef]
68. Faroon, O.; Ashizawa, A.; Wright, S.; Tucker, P.; Jenkins, K.; Ingerman, L.; Rudisill, C. *Toxicological Profile for Cadmium*; U.S. Department of Health and Human Services, Public Health Service Agency for Toxic Substances and Disease Registry: Atlanta, GA, USA, 2012.
69. Canada Health. Product Safety Testing: Chemistry Methods. Available online: https://www.canada.ca/en/health-canada/services/consumer-product-safety/product-safety-testing/chemistry-methods.html (accessed on 22 April 2022).
70. Roberts, C.A.; Clark, J.M. Improved determination of cadmium in blood and plasma by flameless atomic absorption spectroscopy. *Bull. Environ. Contam. Toxicol.* **1986**, *36*, 496–499. [CrossRef] [PubMed]
71. Satzger, R.D.; Clow, C.S.; Bonnin, E.; Fricke, F.L. Determination of background levels of lead and cadmium in raw agricultural crops by using differential pulse anodic stripping voltammetry. *J.-Assoc. Off. Anal. Chem.* **1982**, *65*, 987–991. [CrossRef]

72. Knutsen, H.; Wiech, M.; Duinker, A.; Maage, A. Cadmium in the shore crab *Carcinus maenas* along the Norwegian coast: Geographical and seasonal variation and correlation to physiological parameters. *Environ. Monit. Assess.* **2018**, *190*, 253. [CrossRef] [PubMed]
73. Nissen, L.R.; Bjerregaard, P.; Simonsen, V. Interindividual variability in metal status in the shore crab *Carcinus maenas*: The role of physiological condition and genetic variation. *Mar. Biol.* **2005**, *146*, 571–580. [CrossRef]
74. Nørum, U.; Bondgaard, M.; Pedersen, T.V.; Bjerregaard, P. In vivo and in vitro cadmium accumulation during the moult cycle of the male shore crab *Carcinus maenas*—Interaction with calcium metabolism. *Aquat. Toxicol.* **2005**, *72*, 29–44. [CrossRef]
75. Wold, J.P.; Kermit, M.; Woll, A. Rapid Nondestructive Determination of Edible Meat Content in Crabs (*Cancer pagurus*) by Near-Infrared Imaging Spectroscopy. *Appl. Spectrosc.* **2010**, *64*, 691–699. [CrossRef]
76. Fairfield, E.A.; Richardson, D.S.; Daniels, C.L.; Butler, C.L.; Bell, E.; Taylor, M.I. Ageing European lobsters (*Homarus gammarus*) using DNA methylation of evolutionarily conserved ribosomal DNA. *Evol. Appl.* **2021**, *14*, 2305–2318. [CrossRef] [PubMed]
77. Whiteley, N.M.; Suckling, C.C.; Ciotti, B.J.; Brown, J.; McCarthy, I.D.; Gimenez, L.; Hauton, C. Sensitivity to near-future CO2 conditions in marine crabs depends on their compensatory capacities for salinity change. *Sci. Rep.* **2018**, *8*, 15639. [CrossRef] [PubMed]
78. Bord Iascaigh Mhara. Brown Crab: Handling and Quality Guide. Available online: https://bim.ie/wp-content/uploads/2021/03/BIMBrownCrabHandlingandQualityGuide.pdf (accessed on 23 March 2022).
79. Nugegoda, D.; Rainbow, P.S. The uptake of dissolved zinc and cadmium by the decapod crustacean Palaemon elegans. *Mar. Pollut. Bull.* **1995**, *31*, 460–463. [CrossRef]
80. Blewett, T.A.; Newton, D.; Flynn, S.L.; Alessi, D.S.; Goss, G.G.; Hamilton, T.J. Cadmium bioaccumulates after acute exposure but has no effect on locomotion or shelter-seeking behaviour in the invasive green shore crab (*Carcinus maenas*). *Conserv. Physiol.* **2017**, *5*, cox057. [CrossRef] [PubMed]
81. Rafati Rahimzadeh, M.; Rafati Rahimzadeh, M.; Kazemi, S.; Moghadamnia, A.-A. Cadmium toxicity and treatment: An update. *Casp. J. Intern. Med.* **2017**, *8*, 135–145. [CrossRef]
82. Clark, P.F.; Mortimer, D.N.; Law, R.J.; Averns, J.M.; Cohen, B.A.; Wood, D.; Rose, M.D.; Fernandes, A.R.; Rainbow, P.S. Dioxin and PCB Contamination in Chinese Mitten Crabs: Human Consumption as a Control Mechanism for an Invasive Species. *Environ. Sci. Technol.* **2009**, *43*, 1624–1629. [CrossRef] [PubMed]
83. Zhu, Q.-H.; Zhou, Z.-K.; Tu, D.-D.; Zhou, Y.-L.; Wang, C.; Liu, Z.-P.; Gu, W.-B.; Chen, Y.-Y.; Shu, M.-A. Effect of cadmium exposure on hepatopancreas and gills of the estuary mud crab (*Scylla paramamosain*): Histopathological changes and expression characterization of stress response genes. *Aquat. Toxicol.* **2018**, *195*, 1–7. [CrossRef]
84. Tang, D.; Guo, H.; Shi, X.; Wang, Z. Comparative Transcriptome Analysis of the Gills from the Chinese Mitten Crab (*Eriocheir japonica sinensis*) Exposed to the Heavy Metal Cadmium. *Turk. J. Fish. Aquat. Sci.* **2019**, *20*, 467–479. [CrossRef]
85. Liu, J.; Wang, E.; Jing, W.; Dahms, H.-U.; Murugan, K.; Wang, L. Mitigative effects of zinc on cadmium-induced reproductive toxicity in the male freshwater crab *Sinopotamon henanense*. *Environ. Sci. Pollut. Res.* **2020**, *27*, 16282–16292. [CrossRef]
86. Zhang, Y.; Li, Z.; Kholodkevich, S.; Sharov, A.; Chen, C.; Feng, Y.; Ren, N.; Sun, K. Effects of cadmium on intestinal histology and microbiota in freshwater crayfish (*Procambarus clarkii*). *Chemosphere* **2020**, *242*, 125105. [CrossRef]
87. Wu, H.; Xuan, R.; Li, Y.; Zhang, X.; Jing, W.; Wang, L. Biochemical, histological and ultrastructural alterations of the alimentary system in the freshwater crab *Sinopotamon henanense* subchronically exposed to cadmium. *Ecotoxicology* **2014**, *23*, 65–75. [CrossRef] [PubMed]
88. Xu, P.; Guo, H.; Wang, H.; Xie, Y.; Lee, S.C.; Liu, M.; Zheng, J.; Mao, X.; Wang, H.; Liu, F.; et al. Identification and profiling of microRNAs responsive to cadmium toxicity in hepatopancreas of the freshwater crab *Sinopotamon henanense*. *Hereditas* **2019**, *156*, 34. [CrossRef] [PubMed]
89. Condón-Abanto, S.; Raso, J.; Arroyo, C.; Lyng, J.G.; Condón, S.; Álvarez, I. Evaluation of the potential of ultrasound technology combined with mild temperatures to reduce cadmium content of edible crab (*Cancer pagurus*). *Ultrason. Sonochem.* **2018**, *48*, 550–554. [CrossRef] [PubMed]
90. De Guglielmo, V.; Puoti, R.; Notariale, R.; Maresca, V.; Ausió, J.; Troisi, J.; Verrillo, M.; Basile, A.; Febbraio, F.; Piscopo, M. Alterations in the properties of sperm protamine-like II protein after exposure of *Mytilus galloprovincialis* (Lamarck 1819) to sub-toxic doses of cadmium. *Ecotoxicol. Environ. Saf.* **2019**, *169*, 600–606. [CrossRef] [PubMed]
91. Godt, J.; Scheidig, F.; Grosse-Siestrup, C.; Esche, V.; Brandenburg, P.; Reich, A.; Groneberg, D.A. The toxicity of cadmium and resulting hazards for human health. *J. Occup. Med. Toxicol.* **2006**, *1*, 22. [CrossRef]
92. Ahn, J.; Kim, N.-S.; Lee, B.-K.; Oh, I.; Kim, Y. Changes of Atmospheric and Blood Concentrations of Lead and Cadmium in the General Population of South Korea from 2008 to 2017. *Int. J. Environ. Res. Public Health* **2019**, *16*, 2096. [CrossRef]
93. Lanceleur, L.; Schäfer, J.; Chiffoleau, J.-F.; Blanc, G.; Auger, D.; Renault, S.; Baudrimont, M.; Audry, S. Long-term records of cadmium and silver contamination in sediments and oysters from the Gironde fluvial–estuarine continuum–Evidence of changing silver sources. *Chemosphere* **2011**, *85*, 1299–1305. [CrossRef]
94. Yuan, Z.; Luo, T.; Liu, X.; Hua, H.; Zhuang, Y.; Zhang, X.; Zhang, L.; Zhang, Y.; Xu, W.; Ren, J. Tracing anthropogenic cadmium emissions: From sources to pollution. *Sci. Total Environ.* **2019**, *676*, 87–96. [CrossRef]
95. Andersen, O.; Nielsen, J.B.; Nordberg, G.F. Nutritional interactions in intestinal cadmium uptake–Possibilities for risk reduction. *Biometals* **2004**, *17*, 543–547. [CrossRef]

96. Järup, L.; Berglund, M.; Elinder, C.G.; Nordberg, G.; Vanter, M. Health effects of cadmium exposure—A review of the literature and a risk estimate. *Scand. J. Work Environ. Health* **1998**, *24*, 1–51.
97. Ashraf, M.W. Levels of heavy metals in popular cigarette brands and exposure to these metals via smoking. *Sci. World J.* **2012**, *2012*, 729430. [CrossRef] [PubMed]
98. Keil, D.E.; Berger-Ritchie, J.; McMillin, G.A. Testing for Toxic Elements: A Focus on Arsenic, Cadmium, Lead, and Mercury. *Lab. Med.* **2011**, *42*, 735–742. [CrossRef]
99. Satarug, S.; Moore, M.R. Adverse health effects of chronic exposure to low-level cadmium in foodstuffs and cigarette smoke. *Environ. Health Perspect.* **2004**, *112*, 1099–1103. [CrossRef] [PubMed]
100. Satarug, S.; Vesey, D.A.; Gobe, G.C. Current health risk assessment practice for dietary cadmium: Data from different countries. *Food Chem. Toxicol.* **2017**, *106*, 430–445. [CrossRef] [PubMed]
101. Food Safety Authority of Ireland. Metals of Toxicological Importance in the Irish Diet. Available online: https://www.lenus.ie/handle/10147/609836 (accessed on 29 August 2020).
102. Irish Universities Nutrition Alliance. National Adult Nutrition Survey: Physical Measurements, Physical Activity Patterns and Food Choice Motives. Available online: https://www.iuna.net/surveyreports (accessed on 29 August 2022).
103. Kim, K.; Melough, M.M.; Vance, T.M.; Noh, H.; Koo, S.I.; Chun, O.K. Dietary Cadmium Intake and Sources in the US. *Nutrients* **2019**, *11*, 2. [CrossRef] [PubMed]
104. Lordan, R.; Tsoupras, A.; Zabetakis, I. Chapter 1-The Origin of Chronic Diseases with Respect to Cardiovascular Disease. In *The Impact of Nutrition and Statins on Cardiovascular Diseases*; Zabetakis, I., Lordan, R., Tsoupras, A., Eds.; Academic Press: Cambridge, MA, USA, 2019; pp. 1–21. [CrossRef]
105. Awata, H.; Linder, S.; Mitchell, L.E.; Delclos, G.L. Association of Dietary Intake and Biomarker Levels of Arsenic, Cadmium, Lead, and Mercury among Asian Populations in the United States: NHANES 2011–2012. *Environ. Health Perspect.* **2017**, *125*, 314–323. [CrossRef] [PubMed]
106. Hecht, E.M.; Landy, D.C.; Ahn, S.; Hlaing, W.M.; Hennekens, C.H. Hypothesis: Cadmium explains, in part, why smoking increases the risk of cardiovascular disease. *J. Cardiovasc. Pharmacol. Ther.* **2013**, *18*, 550–554. [CrossRef]
107. Zeng, L.; Ruan, M.; Liu, J.; Wilde, P.; Naumova, E.N.; Mozaffarian, D.; Zhang, F.F. Trends in Processed Meat, Unprocessed Red Meat, Poultry, and Fish Consumption in the United States, 1999–2016. *J. Acad. Nutr. Diet.* **2019**, *119*, 1085–1098.e1012. [CrossRef]
108. Song, Y.; Wang, Y.; Mao, W.; Sui, H.; Yong, L.; Yang, D.; Jiang, D.; Zhang, L.; Gong, Y. Dietary cadmium exposure assessment among the Chinese population. *PLoS ONE* **2017**, *12*, e0177978. [CrossRef]
109. He, P.; Lu, Y.; Liang, Y.; Chen, B.; Wu, M.; Li, S.; He, G.; Jin, T. Exposure assessment of dietary cadmium: Findings from shanghainese over 40 years, China. *BMC Public Health* **2013**, *13*, 590. [CrossRef]
110. Zhao, F.J.; Ma, Y.; Zhu, Y.G.; Tang, Z.; McGrath, S.P. Soil Contamination in China: Current Status and Mitigation Strategies. *Environ. Sci. Technol.* **2015**, *49*, 750–759. [CrossRef] [PubMed]
111. Satarug, S. Dietary Cadmium Intake and Its Effects on Kidneys. *Toxics* **2018**, *6*, 15. [CrossRef] [PubMed]
112. Callan, A.; Hinwood, A.; Devine, A. Metals in commonly eaten groceries in Western Australia: A market basket survey and dietary assessment. *Food Addit. Contam. Part A* **2014**, *31*, 1968–1981. [CrossRef] [PubMed]
113. Calafat, A.M. The U.S. National Health and Nutrition Examination Survey and human exposure to environmental chemicals. *Int. J. Hyg. Environ. Health* **2012**, *215*, 99–101. [CrossRef]
114. Adams, S.V.; Quraishi, S.M.; Shafer, M.M.; Passarelli, M.N.; Freney, E.P.; Chlebowski, R.T.; Luo, J.; Meliker, J.R.; Mu, L.; Neuhouser, M.L.; et al. Dietary cadmium exposure and risk of breast, endometrial, and ovarian cancer in the Women's Health Initiative. *Environ. Health Perspect.* **2014**, *122*, 594–600. [CrossRef]
115. Puerto-Parejo, L.M.; Aliaga, I.; Canal-Macias, M.L.; Leal-Hernandez, O.; Roncero-Martín, R.; Rico-Martín, S.; Moran, J.M. Evaluation of the Dietary Intake of Cadmium, Lead and Mercury and Its Relationship with Bone Health among Postmenopausal Women in Spain. *Int. J. Environ. Res. Public Health* **2017**, *14*, 564. [CrossRef]
116. Lavado-García, J.M.; Puerto-Parejo, L.M.; Roncero-Martín, R.; Moran, J.M.; Pedrera-Zamorano, J.D.; Aliaga, I.J.; Leal-Hernández, O.; Canal-Macias, M.L. Dietary Intake of Cadmium, Lead and Mercury and Its Association with Bone Health in Healthy Premenopausal Women. *Int. J. Environ. Res. Public Health* **2017**, *14*, 1437. [CrossRef]
117. Lin, J.; Zhang, F.; Lei, Y. Dietary intake and urinary level of cadmium and breast cancer risk: A meta-analysis. *Cancer Epidemiol.* **2016**, *42*, 101–107. [CrossRef]
118. Jin, T.; Nordberg, M.; Frech, W.; Dumont, X.; Bernard, A.; Ye, T.-t.; Kong, Q.; Wang, Z.; Li, P.; Lundström, N.-G.; et al. Cadmium biomonitoring and renal dysfunction among a population environmentally exposed to cadmium from smelting in China (ChinaCad). *Biometals* **2002**, *15*, 397–410. [CrossRef]
119. Taylor, W.R. Permeation of barium and cadmium through slowly inactivating calcium channels in cat sensory neurones. *J. Physiol.* **1988**, *407*, 433–452. [CrossRef]
120. Foulkes, E.C. Interactions between metals in rat jejunum: Implications on the nature of cadmium uptake. *Toxicology* **1985**, *37*, 117–125. [CrossRef]
121. Reeves, P.G.; Chaney, R.L. Bioavailability as an issue in risk assessment and management of food cadmium: A review. *Sci. Total Environ.* **2008**, *398*, 13–19. [CrossRef] [PubMed]
122. Fox, M.R.S. Nutritional Factors that May Influence Bioavailability of Cadmium. *J. Environ. Qual.* **1988**, *17*, 175–180. [CrossRef]

123. Bjerregaard, P.; Jensen, L.B.E.; Pedersen, K.L. Effect of size on concentrations and cadmium inducibility of metallothionein in the shore crab *Carcinus maenas*. *Comp. Biochem. Physiol. Part C Toxicol. Pharmacol.* **2021**, *249*, 109146. [CrossRef] [PubMed]
124. Siewicki, T.; Balthrop, J. Comparison of the digestion of oyster tissue containing intrinsically or extrinsically labeled cadmium [Rats]. *Nutr. Rep. Int.* **1983**, *27*, 899–909.
125. Lordan, R.; Tsoupras, A.; Mitra, B.; Zabetakis, I. Dairy fats and cardiovascular disease: Do we really need to be concerned? *Foods* **2018**, *7*, 29. [CrossRef]
126. Reeves, P.G.; Chaney, R.L. Nutritional status affects the absorption and whole-body and organ retention of cadmium in rats fed rice-based diets. *Environ. Sci. Technol.* **2002**, *36*, 2684–2692. [CrossRef] [PubMed]
127. Reeves, P.G.; Chaney, R.L. Marginal nutritional status of zinc, iron, and calcium increases cadmium retention in the duodenum and other organs of rats fed rice-based diets. *Environ. Res.* **2004**, *96*, 311–322. [CrossRef] [PubMed]
128. Reeves, P.G.; Chaney, R.L.; Simmons, R.W.; Cherian, M.G. Metallothionein induction is not involved in cadmium accumulation in the duodenum of mice and rats fed diets containing high-cadmium rice or sunflower kernels and a marginal supply of zinc, iron, and calcium. *J. Nutr.* **2005**, *135*, 99–108. [CrossRef] [PubMed]
129. Flanagan, P.R.; McLellan, J.S.; Haist, J.; Cherian, M.G.; Chamberlain, M.J.; Valberg, L.S. Increased dietary cadmium absorption in mice and human subjects with iron deficiency. *Gastroenterology* **1978**, *74*, 841–846. [CrossRef]
130. Silver, M.K.; Lozoff, B.; Meeker, J.D. Blood cadmium is elevated in iron deficient U.S. children: A cross-sectional study. *Environ. Health* **2013**, *12*, 117. [CrossRef] [PubMed]
131. Gunshin, H.; Mackenzie, B.; Berger, U.V.; Gunshin, Y.; Romero, M.F.; Boron, W.F.; Nussberger, S.; Gollan, J.L.; Hediger, M.A. Cloning and characterization of a mammalian proton-coupled metal-ion transporter. *Nature* **1997**, *388*, 482–488. [CrossRef] [PubMed]
132. Kim, D.-W.; Kim, K.-Y.; Choi, B.-S.; Youn, P.; Ryu, D.-Y.; Klaassen, C.D.; Park, J.-D. Regulation of metal transporters by dietary iron, and the relationship between body iron levels and cadmium uptake. *Arch. Toxicol.* **2007**, *81*, 327–334. [CrossRef] [PubMed]
133. Richens, D.T. *The Chemistry of Aqua Ions*; Wiley Chichester: Chichester, UK, 1997.
134. Zalups, R.K.; Ahmad, S. Molecular handling of cadmium in transporting epithelia. *Toxicol. Appl. Pharmacol.* **2003**, *186*, 163–188. [CrossRef]
135. Bernard, A. Confusion about Cadmium Risks: The Unrecognized Limitations of an Extrapolated Paradigm. *Environ. Health Perspect.* **2016**, *124*, 1–5. [CrossRef]
136. Barbier, O.; Jacquillet, G.; Tauc, M.; Cougnon, M.; Poujeol, P. Effect of Heavy Metals on, and Handling by, the Kidney. *Nephron Physiol.* **2005**, *99*, 105–110. [CrossRef]
137. Aitio, A.; Kiilunen, M.; Santonen, T.; Nordberg, M. *Handbook on the Toxicology of Metals*, 4th ed.; Chapter: Gold and Gold Mining; Elsevier: Amsterdam, The Netherlands, 2015.
138. Bernard, A. Renal dysfunction induced by cadmium: Biomarkers of critical effects. *Biometals* **2004**, *17*, 519–523. [CrossRef]
139. Bernard, A.; Roels, H.; Buchet, J.-P.; Cardenas, A.; Lauwerys, R. Cadmium and health: The Belgian experience. *IARC Sci. Publ.* **1992**, *118*, 15–33.
140. Nordberg, G.F.; Fowler, B.A.; Nordberg, M. *Handbook on the Toxicology of Metals*; Academic Press: Cambridge, MA, USA, 2015.
141. Chaumont, A.; De Winter, F.; Dumont, X.; Haufroid, V.; Bernard, A. The threshold level of urinary cadmium associated with increased urinary excretion of retinol-binding protein and β2-microglobulin: A re-assessment in a large cohort of nickel-cadmium battery workers. *Occup. Environ. Med.* **2011**, *68*, 257–264. [CrossRef] [PubMed]
142. Liang, Y.; Lei, L.; Nilsson, J.; Li, H.; Nordberg, M.; Bernard, A.; Nordberg, G.F.; Bergdahl, I.A.; Jin, T. Renal Function after Reduction in Cadmium Exposure: An 8-Year Follow-up of Residents in Cadmium-Polluted Areas. *Environ. Health Perspect.* **2012**, *120*, 223–228. [CrossRef]
143. Dyck, K.N.; Bashir, S.; Horgan, G.W.; Sneddon, A.A. Regular crabmeat consumers do not show increased urinary cadmium or beta-2-microglobulin levels compared to non-crabmeat consumers. *J. Trace Elem. Med. Biol.* **2019**, *52*, 22–28. [CrossRef] [PubMed]
144. Guan, S.; Palermo, T.; Meliker, J. Seafood intake and blood cadmium in a cohort of adult avid seafood consumers. *Int. J. Hyg. Environ. Health* **2015**, *218*, 147–152. [CrossRef]
145. Lind, Y.; Wicklund Glynn, A.; Engman, J.; Jorhem, L. Bioavailability of cadmium from crab hepatopancreas and mushroom in relation to inorganic cadmium: A 9-week feeding study in mice. *Food Chem. Toxicol.* **1995**, *33*, 667–673. [CrossRef]
146. Maage, A.; Julshamn, K. A comparison of dressed crab and a cadmium salt (CdCl2) as cadmium sources in rat diets. *Comp Biochem. Physiol. C Comp. Pharm. Toxicol.* **1987**, *88*, 209–211. [CrossRef]
147. Ju, Y.-R.; Chen, W.-Y.; Liao, C.-M. Assessing human exposure risk to cadmium through inhalation and seafood consumption. *J. Hazard. Mater.* **2012**, *227–228*, 353–361. [CrossRef]
148. FAO/WHO (Food and Agriculture Organisation/World Health Organization). Joint FAO/WHO Expert Committee on Food Additives. In Proceedings of the Seventy-Third Meeting, Geneva, Switzerland,, 8–17 June 2010; Summary and Conclusions. Issued 24 June 2010. Available online: https://www.who.int/publications/i/item/9789241209601 (accessed on 29 September 2022).
149. Satarug, S.; Gobe, G.C.; Vesey, D.A. Multiple Targets of Toxicity in Environmental Exposure to Low-Dose Cadmium. *Toxics* **2022**, *10*, 472. [CrossRef]
150. Wong, C.; Roberts, S.M.; Saab, I.N. Review of regulatory reference values and background levels for heavy metals in the human diet. *Regul. Toxicol. Pharmacol.* **2022**, *130*, 105122. [CrossRef]

151. The Panel on Contaminants in the Food Chain of the European Food Safety Authority (CONTAM Panel). Statement on tolerable weekly intake for cadmium. *EFSA J.* **2011**, *9*, 1975.
152. Satarug, S.; Vesey, D.A.; Nishijo, M.; Ruangyuttikarn, W.; Gobe, G.C. The inverse association of glomerular function and urinary β2-MG excretion and its implications for cadmium health risk assessment. *Environ. Res.* **2019**, *173*, 40–47. [CrossRef] [PubMed]
153. Mitra, S.; Varghese, A.C.; Mandal, S.; Bhattacharyya, S.; Nandi, P.; Rahman, S.M.; Kar, K.K.; Saha, R.; Roychoudhury, S.; Murmu, N. Lead and cadmium exposure induces male reproductive dysfunction by modulating the expression profiles of apoptotic and survival signal proteins in tea-garden workers. *Reprod. Toxicol.* **2020**, *98*, 134–148. [CrossRef]
154. Wang, Y.X.; Wang, P.; Feng, W.; Liu, C.; Yang, P.; Chen, Y.J.; Sun, L.; Sun, Y.; Yue, J.; Gu, L.J.; et al. Relationships between seminal plasma metals/metalloids and semen quality, sperm apoptosis and DNA integrity. *Environ. Pollut.* **2017**, *224*, 224–234. [CrossRef]
155. Lee, S.; Min, J.-Y.; Min, K.-B. Female Infertility Associated with Blood Lead and Cadmium Levels. *Int. J. Environ. Res. Public Health* **2020**, *17*, 1794. [CrossRef]
156. Upson, K.; O'Brien, K.M.; Hall, J.E.; Tokar, E.J.; Baird, D.D. Cadmium Exposure and Ovarian Reserve in Women Aged 35-49 Years: The Impact on Results From the Creatinine Adjustment Approach Used to Correct for Urinary Dilution. *Am. J. Epidemiol.* **2021**, *190*, 116–124. [CrossRef] [PubMed]
157. Pan, W.; Ye, X.; Zhu, Z.; Li, C.; Zhou, J.; Liu, J. Urinary cadmium concentrations and risk of primary ovarian insufficiency in women: A case-control study. *Environ. Geochem. Health* **2021**, *43*, 2025–2035. [CrossRef]
158. Genchi, G.; Sinicropi, M.S.; Lauria, G.; Carocci, A.; Catalano, A. The Effects of Cadmium Toxicity. *Int. J. Environ. Res. Public Health* **2020**, *17*, 3782. [CrossRef] [PubMed]
159. Awadalla, A.; Mortada, W.I.; Abol-Enein, H.; Shokeir, A.A. Correlation between blood levels of cadmium and lead and the expression of microRNA-21 in Egyptian bladder cancer patients. *Heliyon* **2020**, *6*, e05642. [CrossRef] [PubMed]
160. Wallace, D.R.; Taalab, Y.M.; Heinze, S.; Tariba Lovaković, B.; Pizent, A.; Renieri, E.; Tsatsakis, A.; Farooqi, A.A.; Javorac, D.; Andjelkovic, M.; et al. Toxic-Metal-Induced Alteration in miRNA Expression Profile as a Proposed Mechanism for Disease Development. *Cells* **2020**, *9*, 901. [CrossRef]
161. Patrick, L. Toxic metals and antioxidants: Part II. The role of antioxidants in arsenic and cadmium toxicity. *Altern. Med. Rev.* **2003**, *8*, 106–128. [PubMed]
162. Joseph, P. Mechanisms of cadmium carcinogenesis. *Toxicol. Appl. Pharmacol.* **2009**, *238*, 272–279. [CrossRef] [PubMed]
163. Filipič, M. Mechanisms of cadmium induced genomic instability. *Mutat. Res./Fundam. Mol. Mech. Mutagen.* **2012**, *733*, 69–77. [CrossRef]
164. Liu, J.; Qu, W.; Kadiiska, M.B. Role of oxidative stress in cadmium toxicity and carcinogenesis. *Toxicol. Appl. Pharmacol.* **2009**, *238*, 209–214. [CrossRef] [PubMed]
165. Bimonte, V.M.; Besharat, Z.M.; Antonioni, A.; Cella, V.; Lenzi, A.; Ferretti, E.; Migliaccio, S. The endocrine disruptor cadmium: A new player in the pathophysiology of metabolic diseases. *J. Endocrinol. Investig.* **2021**, *44*, 1363–1377. [CrossRef] [PubMed]
166. Nie, X.; Chen, Y.; Chen, Y.; Chen, C.; Han, B.; Li, Q.; Zhu, C.; Xia, F.; Zhai, H.; Wang, N.; et al. Lead and cadmium exposure, higher thyroid antibodies and thyroid dysfunction in Chinese women. *Environ. Pollut.* **2017**, *230*, 320–328. [CrossRef] [PubMed]
167. Rezaei, M.; Javadmoosavi, S.Y.; Mansouri, B.; Azadi, N.A.; Mehrpour, O.; Nakhaee, S. Thyroid dysfunction: How concentration of toxic and essential elements contribute to risk of hypothyroidism, hyperthyroidism, and thyroid cancer. *Environ. Sci. Pollut. Res. Int.* **2019**, *26*, 35787–35796. [CrossRef]
168. Yu, Y.; Ma, R.; Yu, L.; Cai, Z.; Li, H.; Zuo, Y.; Wang, Z.; Li, H. Combined effects of cadmium and tetrabromobisphenol a (TBBPA) on development, antioxidant enzymes activity and thyroid hormones in female rats. *Chem. Biol. Interact.* **2018**, *289*, 23–31. [CrossRef]
169. Chen, A.; Kim, S.S.; Chung, E.; Dietrich, K.N. Thyroid hormones in relation to lead, mercury, and cadmium exposure in the National Health and Nutrition Examination Survey, 2007–2008. *Environ. Health Perspect.* **2013**, *121*, 181–186. [CrossRef]
170. Jain, R.B.; Choi, Y.S. Interacting effects of selected trace and toxic metals on thyroid function. *Int. J. Environ. Health Res.* **2016**, *26*, 75–91. [CrossRef]
171. Buha, A.; Matovic, V.; Antonijevic, B.; Bulat, Z.; Curcic, M.; Renieri, E.A.; Tsatsakis, A.M.; Schweitzer, A.; Wallace, D. Overview of Cadmium Thyroid Disrupting Effects and Mechanisms. *Int. J. Mol. Sci.* **2018**, *19*, 1501. [CrossRef]
172. Byrne, C.; Divekar, S.D.; Storchan, G.B.; Parodi, D.A.; Martin, M.B. Cadmium—A metallohormone? *Toxicol. Appl. Pharmacol.* **2009**, *238*, 266–271. [CrossRef]
173. Brama, M.; Gnessi, L.; Basciani, S.; Cerulli, N.; Politi, L.; Spera, G.; Mariani, S.; Cherubini, S.; d'Abusco, A.S.; Scandurra, R.; et al. Cadmium induces mitogenic signaling in breast cancer cell by an ERα-dependent mechanism. *Mol. Cell. Endocrinol.* **2007**, *264*, 102–108. [CrossRef]
174. Strumylaite, L.; Kregzdyte, R.; Bogusevicius, A.; Poskiene, L.; Baranauskiene, D.; Pranys, D. Cadmium Exposure and Risk of Breast Cancer by Histological and Tumor Receptor Subtype in White Caucasian Women: A Hospital-Based Case-Control Study. *Int. J. Mol. Sci.* **2019**, *20*, 3029. [CrossRef] [PubMed]
175. Wang, Y.; Shi, L.; Li, J.; Li, L.; Wang, H.; Yang, H. Long-term cadmium exposure promoted breast cancer cell migration and invasion by up-regulating TGIF. *Ecotoxicol. Environ. Saf.* **2019**, *175*, 110–117. [CrossRef] [PubMed]
176. Henson, M.C.; Chedrese, P.J. Endocrine Disruption by Cadmium, a Common Environmental Toxicant with Paradoxical Effects on Reproduction. *Exp. Biol. Med.* **2004**, *229*, 383–392. [CrossRef] [PubMed]
177. Dai, C.; Heemers, H.; Sharifi, N. Androgen signaling in prostate cancer. *Cold Spring Harb. Perspect. Med.* **2017**, *7*, a030452. [CrossRef]

178. Chandrasekaran, B.; Dahiya, N.R.; Tyagi, A.; Kolluru, V.; Saran, U.; Baby, B.V.; States, J.C.; Haddad, A.Q.; Ankem, M.K.; Damodaran, C. Chronic exposure to cadmium induces a malignant transformation of benign prostate epithelial cells. *Oncogenesis* **2020**, *9*, 23. [CrossRef]
179. Kumar, S.; Sharma, A. Cadmium toxicity: Effects on human reproduction and fertility. *Rev. Environ. Health* **2019**, *34*, 327–338. [CrossRef]
180. Imura, J.; Tsuneyama, K.; Ueda, Y. Novel Pathological Study of Cadmium Nephropathy of Itai-itai Disease. In *Cadmium Toxicity: New Aspects in Human Disease, Rice Contamination, and Cytotoxicity*; Himeno, S., Aoshima, K., Eds.; Springer: Singapore, 2019; pp. 39–50.
181. Nishijo, M.; Nakagawa, H.; Suwazono, Y.; Nogawa, K.; Sakurai, M.; Ishizaki, M.; Kido, T. Cancer Mortality in Residents of the Cadmium-Polluted Jinzu River Basin in Toyama, Japan. *Toxics* **2018**, *6*, 23. [CrossRef]
182. Guan, J.; MacGibbon, A.; Fong, B.; Zhang, R.; Liu, K.; Rowan, A.; McJarrow, P. Long-Term Supplementation with Beta Serum Concentrate (BSC), a Complex of Milk Lipids, during Post-Natal Brain Development Improves Memory in Rats. *Nutrients* **2015**, *7*, 4526. [CrossRef]
183. Birgisdottir, B.E.; Knutsen, H.K.; Haugen, M.; Gjelstad, I.M.; Jenssen, M.T.S.; Ellingsen, D.G.; Thomassen, Y.; Alexander, J.; Meltzer, H.M.; Brantsæter, A.L. Essential and toxic element concentrations in blood and urine and their associations with diet: Results from a Norwegian population study including high-consumers of seafood and game. *Sci. Total Environ.* **2013**, *463–464*, 836–844. [CrossRef]

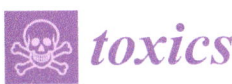

Article

Antibiotics in Raw Meat Samples: Estimation of Dietary Exposure and Risk Assessment

Athina Stavroulaki [1,2], Manolis N. Tzatzarakis [1,*], Vasiliki Karzi [1], Ioanna Katsikantami [1], Elisavet Renieri [1], Elena Vakonaki [1], Maria Avgenaki [1], Athanasios Alegakis [1], Miriana Stan [3], Matthaios Kavvalakis [1], Apostolos K. Rizos [2] and Aristidis Tsatsakis [1,*]

1. Laboratory of Toxicology, Medicine School, University of Crete, 70013 Heraklion, Greece
2. Department of Chemistry, University of Crete and Foundation for Research and Technology—Hellas (FORTH-IESL), 70013 Heraklion, Greece
3. Department of Toxicology, Faculty of Pharmacy, Carol Davila University of Medicine and Pharmacy, 200349 Bucharest, Romania
* Correspondence: tzatzarakis@uoc.gr (M.N.T.); tsatsaka@uoc.gr (A.T.)

Abstract: The extensive use of antibiotics in livestock farming poses increased concerns for human health as residues of these substances are present in edible tissues. The aim of this study was the determination of the levels of four groups of antibiotics (sulfonamides—SAs, tetracyclines—TCs, streptomycines—STr and quinolones—QNLs) in meat samples (muscles, livers and kidneys from beef, chicken and pork) and the estimation of the dietary exposure to antibiotics from meat consumption and the potential hazard for human health. Fifty-four samples of raw meat were randomly collected in 2018 from the Cretan market, Greece and analyzed both with an enzyme-linked immunosorbent assay (ELISA) and liquid chromatography–mass spectrometry (LC–MS). According to the results derived from the ELISA method, only 2% of the meat samples were free from antibiotics, 2% were detected with 4 antibiotics and the great majority of the samples (87%) were detected with 2 to 3 antibiotics. SAs presented the highest detection frequencies for all samples whereas TCs were not detected in any bovine sample. The highest median concentration was detected for STr in bovine muscles (182.10 µg/kg) followed by QNLs (93.36 µg/kg) in pork kidneys whereas the chicken samples had higher burdens of QNLs compared to the other meat samples. LC–MS analysis showed that oxytetracycline (OTC) was the most common antibiotic in all samples. The highest median concentration of all antibiotics was detected for doxycycline (DOX) (181.73 µg/kg in pork kidney) followed by OTC in bovine liver (74.46 µg/kg). Risk characterization was applied for each of the two methods; The hazard quotients (HQ) did not exceed 0.059 for the ELISA method and 0.113 for the LC–MS method for any group of antibiotics, whereas the total hazard indexes (HI) were 0.078 and 0.021, respectively. The results showed the presence of different groups of antibiotics in meat from the Cretan market and that the health risk to antibiotics is low. A risk assessment analysis conducted for meat consumption and corrected for the aggregated exposure revealed no risk for the consumers.

Keywords: tetracyclines; sulfonamides; quinolones; streptomycines; meat; antibiotics; risk assessment

1. Introduction

The aim of antibiotics is to destroy bacteria and they are used in livestock and poultry production for therapeutic purposes to prevent, control and treat infectious diseases in animals, although some producers use antibiotics to improve meat production by increasing the rate of animal growth [1]. Antibiotics as growth promoters are no longer used in European Union countries as there has been a legal ban from January 2006 [2]. The widespread and prolonged use of antibiotics has contributed negatively to their effectiveness and thus the doses have been increased, alternative more powerful antibiotics have to be used and the times of administration have to be extended [3]. In cases where antibiotics are misused

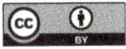

and legal withdrawal periods (the time span from drug administration to animal slaughter and use of meat for human consumption) are not respected, the residues in edible tissues pose an increased risk for consumers [4].

The parent substance of the antibiotics poses the highest toxicity; however, in the human it is metabolized and converted into an inactive and more easily excreted form [5,6]. Allergic reactions and other toxic effects have been observed and the risk is greater for hypersensitive individuals. The most common health effects of quinolones (QNLs) include effects on the central nervous system (CNS), such as anxiety, worry, nervousness and dizziness [7]. In addition to seizures, other serious CNS reactions include delirium, delusions, psychosis, mania, encephalopathy and dysarthria [8]. Recently, pharmacovigilance studies found a possible association between QNLs and peripheral nervous system toxicity [9], including Guillain–Barré syndrome (GBS), a potentially severe form of acute peripheral polyneuropathy [10]. In 2012, a study by a Canadian research team showed an increased risk of retinal detachment associated with the oral administration of QNLs [11]. Gastrointestinal symptoms such as indigestion, nausea, vomiting and diarrhea are common side effects associated with QNL consumption [12].

Allergic reactions associated with sulfonamides (SAs) include the full range of Gell–Coombs hypersensitivity reactions. In addition, there are reactions associated with immunoglobulin E (IgE), such as urticaria, angioedema and anaphylaxis [13]. SAs have been correlated with hepatotoxicity and systemic hypersensitivity reactions [14,15].

Tetracyclines (TCs) can modify the normal intestinal flora, allowing the overproduction of Pseudomonas and Clostridium [16], and cause nausea, diarrhea and even mortality. They are also found in the structure of newly formed teeth, if consumed during certain periods of pregnancy, such as the embryonic period (from the third through the eighth week after conception) [17]. Hepatotoxicity occurs in patients with hepatic impairment or after intravenous administration of TCs and nephrotoxicity when administered concomitantly with diuretics [18].

Streptomycines (STr) belong to the aminoglycosides (AGs) category of antibiotics. Patients receiving AGs may have reversible nephrotoxicity [19] because AGs can enter the proximal tubule through megaline, a multiligand binding receptor. AG excretion from this intracellular compartment occurs very slowly and can take several days [20]. Side effects include cochlear damage of the auditory nerve [21], optic nerve dysfunction [22], peripheral neuropathy [23], arachnoiditis [24] and encephalopathy [25].

Meat and dairy products constitute an important part of the diet. In 2013, global poultry meat production exceeded 109 million tons and global egg production was estimated at over 73 million tons. In 2014, global production of beef and pork was estimated at about 170 million tons [26]. A major review by the Food and Agriculture Organization (FAO) of the United Nations, which makes extensive use of expert judgement, reported an increase of 76% in the total quantity of meat consumed by the mid-century. This includes a doubling in the consumption of poultry, a 69% increase in beef and a 42% increase in pork [27]. In Europe, cheese and pig meat are the preferred animal-based protein sources, followed by poultry, milk and bovine meat. The EU citizen consumed an average of 2.2 kg less bovine meat in 2013 than in 2000 (decreased by 13%), but 3.0 kg more poultry (increased by 15%). Pork consumption remained nearly fixed throughout this period. According to FAOSTAT (Food and Agriculture Organization of the United Nations) [28], in Greece the mean consumption of bovine meat in 2019 was 14.1 kg/capita/year, for pork 28.9 kg/capita/year and for poultry 25.6 kg/capita/year.

As noted by Arsène et al., antibiotic residues in food, such as meat, are likely to induce antibiotic resistance in bacteria and cause allergies and other more severe effects in humans [29]. This fact, combined with the high positivity in food samples, leads to the assumption that increased meat consumption may be associated with a risk of antibiotic contamination. In addition, as the European Medicines Agency (EMA) describes, when the withdrawal period ("The time that must elapse between the last administration of a veterinary medicine and the slaughter or production of food from that animal") is not respected then the antibiotic residues in meat can exceed the maximum residue levels (MRLs) [30].

This study aims at screening the antibiotic residues in bovine, pork and chicken samples (muscle, liver and kidney) from the local Cretan market, assessing the exposure of the Cretan population to certain compounds due to meat consumption and ultimately estimating the risk for human health resulting from the dietary intake of multiple antibiotics through meat consumption, corrected for the aggregated dietary exposure.

2. Materials and Methods

2.1. Reagents

Methanol (99.9%), formic acid ($\geq$95%) and acetonitrile ($\geq$99.9%) were purchased from Honeywell. Ethyl acetate (99.8%), NaCl (99.9%), n-hexane (99%) and phosphate buffer saline (PBS) tablets were from Sigma Aldrich (Saint Louis, MO, USA). Ultrapure water (Direct-Q 3UV), $Na_2HPO_4 \times 2H_2O$ (99.5%) and NaOH (99%) were purchased from Merck (Darmstadt, Germany). ELISA kits (R3505 RIDASCREEN® Tetracyclin, R3004 RIDASCREEN® Sulfonamide, R3104 RIDASCREEN® Streptomycin, R3113 RIDASCREEN® Quinolones) were purchased from R-Biopharm (Darmstadt, Germany).

2.2. Sampling

A total of 54 samples of raw meat were randomly collected on November 2018 from butcheries in Crete, Greece. The samples were collected from the area of Crete but the animals originated from all over the country. Data concerning the age of the animals and the country of origin were collected. The collected samples were 16 (29.6%) bovine samples, 20 (37.0%) chicken and 18 (33.3%) pork. The collected samples consisted of 29 muscles (53.7%), 17 livers (31.5%) and 8 kidneys (14.8%). Out of the 29 samples there were 10 beef muscles, 6 beef livers, 10 pork muscles, 2 pork livers, 6 pork kidneys, 9 chicken muscles, 9 chicken livers and 2 chicken kidneys. Beef kidneys were not found in any Cretan butcher shop. The majority of the samples (81.5 %) came from animals of Greek origin. The average age of cattle was 15.5 $\pm$ 3.3, for pork 4.9 $\pm$ 2.0 and for chicken 2.3 $\pm$ 0.8 months. All samples were weighted and packed in properly labeled conical centrifuge tubes, sealed and kept at -20 °C, until the analysis.

2.3. Sample Preparation

Total SAs, TCs, STr and QNLs residues were detected using an ELISA test kit. The samples were cut into small pieces and then homogenized with a homogenizer of Janke & Kunkel, Ultraturrax T25 (Staufen, Germany). Then, they were placed in 50 mL Falcon tubes and stored in the freezer (-20 °C) until use. The sample preparation and analysis protocols were instructed from the manufacturer. Briefly, for SAs determination, the homogenized samples were weighed (1 g pork/bovine, 2 g chicken) and vortexed with organic solvent (2 mL methanol for pork/bovine, 6 mL acetonitrile/water 84:16 v/v for chicken). The mixture was centrifuged at 4000 rpm for 10 min and an aliquot of 1.5 mL of supernatant was evaporated to dryness. The dry residue was reconstituted in 0.5 mL buffer (provided by the kit) and 1 mL n-hexane was added. An aliquot of 50 μL of the lower phase was used for analysis. For chicken samples, 4 mL of the supernatant were transferred into a new centrifuge vial, 2 mL 2 M NaCl and 7 mL ethyl acetate were added and the mixture was shaken for 10 min. The mixture was centrifuged for 10 min at 3000 rpm (15 °C). The whole supernatant was evaporated to dryness and reconstituted in 1 mL sample buffer and 1 mL n-hexane. An aliquot of 50 μL of the lower phase was used for analysis.

For STr, 5 g of homogenized sample were mixed with 20 mL of wash buffer, vortexed for 10 s and shaken for 30 min. The mixture was centrifuged (10 min, 4000 rpm, 25 °C), the supernatant was diluted with wash buffer (1:10) and 50 μL were used for analysis.

For TCs, 1 g of homogenized sample and 9 mL 20 mM PBS buffer pH 7.4 were transferred into a centrifuge vial and shaken 10 min for extraction. Then, the mixture was centrifuged (10 min, 4000 rpm, 25 °C) and 1 mL of supernatant was transferred and mixed with 2 mL of n-hexane. An aliquot of 50 µL of the lower aqueous phase was used per well in the assay.

For QNLs, 1 g of homogenized sample and 4 mL methanol/water (70/30, v/v) were mixed vigorously for 10 min and centrifuged (10 min, 4000 rpm, 25 °C). The supernatant was diluted with washing buffer (1:2) and 50 µL were used for analysis.

After samples/standards were loaded, 50 µL of antibody solution were added in each well and plates were incubated for 1 h at room temperature. The wells were washed with 250 µL buffer three times, 100 µL of substrate/chromogen was added and incubated for 15 min at room temperature in the dark. Finally, 100 µL of the stop solution were added to each well and the absorbance was measured at 450 nm.

The LC–MS-based methodology for the detection of antibiotics residues was carried out according to a previously published method [31]. Briefly, 500 µL of EDTA 150 mM were added in 5 g of homogenized meat and vortexed for 10 minutes. Extraction was carried out with 5 mL acidified acetonitrile (0.1% formic acid) for 10 minutes and then the mixtures were placed in the freezer (−20 °C) for 30 minutes. Then extracts were centrifuged (10 min, 4000 rpm), the supernatant was collected and the extraction was repeated. The combined supernatants were evaporated to dryness and the dry residue was reconstituted in 500 µL of the mobile phase.

2.4. Instrumental Analysis

A Shimadzu LC-MS-2010EV (Kyoto, Japan) was used for the detection and quantification of the analytes after the separation of the analytes on a Supelco Discovery C18 column (25 cm × 4.6 mm, 5 µm) (Sigma-Aldrich, Saint Louis, MO, USA). The oven was set at 30 °C and the flow rate was 0.6 mL/min. The mobile phase was water with 0.1% formic acid (Solvent A) and acetonitrile with 0.1% formic acid (Solvent B). The mass spectrometer was coupled with an ESI (electrospray ionization) ion source and the detection was achieved in selected ion monitoring (SIM) in positive mode. The retention times and m/z ions were for MBX: 8.66 min and m/z 362.1, for OTC: 8.90 min and m/z 461.15, for ENR: 9.21 min and m/z 360.1, for DOX: 10.48 min and m/z 445.05, for SDZ: 8.01 min and m/z 251.0/272.9 and for SMX: 11.11 min and m/z 254.0/275.9, respectively

2.5. Exposure Assessment

Exposure of the general population was assessed for each one of the four antibiotic groups (SAs, TCs, QNLs and STr). The daily dietary intake of antibiotics derives from the antibiotic concentration in food consumed and the daily food consumption.

Consumption data for the Greek population for all food items were retrieved from the FAOSTAT database [28] and 2019 data are represented (Table 1). The estimated daily intake of antibiotics from meat, and specifically bovine meat, pig meat and poultry meat (EDImeat) (µg/kg body weight/day), was calculated using the following equation:

$$\text{EDImeat} = \text{Cantibiotic} \times \text{Wfood}/\text{BW} \qquad (1)$$

where cantibiotic is the concentration of antibiotics in meat tissue determined in this study (bovine meat, pig meat and poultry meat), expressed as the median concentration (µg/kg meat, on fresh weight basis), Wmeat (g meat/capita) represents the daily average consumption of meat (bovine meat, pig meat and poultry meat) per person and BW is the mean body weight for an adult consumer (70 kg).

Table 1. Consumption data of food items contributing to the antibiotic dietary exposure, the respective MRLs and the calculated maximum "permitted" daily exposure for each food item (MPDI), for all food items (aggregated (MPDIA)), for meat items estimated (bovine, pig meat and poultry meat) (MPDIm) and correction factor calculated (CF).

Food Item	Consumption Data	Sulfonamides (SAs)		Tetracyclines (TCs)		Quinolones (QNLs)		Streptomycines (STr)	
		MRL	MPDI	MRL	MPDI	MRL	MPDI	MRL	MPDI
	g food/kg bw/day	μg/kg	(μg/kg bw/day)	μg/kg	(μg/kg bw/day)	μg/kg	(μg/kg bw/day)	μg/kg	(μg/kg bw/day)
Honey	0.0650	100	0.0065	100	0.0065	100	0.0065		<0.0001
Bovine Meat	0.5859	100	0.0586	200	0.1172	100	0.0586	600	0.3515
Mutton and Goat Meat	0.3323	100	0.0332	200	0.0665	100	0.0332	600	0.1994
Pig meat	1.1299	100	0.1130	200	0.2260	100	0.1130	600	0.6780
Poultry Meat	1.0023	100	0.1002	200	0.2005	100	0.1002	600	0.6014
Meat, Other	0.0767	100	0.0077	100	0.0077	100	0.0077		<0.0001
Offals, Edible	0.1335	100	0.0133	100	0.0133	100	0.0133		<0.0001
Butter, Ghee	0.0391	100	0.0039	100	0.0039	100	0.0039		<0.0001
Cream	0.0595	100	0.0059	100	0.0059	100	0.0059		<0.0001
Eggs	0.3299	100	0.0330	200	0.0660	100	0.0330		<0.0001
Milk—Excluding Butter	8.9941	100	0.8994	100	0.8994	100	0.8994	200	1.7988
Freshwater Fish	0.0779	100	0.0078	200	0.0156	100	0.0078		<0.0001
Demersal Fish	0.1718	100	0.0172	200	0.0344	100	0.0172		<0.0001
Pelagic Fish	0.1710	100	0.0171	200	0.0342	100	0.0171		<0.0001
Marine Fish, Other	0.0196	100	0.0020	200	0.0039	100	0.0020		<0.0001
MDPIA (μg/kg bw/day)			1.3189		1.7009		1.3189		3.6291
MPDImeat (μg/kg bw/day)			0.2718		0.5436		0.2718		1.6309
CFmeat			0.2061		0.3196		0.2061		0.4494

2.6. Risk Characterization

Risk characterization was conducted following the approach of the source-related hazard quotient (HQ) and hazard index (HI) initially proposed in Goumenou and Tsatsakis [32], and application of the methodology is presented in details in relevant case studies [33–37]. Using this approach, the source-related hazard quotient (HQ) is assessed, after accounting for the correction factor for meat (CFm). The CFm expresses the contribution of meat to the total antibiotic dietary daily intake and it is equal with the ratio of the maximum permitted daily intake through meat consumption MPDIm (meat consumption × maximum residue level (MRL) in meat) to the maximum permitted daily intake through the whole diet, MPDIA (SUM of MPDIi = SUM (food$_i$ consumption × MRL in the food$_i$), where food$_i$ represents each food item with considerable contribution in the overall exposure).

$$\text{MPDIA} = \Sigma \text{MPDIi} \tag{2}$$

$$\text{CFm} = \text{MPDIm}/\text{MPDIA} \tag{3}$$

More specifically, CFm = (consumption data for the meat × MRL for meat)/SUM (consumption data for relevant food$_i$ × MRL in relevant food$_i$).

The corrected EDImeat is calculated with the formula:

$$\text{cEDImeat} = \text{EDImeat}/\text{CFm} \tag{4}$$

ADI and MRL values in relevant food items were extracted from official databases, such as the European Commission [38] and FAO/WHO [39]. According to FAO/WHO, the ADI for SAs and STr is 50 µg/kg bw/day whereas the corresponding value for tetracyclines is 30 µg/kg bw/day. The ADI for quinolones is referred to as 6.2 µg/kg bw/day and specifically for enrofloxacin, selected as the most conservative value [40]. MRLs for TCs, SAs and QNLs were set to be 100 µg/kg, whereas for STr the MRL is 600 µg/kg. The food groups contributing the most to the dietary antibiotic intake we considered from the FAOSTAT database [28] were: honey, bovine meat, mutton and goat meat, pig meat, poultry meat, meat, other, offals, edible butter, ghee, cream, eggs, milk—excluding butter, freshwater fish, demersal fish, pelagic fish, marine fish, other.

Finally, the source-related hazard quotients (HQs) for each antibiotic group (SAs, TCs, QNLs and STr) were calculated with the following formula

$$\text{HQ} = \text{cEDImeat}/\text{ADI} \tag{5}$$

and the HI was calculated as the sum of all HQs.

For considering no risk it should be: CFmi > Hqi, where i is the respective antibiotic group/antibiotic.

3. Results

3.1. Method Performance

For LC–MS analysis, standard solutions of SMX, SDZ, OTC, DOX, MBX and ENR were prepared at concentrations of 0, 50, 100, 250 and 500 ng/mL. Samples of blank raw meat were used for the preparation of spiked samples at concentrations of 0, 10, 25, 50 and 100 µg/kg. The calibration curves were created by the spiked samples and the coefficient of determination (r^2) showed good method linearity for all compounds. The mean accuracy ranged from 92.2% (SMX) to 108.9% (OTC). Limits of detection (LODs) were calculated from the signal-to-noise ratio (S/N) which was S/N > 3 and the achieved values ranged from 0.04 µg/kg (ENR) to 2.54 µg/kg (SDZ) depending on the tissue. Likewise, limits of quantification (LOQs) were calculated as S/N > 10 and the values ranged from 0.13 µg/kg (ENR) to 8.38 µg/kg (SDZ) (Table 2).

Table 2. Analytical parameters for the applied LC–MS protocol.

	Linearity (r²)	LOD (µg/kg)	LOQ (µg/kg)	% Accuracy
MBX	0.999	0.06–0.32 *	0.20–1.06 *	101.4
OTC	0.967	0.67–1.43 *	2.21–4.72 *	108.9
ENR	0.999	0.04–0.14 *	0.13–0.46 *	98.5
DOX	0.996	1.02–2.16 *	3.37–7.13 *	94.8
SDZ	0.998	2.54	8.38	96.5
SMX	0.994	1.15	3.80	92.2

* Depends on the tissue.

3.2. Antibiotic Concentrations Determined with LC–MS

The concentrations of antibiotics that were detected in meat samples by LC–MS are presented in Table 3. The highest median concentrations were detected for DOX at pork kidney (181.73 µg/kg), and OTC at bovine liver (74.46 µg/kg) and chicken liver (64.74 µg/kg). SMX, DOX and MBX were not detected in any bovine liver sample although they were detected in bovine muscle samples. ENR was the one and only antibiotic that was detected in kidneys from chicken at a median concentration of 2.10 µg/kg and it was positive in 100% of the samples. The use of ENR in poultry has been banned by the FDA since 2005 [31], the EU MRL is 100 µg/kg and the detected levels in the present study are lower. According to the results obtained using the ELISA method, only 2% of the meat samples were free from antibiotics, 2% were detected with 4 antibiotics and the great majority of the samples (87%) were detected with 2 to 3 antibiotics (Figure 1).

Table 3. Monitoring results (µg/kg) of antibiotics in all meat samples by LC–MS analysis.

Compounds	µg/kg	Bovine		Pork			Chicken		
		Muscle	Liver	Muscle	Liver	Kidney	Muscle	Liver	Kidney
SMX	% Positive	40	0	60	50	33	89	22	0
	Mean ± SD	22.42 ± 29.78	ND	12.73 ± 5.44	4.49	7.93 ± 4.34	8.23 ± 6.31	4.75 ± 1.12	ND
	Median	9.16	ND	12.39	4.49	7.93	5.58	4.75	ND
	Range	4.40–66.95	ND	7.23–21.68	ND	4.86–11.00	4.51–22.60	3.96–5.54	ND
OTC	% Positive	30	83	60	100	100	22	100	0
	Mean ± SD	10.1 ± 6.53	77.47 ± 14.37	4.75 ± 2.35	34.80 ± 15.13	10.38 ± 5.13	6.39 ± 1.68	68.57 ± 20.55	ND
	Median	8.83	74.46	4.56	34.80	9.08	6.39	64.74	ND
	Range	4.31–17.17	66.60–102.06	2.32–8.54	24.10–45.50	5.46–16.69	5.20–7.57	50.16–94.64	ND
DOX	% Positive	20	0	30	50	50	11	11	0
	Mean ± SD	13.28 ± 11.50	ND	53.14 ± 45.51	26.98	99.91 ± 84.81	12.17	31.72	ND
	Median	13.28	ND	44.10	26.98	181.73	ND	ND	ND
	Range	5.15–21.41	ND	12.84–102.50	ND	12.39–181.73	ND	ND	ND
ENR	% Positive	30	83	30	50	50	44	33	100
	Mean ± SD	3.41 ± 4.24	2.66 ± 1.56	0.56 ± 0.26	1.89	15.63 ± 12.68	3.38 ± 4.20	7.82 ± 1.59	2.10 ± 0.95
	Median	3.41	2.66	0.56	ND	21.13	1.88	7.60	2.10
	Range	0.41–6.41	0.86–4.69	0.37–0.74	ND	1.12–24.63	0.42–9.34	6.35–9.50	1.43–2.77
MBX	% Positive	20	0	20	0	100	33	22	0
	Mean ± SD	14.71 ± 20.42	ND	0.36	ND	0.86 ± 0.23	1.29	9.12	ND
	Median	14.71	ND	ND	ND	0.78	1.29	9.12	ND
	Range	0.27–29.15	ND	ND	ND	0.72–1.33	ND	ND	ND

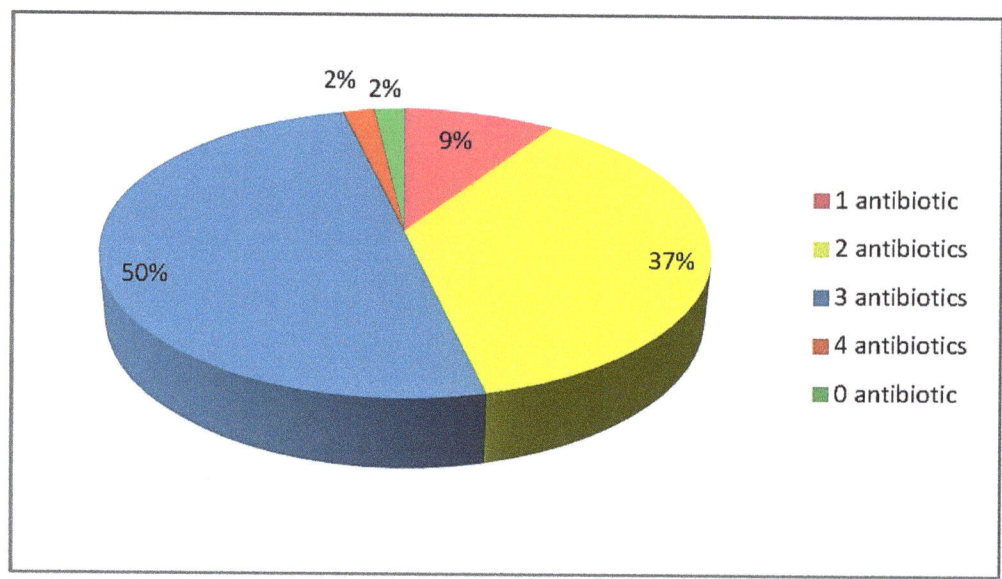

Figure 1. Percentage detection of the investigated antibiotics in all meat samples.

3.3. Antibiotic Concentrations Determined with ELISA

The concentrations of antibiotics that were detected in all meat samples with the ELISA protocol are presented in Table 4 and Figure 2. SAs were the most frequently detected antibiotics in all meat samples, as percentage detection frequency ranged from 83% to 100%. The highest median concentrations were detected in bovine muscles for STr and QNLs at 182.10 µg/kg and 50.78 µg/kg, respectively, and QNLs in pork kidney at 93.36 µg/kg. STr were not detected in any muscle and liver sample from pork and chicken, but it was detected in pork and chicken kidneys. TCs were detected only in pork kidney samples (50%) at a median concentration of 6.89 µg/kg and muscle and liver from chicken at low frequencies (11%).

Table 4. Monitoring results (in µg/kg) of antibiotics in all meat samples by ELISA analysis.

Compounds	µg/kg	Bovine		Pork			Chicken		
		Muscle	Liver	Muscle	Liver	Kidney	Muscle	Liver	Kidney
SAs	% Positive	90	100	100	100	83	89	100	100
	Mean ± SD	7.38 ± 8.68	23.78 ± 30.11	6.31 ± 4.72	47.22 ± 54.88	14.00 ± 15.19	5.17 ± 4.63	4.82 ± 1.55	4.97 ± 0.89
	Median	4.20	9.76	4.40	47.22	3.17	3.60	4.36	4.97
	Range	2.52–30.04	2.10–77.51	2.84–18.9	8.41–86.03	2.51–31.89	1.78–15.70	2.54–7.18	4.35–5.60
STr	% Positive	30	17	0	0	17	0	0	50
	Mean ± SD	169.76 ± 29.94	92.47	ND	ND	151.71	ND	ND	53.44
	Median	182.10	ND	ND	ND	ND	ND	ND	ND
	Range	135.62–191.55	ND	ND	ND	ND	ND	ND	ND
TCs	% Positive	0	0	0	0	50	11	11	0
	Mean ± SD	ND	ND	ND	ND	5.92 ± 1.77	1.97	4.05	ND
	Median	ND	ND	ND	ND	6.89	ND	ND	ND
	Range	ND	ND	ND	ND	3.88–6.99	ND	ND	ND
QNLs	% Positive	20	0	0	0	50	44	33	100
	Mean ± SD	50.78 ± 40.19	ND	ND	ND	146.82 ± 94.00	52.92 ± 46.54	20.82 ± 10.39	13.44 ± 2.09
	Median	50.78	ND	ND	ND	93.36	45.56	20.84	13.44
	Range	22.36–79.20	ND	ND	ND	91.74–255.35	12.76–107.80	10.42–31.20	11.96–14.92

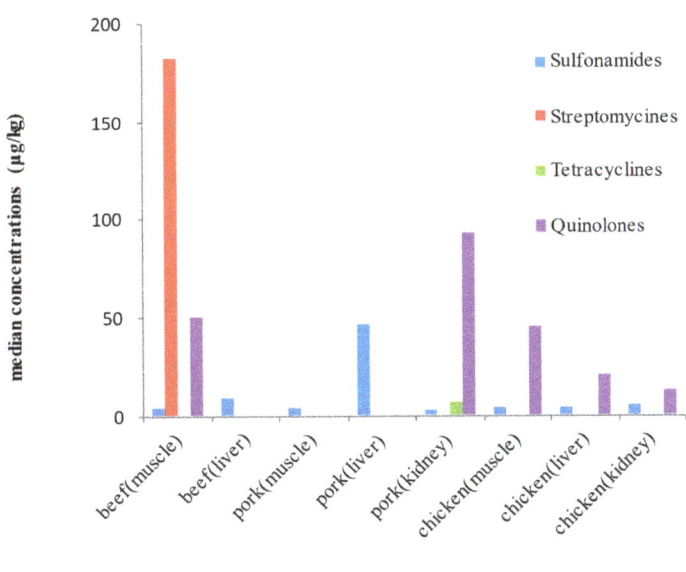

Figure 2. Median concentrations of the investigated antibiotics (μg/kg) determined by the ELISA protocol in all meat samples.

3.4. Exposure Assessment and Risk Characterization

For exposure assessment, we calculated the EDI based on the levels of antibiotics (SAs, TCs, QNLs and STr) in meat samples of three different kinds (pork, bovine and chicken). The daily consumptions per person for Greeks are 41.0 g for bovine, 79.1 g for pork and 70.2 g for poultry meat, according to FAOSTAT. The body weight was considered to be 70 kg [41]. Our results were presented for both methods of analysis used. The EDI through meat consumption (EDIm) of SAs, TCs, QNLs and STr for the Greek population are presented in Table 5 for ELISA values and Table 6 for LC–MS values determined in each kind of meat and total. EDIm did not exceed ADI values either by the type of antibiotic.

Table 5. Estimation of the corrected exposure (cEDI) and hazard quotients (HQs) by ELISA detected levels, ADIs and calculated CFs *.

	Quinolones (QNLs)			Sulfonamides (SAs)			Streptomycines (STr)		
	EDI	cEDI	HQ	EDI	cEDI	HQ	EDI	cEDI	HQ
	μg/kg bw/day	μg/kg bw/day		μg/kg bw/day	μg/kg bw/day		μg/kg bw/day	μg/kg bw/day	
Bovine Meat	0.0298	0.1444	0.0233	0.0025	0.0119	0.0002	0.1067	0.2374	0.0047
Pig Meat	0	0	0	0.0533	0.2589	0.0052	0	0	0
Poultry Meat	0.0457	0.2216	0.0357	0.0036	0.0175	0.0004	0	0	0
cEDIm		0.3659			0.2883			0.2374	
HI			0.0590			0.0058			0.0047
HI total					0.078				

* $CF_{QNLs} = 0.2061$, $CF_{SAs} = 0.2061$, $CF_{Str} = 0.4494$, $ADI_{QNLs} = 6.2$, $ADI_{SAs} = 50$, $ADI_{TCs} = 30$, $ADI_{Str} = 50$ μg/kg bw.

Table 6. Estimation of the corrected exposure(cEDI) and hazard quotients (HQs) by LC-MS detected levels (DL), ADIs and calculated CFs *.

	Quinolones (QNLs)						Sulfonamides (SAs)			Tetracyclines (TCs)					
	ENR			MBX			SMX			OTC			DOX		
	EDI	cEDI	HQ	EDI	cEDI	HQ	EDI	cEDI	HQ	EDI	cEDI	HQ	EDI	cEDI	HQ
	μg/kg bw/day	μg/kg bw/day		μg/kg bw/day	μg/kg bw/day		μg/kg bw/day	μg/kg bw/day		μg/kg bw/day	μg/kg bw/day		μg/kg bw/day	μg/kg bw/day	
Bovine Meat	0.0020	0.0097	0.0016	0.0086	0.0418	0.0067	0.0054	0.0260	0.0005	0.0051	0.0162	0.0005	0.0078	0.0243	0.0008
Pig meat	0.0006	0.0031	0.0005	0	0	0	0.0140	0.0679	0.0014	0.0052	0.0161	0.0005	0.0498	0.1559	0.0052
Poultry Meat	0.0019	0.0091	0.0015	0.0013	0.0063	0.0010	0.0056	0.0271	0.0005	0.0064	0.0200	0.0007	0	0	0
HI				0.0113				0.0024					0.0078		
HI total							0.021								

* CF_{QNLs} = 0.2061, CF_{SAs} = 0.2061, CF_{TCs} = 0.3196, CF_{Str} = 0.4494, ADI_{QNLs} = 6.2, ADI_{SAs} = 50, ADI_{TCs} = 30, ADI_{Str} = 50 μg/kg bw.

Risk characterization methodology, as described by Goumenou and Tsatsakis [31], was applied, in order to assess the risk of exposure to antibiotics (Table 1). Official data were used for the needed calculations. For the risk assessment, we calculated the HQ for each kind of meat and antibiotic (Tables 5 and 6).

For the ELISA method, the HI was calculated to be 0.059 for QNLs, 0.006 for SAs and 0.005 for STr, lower than the corresponding ADI. We had no detected levels for TCs in the ELISA method. LC–MS results led to the calculation of the HI as 0.011 for ENR and MBX, 0.002 for SMX and 0.0078 for OTC and DOX, still far lower than the corresponding ADIs. Admittedly, there is a big difference between the HI of the two methods applied, proportional to the difference in levels and EDIs.

Risk characterization parameters presented in Tables 7 and 8 for both methods, reveal that the ratios of cEDIm to ADI are well below the respective CFs for each antibiotic group indicating no risk for the Greek population, with higher values determined for quinolones by ELISA (Table 7). More specifically, normalized results with CF equal to 1, reach a cEDIm/ADI ratio of 0.2863 corresponding to 28.63% risk, expressing the HQ as a percentage of CF.

Table 7. Hazard characterization parameters (by ELISA analysis).

	Sulfonamides (SAs)	Tetracyclines (TCs)	Quinolones (QNLs)	Streptomycines (STr)
cEDIm (μg/kg bw/day)	0.288	0.250	0.366	0.237
ADI (μg/kg bw/day)	50.000	30.000	6.200	50.000
HQ (=cEDIm/ADI)	0.006	0.008	0.059	0.005
MPDIm (μg/kg bw/day)	0.272	0.544	0.272	1.631
MPDIA (μg/kg bw/day)	1.319	1.701	1.319	3.629
CF	0.206	0.320	0.206	0.449
Risk %	2.798	2.605	28.637	1.111

Table 8. Hazard characterization parameters (by LC–MS analysis).

	Quinolones (QNLs)		Tetracyclines (TCs)		Sulfonamides (SAs)
	ENR	MBX	OTC	DOX	SMX
cEDIm (μg/kg bw/day)	0.022	0.048	0.052	0.180	0.121
ADI (μg/kg bw/day)	6.200	6.200	30.000	30.000	50.000
HQs (=cEDIm/ADI)	0.004	0.008	0.002	0.006	0.002
HQ	0.011		0.008		0.002
MPDIm (μg/kg bw/day)	0.272		0.544		0.272
MPDIA (μg/kg bw/day)	1.319		1.701		1.319
CF	0.206		0.320		0.206
Risk %	5.478		2.426		0.970

4. Discussion

The results of the present study are compared with similar data in literature in Table 9. A study conducted in southern Italy determined OTC levels in beef muscle and liver samples, using LC–MS [42]. Although the number of samples was greater than the present study, very low frequencies were reported (3% in muscle, 7% in liver). The more positive liver samples compared to muscle and the higher liver concentrations of 31.5 µg/kg (23.9–40.2 µg/kg) compared to muscle concentrations of 15.9 µg/kg (15.0–28.6 µg/kg), show a similar trend that was observed in the present study (83% positive bovine liver samples, range: 66.60–102.1 µg/kg and 30% bovine muscle samples, range: 4.31–17.17 µg/kg).

Higher frequencies as well as higher concentrations may be due to inappropriate use of antibiotics and may depend on the rate of drug administration and amounts used. Oxytetracycline is used for pneumonia and some mouth infections. It has been reported that disease burden can vary between seasons depending on humidity [43]. Furthermore, the rate of metabolism of drugs from the body depends on weather and seasonal variations [44]. It should be noted that the seasons when the samples were collected for the present study were autumn and winter.

Panzenhagen et al. screened ENR in muscles, livers and kidneys from chickens with liquid chromatography [45]. Based on their results, 23% of the muscle samples (mean: 12.3 µg/kg), 17% of liver samples (mean: 45.4 µg/kg) and 17% of kidney samples (mean: 17.4 µg/kg) were positive for ENR. Although higher frequencies of detection (44% in muscle, 33% in liver and 100 in kidney samples) were depicted in the current study, the detected mean values of all type of samples were much lower than those reported in the above study.

In South Africa, Ramatla et al. measured sulfonamide residues in pork samples (muscle, liver and kidney) using the ELISA [46]. No sulfonamides were detected in the pork muscle samples, whereas 9% of pork liver samples and 36% of pork kidney samples were positive. The mean concentrations were 58.5 µg/kg (48.2–69.9 µg/kg) and 72.7 µg/kg (52.8–92.8 µg/kg), respectively. The results of the present study are in agreement with Ramatla et al., as higher concentrations of SAs in pork liver/kidney were found compared to pork muscle. In contrast with the literature, higher detection frequencies were found in the present study and particularly all samples of pork muscle were positive.

Table 9. Comparison between current results and data from other monitoring studies in literature.

Reference	Country	Method	N	Samples	Compounds	Mean (µg/kg)	Range	% Positive Samples
Present study	Greece	LC–MS	16 beef	Muscle	OTC	10.1	4.3–17.2	30
				Liver		77.5	66.6–102.1	83
Cammilleri et al., 2019 [42]	Italy	LC–MS	369 beef	Muscle	OTC	15.9	15.0–28.6	3
				Liver		31.5	23.9–40.2	7
Present study	Greece	ELISA	18 pork	Muscle	SAs	6.3	2.8–18.9	100
				Liver		47.2	8.4–86.0	100
				Kidney		14.0	2.5–31.9	83
			20 chicken	Muscle		22.9	1.8–157.3	89
				Liver		4.8	2.5–7.2	100
			16 beef	Muscle		7.4	2.5–30.0	90
				Liver		23.8	2.1–77.5	100
Ramatla et al., 2017 [46]	Africa	ELISA	50 pork	Muscle	SAs	0	-	0
				Liver		58.5	48.2–69.9	9
				Kidney		72.7	52.8–92.8	36
			50 chicken	Muscle		47.5	32.5–65.9	12
				Liver		73.4	45.8–81.6	28
			32 beef	Muscle		65.3	-	7
				Liver		51.6	19.8–87.9	29
Present study	Greece	LC–MS	20 chicken	Muscle	ENR	3.4	0.4–9.3	44
				Liver		7.8	6.4–9.5	33
				Kidney		2.1	1.4–2.8	100
Panzenhagen et al., 2016 [45]	Brazil	LC–MS	72 chicken	Muscle	ENR	12.3	0.96–35.8	23
				Liver		45.4	-	17
				Kidney		17.4	-	17
Present study	Greece	ELISA	16 Beef	Muscle	STr	169.8	135.6–191.5	30
Abdullah et al., 2012 [47]	Iraq	ELISA	23 Beef	Muscle	STr	59.6	26.0–282.2	61

In a study in Iraq, STr levels in 23 beef muscle samples were determined by ELISA [47]. A total of 61% of the samples were positive with a mean concentration of 59.60 μg/kg (26.0–282.2 μg/kg). However, in our study the results differ significantly as 30% of the samples were positive with a mean concentration of 169.76 μg/kg (135.62–191.5 μg/kg).

The observed differences between the results of the present study and others in literature [46,47] may be due to the way that antibiotics were administered, for example intramuscularly, intravenously or administration via food and drinking water. Furthermore, the long-term use of antibiotics before sampling and the short time between last antibiotic administration and slaughter may be significant parameters for the detection rate of the compounds. According to Yamaguchi et al. [48], the sampling period affected significantly the detected concentrations of antibiotics in chicken samples. Higher or lesser amounts were detected during five separate occasions.

Exposure and risk assessment analysis in the present study showed that the antibiotics levels in chicken, pork and beef from the Cretan market pose no actual risk for human health. To the best of our knowledge, this is the first study for antibiotics in meat from the Greek market although there are others similar in literature. A recent work by Oyedeji et al. [49] presented the concentrations of nineteen antibiotic residues in imported poultry products (turkey muscle and gizzard and chicken muscle) in Nigeria. The risk assessment analysis with the conventional method showed that the dietary exposure to antibiotics per meat type was within safe levels for adults and children. Vragovic et al. examined streptomycin and tetracyclines presence in meat samples of the Croatian market [50]. Similar to the present study, EDI was significantly higher for streptomycin (5.56 μg/person/day or 0.080 μg/kg bw/day) than TCs (0.21 μg/person/day or 0.003 μg/kg bw/day). The same trend was observed in our results too, as performing the LC–MS method for TCs led to EDI approximately two orders of magnitude lower than STr.

In 2017, Wang et al. investigated livestock and poultry meat samples from Shanghai for TCs, QNLs and SAs presence [51]. Estimated daily exposure dose was below 1 μg/kg bw/day, whereas according to the authors aquatic products were a more importance source of these antibiotics than meat or milk. Kyriakides et al. examined the differences in exposure to antibiotics between children and adolescents in Cyprus from the consumption of pork meat for the years from 2012 to 2017 [52]. EDI values were far below ADI and notably higher in children aged 6–9 years old compared to adolescents aged 10–17 years old. All HI values were below 0.056 and indicated low risk exposure for all participants.

A different approach was followed by Zhang et al. [53], who calculated EDI from the urinary levels of the excreted antibiotics to estimate initial exposure of the Chinese. They found that 14.7% of the children had HI greater than 1 as well as 23.6% of the parents and 11.8% of the grandparents, with ciprofloxacin being the major contributor to exposure among all participants. Lately, researchers aimed to describe the antibiotic exposure in Shanghai primary school students [54]. Fluoroquinolones, lincosamides, sulfonamides and tetracyclines were examined and the totally daily exposure dose was found to be below 1 μg/kg bw/day. Finally, the study concluded that intake frequency of white meat (poultry meat) is positively associated with TCS and intake frequency of dairy products with enrofloxacin (QNLs).

5. Conclusions

To the best of our knowledge, this is the first study that screened antibiotic residues in bovine, pork and chicken samples (muscle, liver and kidney) from the Greek Cretan market. Only 2% of the samples were free from antibiotics, 2% were detected with 4 antibiotics and the great majority of the samples (87%) were detected with 2 to 3 antibiotics. The risk assessment analysis indicated that there is no risk from beef, pork and chicken consumption corrected for the aggregated exposure. Although intake was estimated to be low and exposure can be considered safe, the dietary habits among consumers vary and increased consumption of several foods that are burdened with antibiotics can raise the risk. Furthermore, low and long-term exposure can have severe effects for gut microbiota which in turn is related with severe consequences for health and diseases that sometimes are not directly correlated with antibiotics exposure.

6. Limitations

In the current study, we aimed to determine the levels of four groups of antibiotics in meat samples and to estimate the dietary exposure to antibiotics from meat consumption as well as the potential hazard for human health. Although we tried to address the issue of aggregated exposure through the applied methods, we still have not approached the cumulative exposure issue. Additionally, the local market sampling as well as the consumption data, which were derived from one specific database, limited the scope of objectivity. Finally, each of the two applied methods had its own limitations; the ELISA method provided us with concentration data for a whole group of compounds. In contrast, the LC—MS method offered results for specific compounds, but it was not possible to detect all the compounds of each group.

Author Contributions: Investigation, Validation, Formal analysis, Writing—original draft, A.S.; Investigation, Resources, Data curation, Writing—original draft, V.K.; Resources, Methodology, Writing—original draft, I.K.; Methodology, Data curation, E.R.; Resources, Methodology, E.V., M.A., M.S. and M.K.; Formal analysis, Data curation, A.A.; Conceptualization, Methodology, Validation, Supervision, Writing—review and editing, M.N.T., A.K.R. and A.T. All authors have read and agreed to the published version of the manuscript.

Funding: This research received no external funding.

Institutional Review Board Statement: Not applicable.

Informed Consent Statement: Not applicable.

Data Availability Statement: Not applicable.

Conflicts of Interest: The authors declare no conflict of interest.

References

1. Diaz-Sanchez, S.; Moscoso, S.; Solís de los Santos, F.; Andino, A.; Hanning, I. Antibiotic use in poultry; A driving force for organic poultry production. *Food Prot. Trends* **2015**, *35*, 440–447.
2. Regulation (EC) No 1831/2003 of the European Parliament and of the Council of 22 September 2003 on Additives for Use in Animal Nutrition. Available online: https://eur-lex.europa.eu/legal-content/EN/TXT/?uri=CELEX%3A32003R1831 (accessed on 29 November 2018).
3. Baynes, R.E.; Dedonder, K.; Kissell, L.; Mzyk, D.; Marmulak, T.; Smith, G.; Riviere, J.E. Health concerns and management of select veterinary drug residues. *Food Chem. Toxicol.* **2016**, *88*, 112–122. [CrossRef]
4. Directive 2004/28/EC of the European Parliament and of the Council of 31 March 2004 Amending Directive 2001/82/EC on the Community Code Relating to Veterinary Medicinal Products. Available online: https://eur-lex.europa.eu/legal-content/EN/TXT/?uri=celex%3A32004L0028 (accessed on 29 November 2018).
5. Kuriyama, T.; Karasawa, T.; Williams, D.W. Chapter Thirteen-Antimicrobial Chemotherapy: Significance to Healthcare. In *Biofilms in Infection Prevention and Control*; Steven, L., David, P., Williams, W., Randle, J., Cooper, T., Eds.; Academic Press: Cambridge, MA, USA, 2014; pp. 209–244. ISBN 9780123970435.
6. Toldr, F.; Reig, M. Chemical Origin Toxic Compounds. In *Handbook of Fermented Meat and Poultry*; Blackwell: Ames, IA, USA, 2007; pp. 469–475.
7. Sarro, A.; Sarro, G. Adverse Reactions to Fluoroquinolones. An Overview on Mechanistic Aspects. *Curr. Med. Chem.* **2001**, *8*, 371–384. [CrossRef] [PubMed]
8. Grill, M.F.; Maganti, R.K. Neurotoxic effects associated with antibiotic use: Management considerations. *Br. J. Clin. Pharmacol.* **2011**, *72*, 381–393. [CrossRef] [PubMed]
9. Estofan, L.J.F.; Naydin, S.; Gliebus, G. Quinolone-Induced Painful Peripheral Neuropathy: A Case Report and Literature Review. *J. Investig. Med. High Impact Case Rep.* **2018**, *6*, 232470961775273. [CrossRef] [PubMed]
10. Ali, A.K. Peripheral neuropathy and Guillain-Barré syndrome risks associated with exposure to systemic fluoroquinolones: A pharmacovigilance analysis. *Ann. Epidemiol.* **2014**, *24*, 279–285. [CrossRef] [PubMed]
11. Etminan, M.; Forooghian, F.; Brophy, J.M.; Bird, S.T.; Maberley, D. Oral fluoroquinolones and the risk of retinal detachment. *JAMA* **2012**, *307*, 1414–1419. [PubMed]

12. Hsu, S.-C.; Chang, S.-S.; Lee, M.-T.G.; Lee, S.-H.; Tsai, Y.-W.; Lin, S.-C.; Chen, S.-T.; Weng, Y.-C.; Porta, L.; Wu, J.Y.; et al. Risk of gastrointestinal perforation in patients taking oral fluoroquinolone therapy: An analysis of nationally representative cohort. *PLoS ONE* **2017**, *12*, e0183813. [CrossRef]
13. Brackett, C.C. Sulfonamide allergy and cross-reactivity. *Curr. Allergy Asthma Rep.* **2007**, *7*, 41–48. [CrossRef]
14. Slim, R.; Asmar, N.; Yaghi, C.; Honein, K.; Sayegh, R.; Chelala, D. Trimethoprim-sulfamethoxazole-induced hepatotoxicity in a renal transplant patient. *Indian J. Nephrol.* **2017**, *27*, 482. [CrossRef]
15. Yang, J.-J.; Huang, C.-H.; Liu, C.-E.; Tang, H.-J.; Yang, C.-J.; Lee, Y.-C.; Lee, K.-Y.; Taai, M.-S.; Lin, S.-W.; Chen, Y.-H.; et al. Multicenter Study of Trimethoprim/Sulfamethoxazole-Related Hepatotoxicity: Incidence and Associated Factors among HIV-Infected Patients Treated for Pneumocystis jirovecii Pneumonia. *PLoS ONE* **2014**, *9*, e106141. [CrossRef] [PubMed]
16. Heta, S.; Robo, I. The Side Effects of the Most Commonly Used Group of Antibiotics in Periodontal Treatments. *Med. Sci.* **2018**, *6*, 6. [CrossRef] [PubMed]
17. Vennila, V.; Madhu, V.; Rajesh, R.; Ealla, K.K.; Velidandla, S.R.; Santoshi, S. Tetracycline-induced discoloration of deciduous teeth: Case series. *J. Int. Oral Health JIOH* **2014**, *6*, 115–119.
18. Cervelli, M.J.; Russ, G.R. *Comprehensive Clinical Nephrology*, 4th ed.; Elsevier: Amsterdam, The Netherlands, 2010; p. 870.
19. Oliveira, J.F.P.; Cipullo, J.P.; Burdmann, E.A. Nefrotoxicidade dos aminoglicosídeos. *Braz. J. Cardiovasc. Surg.* **2006**, *21*, 444–452. [CrossRef]
20. Nagai, J.; Takano, M. Entry of aminoglycosides into renal tubular epithelial cells via endocytosis-dependent and endocytosis-independent pathways. *Biochem. Pharmacol.* **2014**, *90*, 331–337. [CrossRef] [PubMed]
21. Selimoglu, E. Aminoglycoside-Induced Ototoxicity. *Curr. Pharm. Des.* **2007**, *13*, 119–126. [CrossRef]
22. Hancock, H.A.; Guidry, C.; Read, R.W.; Ready, E.L.; Kraft, T.W. Acute Aminoglycoside Retinal Toxicity In Vivo and In Vitro. *Investig. Opthalmology Vis. Sci.* **2005**, *46*, 4804. [CrossRef] [PubMed]
23. Mitolo-Chieppa, D.; Carratù, M.R. Aminoglycoside Antibiotics: A Study of Their Neurotoxic Effects at Peripheral Nerve Fibres. In *Disease, Metabolism and Reproduction in the Toxic Response to Drugs and Other Chemicals*; Archives of Toxicology (Supplement); Chambers, P.L., Preziosi, P., Chambers, C.M., Eds.; Springer: Berlin/Heidelberg, Germany, 2019; Volume 7.
24. Morcamp, D.; Mizon, J.; Rosa, A. Toxicity of the intrathecal administration of aminoglycosides. 3 cases of paraplegia. In *Agressologie: Revue Internationale de Physio-Biologie et de Pharmacologie Appliquées aux Effets De L'agression*; Springer: Berlin/Heidelberg, Germany, 1983; Volume 24, pp. 187–189.
25. Wadlington, W.; Hatcher, H.; Turner, D.J. Osteomyelitis of the patella: Gentamicin therapy associated with encephalopathy. *Clin. Pediatrics* **1977**, *10*, 577–580. [CrossRef] [PubMed]
26. USDA-FAS. Foreign Agriculture Service–USDA. Available online: https://www.fas.usda.gov/ (accessed on 6 October 2019).
27. Godfray, H.C.J.; Aveyard, P.; Garnett, T.; Hall, J.W.; Key, T.J.; Lorimer, J.; Pierrehumbert, R.T.; Scarborough, P.; Springmann, M.; Jebb, S.A. Meat consumption, health, and the environment. *Science* **2018**, *361*, eaam5324. [CrossRef]
28. FAOSTAT. Available online: http://www.fao.org/faostat/en/ (accessed on 10 November 2021).
29. Arsène, M.M.J.; Davares, A.K.L.; Viktorovna, P.I.; Andreevna, S.L.; Sarra, S.; Khelifi, I.; Sergueïevna, D.M. The public health issue of antibiotic residues in food and feed: Causes, consequences, and potential solutions. *Vet. World* **2022**, *15*, 662–671. [CrossRef]
30. Federal Register 70 FR 44105–Enrofloxacin for Poultry; Final Decision on Withdrawal of New Animal Drug Application Following Formal Evidentiary Public Hearing. Available online: https://www.federalregister.gov/documents/2005/08/01/05-15224/enrofloxacin-for-poultry-final-decision-on-withdrawal-of-new-animal-drug-application-following (accessed on 15 February 2019).
31. Martins, M.T.; Barreto, F.; Hoff, R.B.; Jank, L.; Arsand, J.B.; Feijó, T.C.; Schapoval, E.E.S. Determination of quinolones and fluoroquinolones, tetracyclines and sulfonamides in bovine, swine and poultry liver using LC-MS/MS. *Food Addit. Contam. Part A* **2015**, *32*, 1–9. [CrossRef] [PubMed]
32. Goumenou, M.; Tsatsakis, A. Proposing new approaches for the risk characterization of single chemicals and chemical mixtures: The source related Hazard Quotient (HQS) and Hazard Index (HIS) and the adversity specific Hazard Index (HIA). *Toxicol. Rep.* **2019**, *6*, 632–636. [CrossRef] [PubMed]
33. Taghizadeh, S.F.; Davarynejad, G.; Asili, J.; Nemati, S.H.; Rezaee, R.; Goumenou, M.; Tsatsakis, A.M.; Karimi, G. Health risk assessment of heavy metals via dietary intake of five pistachio (*Pistacia vera* L.) cultivars collected from different geographical sites of Iran. *Food Chem. Toxicol.* **2017**, *107*, 99–107. [CrossRef]
34. Taghizadeh, S.F.; Goumenou, M.; Rezaee, R.; Alegakis, T.; Kokaraki, V.; Anesti, O.; Sarigiannis, D.A.; Tsatsakis, A.; Karimi, G. Cumulative risk assessment of pesticide residues in different Iranian pistachio cultivars: Applying the source specific HQS and adversity specific HIA approaches in Real Life Risk Simulations (RLRS). *Toxicol. Lett.* **2019**, *313*, 91–100. [CrossRef] [PubMed]
35. Renieri, E.A.; Goumenou, M.; Kardonsky, D.A.; Veselov, V.V.; Alegakis, A.; Buha, A.; Tzatzarakis, M.N.; Nosyrev, A.E.; Rakitskii, V.N.; Kentouri, M.; et al. Indicator PCBs in farmed and wild fish in Greece-Risk assessment for the Greek population. *Food Chem. Toxicol.* **2019**, *127*, 260–269. [CrossRef] [PubMed]
36. Tzatzarakis, M.; Kokkinakis, M.; Renieri, E.; Goumenou, M.; Kavvalakis, M.; Vakonaki, E.; Chatzinikolaou, A.; Stivaktakis, P.; Tsakiris, I.; Rizos, A.; et al. Multiresidue analysis of insecticides and fungicides in apples from the Greek market. Applying an alternative approach for risk assessment. *Food Chem. Toxicol.* **2020**, *140*, 111262. [CrossRef] [PubMed]

37. Năstăsescu, V.; Mititelu, M.; Goumenou, M.; Docea, A.O.; Renieri, E.; Udeanu, D.I.; Oprea, E.; Arsene, A.L.; Dinu-Pîrvu, C.E.; Ghica, M. Heavy metal and pesticide levels in dairy products: Evaluation of human health risk. *Food Chem. Toxicol.* **2020**, *146*, 111844. [CrossRef]
38. EU. Commission Regulation (of 22 December 2009) on Pharmacologically Active Substances and Their Classification Regarding Maximum Residue Limits in Foodstuffs of Animal Origin. (EU) No 37/2010. 2010. Available online: https://eur-lex.europa.eu/legal-content/EN/TXT/?uri=celex%3A32010R0037 (accessed on 24 January 2019).
39. FAO/WHO. Maximum Residue Limits (MRLs) and Risk Management Recommendations (RMRs) for Residues of Veterinary Drugs in Foods. CX/MRL 2–2018. 2018. Available online: https://www.fao.org/fao-who-codexalimentarius/codex-texts/maximum-residue-limits/en/ (accessed on 1 May 2019).
40. Hanna, N.; Sun, P.; Sun, Q.; Li, X.; Yang, X.; Ji, X.; Zou, H.; Ottoson, J.; Nilsson, L.E.; Berglund, B.; et al. Presence of antibiotic residues in various environmental compartments of Shandong province in eastern China: Its potential for resistance development and ecological and human risk. *Environ. Int.* **2018**, *114*, 131–142. [CrossRef]
41. WHO. *Guidelines for Drinking-Water Quality*; First Addendum to Third Edition; World Health Organization: Geneva, Switzerland, 2006; Volume 1.
42. Cammilleri, G.; Pulvirenti, A.; Vella, A.; Macaluso, A.; Dico, G.L.; Giaccone, V.; Ferrantelli, V. Tetracycline Residues in Bovine Muscle and Liver Samples from Sicily (Southern Italy) by LC-MS/MS Method: A Six-Year Study. *Molecules* **2019**, *24*, 695. [CrossRef]
43. Aalipour, F.; Mirlohi, M.; Jalali, M. Prevalence of antibiotic residues in com- mercial milk and its variation by season and thermal processing methods. *Int. J. Environ. Health Eng.* **2013**, *2*, 41.
44. Cerveny, D.; Fick, J.; Klaminder, J.; McCallum, E.S.; Bertram, M.G.; Castillo, N.A.; Brodin, T. Water temperature affects the biotransformation and accumulation of a psychoactive pharmaceutical and its metabolite in aquatic organisms. *Environ. Int.* **2021**, *155*, 106705. [CrossRef] [PubMed]
45. Panzenhagen, P.H.N.; Aguiar, W.S.; Gouvêa, R.; Oliveira, A.M.G.D.; Barreto, F.; Pereira, V.L.A.; Aquino, M.H.C. Investigation of enrofloxacin residues in broiler tissues using ELISA and LC-MS/MS. *Food Addit. Contam. Part A* **2016**, *33*, 1–5. [CrossRef]
46. Ramatla, T.; Ngoma, L.; Adetunji, M.; Mwanza, M. Evaluation of Antibiotic Residues in Raw Meat Using Different Analytical Methods. *Antibiotics* **2017**, *6*, 34. [CrossRef] [PubMed]
47. Abdullah, O.A.; Shareef, A.M.; Sheet, O.H. Detection of streptomycin residues in local meat of bovine and ovine. *Iraqi J. Vet. Sci.* **2012**, *26*, 43–46. [CrossRef]
48. Yamaguchi, T.; Okihashi, M.; Harada, K.; Konishi, Y.; Uchida, K.; Hoang, M.; Nguyen, T.D.; Nuyen, P.D.; Chau, V.V.; Dao, K.T.V.; et al. Antibiotic Residue Monitoring Results for Pork, Chicken, and Beef Samples in Vietnam in 2012–2013. *J. Agric. Food Chem.* **2015**, *63*, 5141–5145. [CrossRef]
49. Oyedeji, A.O.; Msagati, T.A.M.; Williams, A.B.; Benson, N.U. Determination of Antibiotic Residues in Frozen Poultry by a Solid-Phase Dispersion Method Using Liquid Chromatography-Triple Quadrupole Mass Spectrometry. *Toxicol. Rep.* **2019**, *6*, 951–956. [CrossRef] [PubMed]
50. Vragović, N.; Bazulić, D.; Njari, B. Risk assessment of streptomycin and tetracycline residues in meat and milk on Croatian market. *Food Chem. Toxicol.* **2011**, *49*, 352–355. [CrossRef] [PubMed]
51. Wang, H.; Ren, L.; Yu, X.; Hu, J.; Chen, Y.; He, G.; Jiang, Q. Antibiotic residues in meat, milk and aquatic products in Shanghai and human exposure assessment. *Food Control* **2017**, *80*, 217–225. [CrossRef]
52. Kyriakides, D.; Lazaris, A.C.; Arsenoglou, K.; Emmanouil, M.; Kyriakides, O.; Kavantzas, N.; Panderi, I. Dietary exposure assessment of veterinary antibiotics in pork meat on children and adolescents in Cyprus. *Foods* **2020**, *9*, 1479. [CrossRef] [PubMed]
53. Zhang, J.; Liu, X.; Zhu, Y.; Yang, L.; Sun, L.; Wei, R. Ecotoxicology and Environmental Safety Antibiotic exposure across three generations from Chinese families and cumulative health risk. *Ecotoxicol. Environ. Saf.* **2020**, *191*, 110237. [CrossRef]
54. Zhang, Y.; Tang, W.; Wang, Y.; Nian, M.; Jiang, F.; Zhang, J.; Chen, Q. Environmental antibiotics exposure in school-age children in Shanghai and health risk assessment: A population-based representative investigation. *Sci. Total Environ.* **2022**, *824*, 153859. [CrossRef] [PubMed]

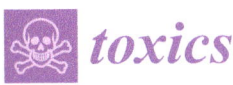

Article

Bisphenol S Impairs Oestradiol Secretion during In Vitro Basal Folliculogenesis in a Mono-Ovulatory Species Model

Claire Vignault [1,2], Véronique Cadoret [1,2], Peggy Jarrier-Gaillard [1], Pascal Papillier [1], Ophélie Téteau [1], Alice Desmarchais [1], Svetlana Uzbekova [1], Aurélien Binet [1,3], Fabrice Guérif [1,2], Sebastien Elis [1] and Virginie Maillard [1,*]

1. CNRS, IFCE, INRAE, Université de Tours, PRC, 37380 Nouzilly, France; claire.vignault@inrae.fr (C.V.); veronique.cadoret@inrae.fr (V.C.); peggy.jarrier-gaillard@inrae.fr (P.J.-G.); pascal.papillier@inrae.fr (P.P.); teteau.ophelie@orange.fr (O.T.); alice.desmarchais@inrae.fr (A.D.); svetlana.uzbekova@inrae.fr (S.U.); aurelien.binet@inrae.fr (A.B.); fabrice.guerif@univ-tours.fr (F.G.); sebastien.elis@inrae.fr (S.E.)
2. Service de Médecine et Biologie de la Reproduction, CHRU de Tours, 37000 Tours, France
3. Service de Chirurgie Pédiatrique Viscérale, Urologique, Plastique et Brûlés, CHRU de Tours, 37000 Tours, France
* Correspondence: virginie.maillard@inrae.fr

Abstract: Bisphenol S (BPS) affects terminal folliculogenesis by impairing steroidogenesis in granulosa cells from different species. Nevertheless, limited data are available on its effects during basal folliculogenesis. In this study, we evaluate in vitro the effects of a long-term BPS exposure on a model of basal follicular development in a mono-ovulatory species. We cultured ovine preantral follicles (180–240 µm, n = 168) with BPS (0.1 µM (possible human exposure dose) or 10 µM (high dose)) and monitored antrum appearance and follicular survival and growth for 15 days. We measured hormonal secretions (oestradiol (at day 13 [D13]), progesterone and anti-Müllerian hormone [D15]) and expression of key follicular development and redox status genes (D15) in medium and whole follicles, respectively. BPS (0.1 µM) decreased oestradiol secretion compared with the control (−48.8%, p < 0.001), without significantly impairing antrum appearance, follicular survival and growth, anti-Müllerian hormone and progesterone secretion and target gene expression. Thus, BPS could also impair oestradiol secretion during basal folliculogenesis as it is the case during terminal folliculogenesis. It questions the use of BPS as a safe BPA substitute in the human environment. More studies are required to elucidate mechanisms of action of BPS and its effects throughout basal follicular development.

Keywords: ovary; endocrine disruptors; follicular growth; hormonal secretions; gene expression; bisphenols; plasticiser; ewe

1. Introduction

Folliculogenesis is a long and discontinuous developmental process that leads to the ovarian follicle growth and that requires constant tight communications between oocyte and somatic follicle cells (granulosa, cumulus and theca cells) [1,2]. From a functional perspective, follicular development is divided into two successive phases: basal folliculogenesis corresponds to the initial development of primordial follicles released from the ovarian reserve to an antral follicle. It is a gonadotrophin hormone independent phase during which granulosa cells have an intense mitotic activity and the ability to produce Anti-Müllerian Hormone (AMH) and some steroid hormones. In contrast, terminal folliculogenesis, which leads to ovulation of a mature and competent oocyte, is strictly dependent on Follicle-Stimulating Hormone (FSH) and Luteinising Hormone (LH) presence. During this phase, granulosa cell proliferation and AMH production decrease, whereas steroidogenesis activity drastically increases. Folliculogenesis is regulated by endogenous growth factors, cytokines, gonadotropins and steroid hormones as well as exogenous factors, such

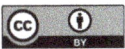

as nutrients and environmental factors [3]. Thus, several environmental pollutants (e.g., the pesticide dichlorodiphenyltrichloroethane (DDT), the fungicide vinclozolin, the synthetic oestrogen Diethylstilbestrol (DES), the plasticiser bisphenol A (BPA), etc.) that present endocrine-disrupting properties can indeed affect female fertility by altering ovarian development and functions [4].

Over the last 20 years, BPA has become one of the most studied endocrine disruptors due to its massive worldwide use in many everyday plastic materials, mainly in polycarbonate plastics (for food containers, cosmetics, electronics, etc.) and epoxy resins (as a protective coating for food cans, pipes, floors and as composite in paints, etc.) [5]. Therefore, BPA human exposure occurs mainly through contaminated diet [6,7] but also through inhalation of plastic dust [8,9] and percutaneous absorption [10,11]. Based on its endocrine-disrupting properties and its possible involvements in the development of human pathologies (metabolic and reproductive disorders and cardiovascular diseases, among others) [12–16], BPA use has been regulated in some countries from the European Union and in Canada [17,18]. Consequently, BPA has been replaced with several structural analogues, with bisphenol S (BPS) being the most used [19,20].

Similar to BPA, BPS is nowadays detected in the environment [9,19] and in several human body fluids and tissue, including urine [21–23], plasma or serum, [24,25], hair [26] and in follicular fluid [27]. Thus, BPS can be in contact with ovarian follicular cells and can induce female mammalian reproductive dysfunctions [28,29]. Indeed, BPS altered oocyte quality and/or embryo development in sows [30], cows [31,32], mice [33–35] and ewes [36]. Furthermore, BPS impaired ovarian steroidogenesis in vivo or in vitro from granulosa cells of both mono-ovulatory species (bovine [31], ovine [37] and human [27]) and polyovulatory species (swine [38,39] and rodents [40,41]). Most of these studies have focussed on terminal folliculogenesis and have highlighted differences in BPS effects depending on species, BPS doses and exposure time. There are few studies on the effects of BPS on basal folliculogenesis. These studies have been conducted in rodent models after in vivo BPS exposure; one of them has shown an increased number of primordial follicles [35] and others have reported a decreased number of preantral and/or antral follicles [33,35,42,43]. These data suggest a potential action of BPS on primordial follicle and antrum formation in rodents, but no data are available in other species or in mono-ovulatory species in particular.

The mechanisms of action of bisphenols are not yet fully understood in the gonads. Studies have shown that bisphenols could interact with several receptor-mediated signalling pathways in different cell types—for example, nuclear Estrogen Receptors (ERα and ERβ), Estrogen-Related Receptors (ERRγ) and Aryl hydrocarbon Receptor (AhR) [44–47]. They could also act by altering DNA methylation in different cells [48–51]. Finally, bisphenols could also enhance oxidative stress in different cells [52–54], including granulosa cells [38,55]. However, to date there is scarce information regarding the potential mechanisms of action of BPS during basal folliculogenesis.

We hypothesized that BPS could impair basal follicular growth and antrum appearance in a mono-ovulatory species. We aimed then to study BPS effects on follicular development and hormonal secretions during basal folliculogenesis (especially in the antrum-appearance phase), as it has already been described for terminal folliculogenesis. We chose the ewe as a study model because its ovarian development and folliculogenesis duration present similarities with those of the human species [2,56,57]. Thus, we studied the effects of two concentrations of BPS on ewe basal follicular development in vitro, especially on follicular growth and survival, antral cavity appearance, follicle hormonal secretions (oestradiol, progesterone and Anti-Müllerian Hormone (AMH)) and the expression of key genes in follicular development and redox status.

2. Materials and Methods

Unless stated otherwise, all culture media and chemicals used in the present study were purchased from Merck Sigma-Aldrich (Saint-Quentin-Fallavier, France).

2.1. Collection of Ovaries and Isolation and In Vitro Culture of Preantral Follicles

Over 300 ovaries were recovered from peri-pubertal ewes (over 150 animals) at a local commercial slaughterhouse to collect all 168 healthy follicles used in the seven independent experiments of this study. Ovaries were washed with sterile 0.9% NaCl supplemented with 52.35 µM gentamicin, and then transported to the laboratory within 2 h after collection in tubes containing HEPES-buffered tissue culture medium 199 supplemented with 6 µM bovine serum albumin (BSA) and 52.35 µM gentamicin (TCM199+). The ovaries were cut into thin slices using a sterile surgical blade. These slices were incubated at 37 °C for 1 h in a cell dissociation phosphate-buffered saline (PBS)-based solution containing 0.1% collagenase IA (m/v) and 0.01% DNase I (m/v), and then in a stop solution of PBS containing 0.3 mM BSA. After rinsing in warm TCM199+ medium, follicles were mechanically isolated from the cortical ovary slices by micro-dissection under a stereomicroscope using two 30-gauge needles fitted to 1 mL syringe barrels. Subsequently, the follicles were stored in Petri dishes containing TCM199+ medium. On this day 0 (D0), the initial diameter of all follicles was measured on the perpendicular axes with a stereomicroscope equipped with a calibrated ocular micrometer. Only healthy preantral follicles between 180 µm and 240 µm in diameter, with no apparent damage to the basal membrane, no visible signs of degeneration (darkness of the oocyte and follicular cells) and no antral cavity were selected for culture.

The follicle culture was adapted from a previously described protocol [58]. The culture medium (MEM+) was prepared the day prior to the culture (or medium renewal) with sodium-bicarbonate-buffered Minimum Essential Medium Eagle (MEM; alpha modification) supplemented with 2 mM glutamine, 2 mM hypoxanthine, 0.28 mM ascorbic acid and ITS+ Universal Culture Supplement Pre-mix (1.08 µM insulin, 81.1 nM transferrin, 48.5 nM selenium, 18.8 µM BSA and 19.1 µM linoleic acid; Corning, D. Dutscher, Issy-les-Moulineaux, France) and with different concentrations of BPS (0, 0.1 or 10 µM). The 0.1 µM dose was chosen, because such concentrations were reported in human biological fluids (urine and plasma) for some people in several studies [19,25,59]. Thus, we decided to name this concentration a possible human exposure dose. The 10 µM dose, defined as a high dose, was tested as a reference to the concentration used in several in vitro studies that observed BPS effects with it for acute exposure in ovarian follicular cells [27,37]. On the other hand, all conditions in our study (including the control condition) contained the same ethanol concentration (1/10,000 = 0.01%). For each culture, Petri dishes containing droplets of 100 µL of culture medium covered with mineral oil were pre-equilibrated overnight at 38.5 °C in 5% CO_2 in air under 95% relative humidity. Isolated measured healthy follicles were washed twice in TCM199+ and then randomly allocated into the three treatment groups. Follicles were individually placed into each 100 µL droplet and incubated for up to 15 days. At days D6 and D13, 50% of the culture medium in each droplet was replaced with fresh pre-incubated medium, and the medium removed from each droplet was individually frozen at −20 °C for the hormone assays, as described below. The 15-day culture period was optimal for studying in vitro basal follicular growth of early antral follicles and the antrum appearance in this in vitro model [58]. Indeed, in this model, the antral cavity appears in follicles with a diameter ≥320 µm, a size obtained after 6 days of culture. Furthermore, at D15 the follicles reach a size of about 550 µm and about 80% of these follicles have an antrum.

2.2. Morphological Evaluation of Follicles

Morphological evaluation occurred at D6, D13 and D15, while manipulating follicles on a heating plate (38 °C) for the least amount of time. Follicle morphology was assessed on seven independent experiments (each with eight follicles per condition) using three criteria: (1) follicular survival, (2) follicular growth determined by their diameter and (3) the formation of an antral cavity, defined as a visible, translucent area within the follicular cell mass. These parameters were measured only in healthy follicles: a follicle was considered healthy when it was an intact follicle (no breakdown of the basal lamina and extrusion of the oocyte) with a light oocyte and a measurable growth within one week.

2.3. In Vitro Follicular Hormonal Secretion Assays

For hormonal quantification, 50 µL and 70 µL of culture medium on the 100 µL of each droplet (in which individual follicle was cultured) was recovered at D13 and D15 respectively from each alive follicle, meaning it had maintained structural integrity and growth. The concentrations of AMH, oestradiol and progesterone in the culture medium were determined for 32–37 individual follicles per treatment at either D13 or D15 (as described below).

2.3.1. Anti-Müllerian Hormone

The AMH concentration in the culture media at D15 was determined in 50 µL of culture medium diluted to 1/15 (in MEM+) using the AMH Gen II ELISA kit (Beckman Coulter, Villepinte, France), which had previously been validated for the analysis of ovine samples [60]. In our working conditions, the limit of detection of the assay was 78 pg/mL and the intra-assay coefficients of variation (CV) were 11.1% for an AMH concentration of 78 pg/mL and <5% for AMH concentrations >1250 pg/mL.

2.3.2. Oestradiol

The oestradiol concentration in the culture media at D13 was determined using the E2-EASIA immunoassay kit (DIAsource, Louvain-la-Neuve, Belgium) from the 50-µL aliquots of culture medium, diluted to 1/5 or to 1/10, as described previously [58]. For the present assay, the limit of detection was 3 pg/mL and the intra-assay CVs were <3.5% for oestradiol concentrations ranging from 3 to 100 pg/mL.

2.3.3. Progesterone

The progesterone concentration was determined in 50 µL of undiluted culture medium at D15 using a previously described ELISA protocol [61]. The limit of detection of the assay was 0.25 ng/mL for a 10 µL deposit volume and the intra-assay CVs averaged 7.1% for progesterone concentrations ranging from 0.25 to 32 ng/mL.

2.4. Gene Expression Analysis

2.4.1. RNA Extraction and Reverse Transcription

A total of 64 alive follicles at D15 (from four independent experiments, 18–24 follicles per conditions) were used for the evaluation of gene expression and individually stored in 20 µL lysis buffer for RNA extraction at −80 °C until use. The diameter of these follicles was 300–870 µm; 46 presented an antrum and 18 did not.

Total RNA was extracted using the Nucleospin RNA XS kit (Macherey Nagel, Hoerdt, France), according to the manufacturer's instructions, including on-column DNase treatment. Total RNA was quantified using a NanoDrop ND-1000 spectrophotometer (Nyxor Biotech, Paris, France). Reverse transcription was performed with 50 ng of total extracted follicle RNA using the Maxima First Strand cDNA Synthesis Kit (Thermo-Fisher Scientific, Illkirch-Graffenstaden, France), according to the manufacturer's recommendations.

2.4.2. Quantitative PCR Amplification

Real time polymerase chain reaction (qPCR) was performed on 2 ng of cDNA, as described previously [62]. The expression of 19 genes (Table 1) was assessed; they are involved in follicle functionality (Cytochrome P450 Family 19 Subfamily A Member 1 (*CYP19A1*), Estrogen Receptor 1 (*ESR1*), Estrogen Receptor 2 (*ESR2*), Follicle-Stimulating Hormone Receptor (*FSHR*), Hydroxy-Delta-5-Steroid Dehydrogenase (*HSD3B1*), Bone Morphogenetic Protein 15 (*BMP15*) and Aryl Hydrocarbon Receptor (*AHR*), or involved in redox status (Catalase (*CAT*), Cytochrome C Oxidase Subunit 4I1 (*COX4I1*), Cytochrome C Oxidase Subunit 5B (*COX5B*), Glutathione Peroxidase 3 (*GPX3*), Glutathione Peroxidase 8 (*GPX8*), NADH Dehydrogenase Ubiquinone 1 Beta Subcomplex Subunit 4 (*NDUFB4*), NADH Dehydrogenase Ubiquinone 1 Beta Subcomplex Subunit 5 (*NDUFB5*), NADH Ubiquinone Oxidoreductase Core Subunit V2 (*NDUFV2*), NADH Ubiquinone Oxidoreductase Complex Assembly Factor 2 (*NDUFAF2*), Succinate Dehydrogenase Complex Flavoprotein Subunit A (*SDHA*), Superoxide Dismutase 1 (*SOD1*) and Superoxide Dismutase 2 (*SOD2*)). The efficiency of the primers (Table 1) and the standard curve was determined for each gene. The expression level of each candidate gene was normalized using the geometric mean of two housekeeping genes (ribosomal protein L19 (*RPL19*) and beta-actin (*ACTB*)). The relative amounts of gene transcripts (*R*) were calculated according to the following equation:

$$R = \frac{(E_{gene}^{-Ct\ gene})}{\left(geometric\ mean\ (E_{RPL19}^{-Ct\ RPL19};\ E_{ACTB}^{-Ct\ ACTB})\right)} \quad (1)$$

where *E* is the primer efficiency of each primer pair and *Ct* is the cycle threshold.

Table 1. Primer sequences for real time reverse transcription polymerase chain reaction used in this study.

Abbrev.	Gene Name	Transcript Accession Number (Ensembl)	Forward Primer (5′→3′)	Reverse Primer (5′→3′)	Size (bp)	E (%)
Specific genes of follicle functionality						
AHR	Aryl Hydrocarbon Receptor	ENSOART00020003479.1	TGGGGCTGTTTCAATGTACC	TACAGGAATCCACCGGATGT	233	81.8
BMP15	Bone morphogenetic protein 15	ENSOART00020018955.1	TCTATTGCCCACCTGCCTGAG	TGAAGCTGATGGCCGTAAACC	326	89.2
CYP19A1	Cytochrome P450 Family 19 Subfamily A Member 1	ENSOART00020040485.1	GGTCATCCTGGTCACCCTTCTG	GCCGGTCGCTGGTCTCGTCTGG	119	100
ESR1	Estrogen receptor 1	ENSOART00020034283.1	CCAGTTCCTCCTCCTCCTCT	GGCTCTGATTCACGTCTTCC	158	87.2
ESR2	Estrogen receptor 2	ENSOART00020022015.1	ACTATGGAGTCTGGTCAT	GTCGGTTCTTATCTATGGTA	114	97.3
FSHR	Follicle-stimulating hormone receptor	ENSOART00000004728.	GGGCCAAGTCAACTTACCACT	TGCAAATTGGATGAAGGTCA	144	88.5
HSD3B1	Hydroxy-Delta-5-Steroid Dehydrogenase	ENSOART00020002039.1	TCATTGACGTCAGGAATGCT	CTCTATGGTGCTGGTGTGGA	128	84
Specific genes of redox status						
CAT	Catalase	ENSOART00020018520.1	GAAACGCTGTGTGAGAACA	AGCTTTCTCCCTTGCAGACA	208	91.2
COX4I1	Cytochrome C Oxidase Subunit 4I1	ENSOART00020014820.1	AGAGCTTTGCCGAGATGAAC	TCATGTCGAGCATCCTCTTG	182	88.3
COX5B	Cytochrome C Oxidase Subunit 5B	ENSOART00000014875.1	GGGCTAGAGAGGGAGGTCAT	CAGCCAGAACCAGATGACAG	180	91.2
GPX3	Glutathione Peroxidase 3	ENSOART00020022210.1	GATGTGAACGGGGAGAAAGA	CCCACCAGGAACTTCTCAAA	152	90.4
GPX8	Glutathione Peroxidase 8	ENSOART00020019722.1	AAGGCATTTGCAGTCTTGCT	GACCTTCAGGGTTGACCAGA	101	85.3
NDUFB4	NADH Dehydrogenase Ubiquinone 1 Beta Subcomplex Subunit 4	ENSOART00020003605.1	GGCCAGCCTACCTACTACCC	TGCATAGGTCAACGAATCA	181	90.7
NDUFB5	NADH Dehydrogenase Ubiquinone 1 Beta Subcomplex Subunit 5	ENSOART00020014020.1	GATTGCCCGAACTTCTTTG	AGTGCCTTATCGATGGTTGG	174	82.1
NDUFV2	NADH Ubiquinone Oxidoreductase Core Subunit V2	ENSOART00020029984.1	TCGAAAGCCTGTTGGAAAGT	ACACCAAACCAGGTCCTTT	205	60.8
NDUFAF2	NADH Ubiquinone Oxidoreductase Complex Assembly Factor 2	ENSOART00020010561.1	AACAGAATGGGAAGCTTGGA	AGAGGCGTGCCCTTTAATCT	196	84.2
SDHA	Succinate Dehydrogenase Complex Flavoprotein Subunit A	ENSOART00000016992.1	AGCAGAAGAAGCCGTTTGAG	TCGGTCTCGTTCAAAGTCCT	121	93.3
SOD1	Superoxide Dismutase 1	ENSOART00020002019.1	CAAAAATTGGTGTTGCCATTG	CCAGCGTTTCCAGTCTTTGT	153	94.0
SOD2	Superoxide Dismutase 2	ENSOART00020009379.1	GGTTGGCTTGGCCTTCAATAA	ACATTCCAAATGGCCTTCAG	178	90.6
Housekeeping genes						
ACTB	Beta Actin	ENSOART00020013384.1	CCAGCACGATGAAGATCAAG	ACATCTGTGAAGGTGGAC	102	97.2
RPL19	Ribosomal Protein L19	ENSOART00020024842.1	CACAAGCTGAAGGCAGACAA	TGATGATTTCCTCCTTCTTGG	129	95.3

Abbrev: gene name abbreviation; bp: base pair; E: efficiency.

2.5. Statistical Analysis

GraphPad Prism 9 (Version 9.3.1, GraphPad Software, Ritme, Paris, France) was used to carry out statistical analyses. Except for the results for the follicular survival and antrum appearance data that are presented as percentages, all results are expressed as mean +/− standard error of the mean (SEM). The data were tested for normality and the homogeneity of variances with the D'Agostino and Pearson test and the Brown–Forsythe test, respectively. Based on these tests, the effects of treatments on oestradiol, progesterone and AMH secretions were analysed with the non-parametric Kruskal–Wallis test followed by a Dunn's multiple comparison post hoc test when a significant global difference was observed. The effects of treatment on follicular diameter growth and gene expressions were analysed with the parametric Brown–Forsythe ANOVA test, and when a significant global difference was observed, Dunnett's T3 multiple comparison test was executed. Nonparametric Spearman correlation coefficients were used to assess the correlation between gene expressions, follicle diameter at D15, antrum presence at D15, oestradiol secretion at D13 and progesterone and AMH secretions at D15. Correlations were considered significant when $|r| \geq 0.70$ and $p < 0.0001$. Lastly, the differences in the percentage of follicles that presented an antrum were compared between experimental groups at D6, D13 and D15 using a multiple logistic regression analysis. The Kaplan–Meier survival curves were drawn for the three conditions throughout the experiment and compared using the log-rank (Mantel–Cox) test. Differences were considered significant when $p < 0.05$.

3. Results

3.1. BPS Effects on Ovine Follicular Survival, Follicular Growth and Antrum Appearance

The percentage of control alive follicles decreased from 85.7% at D6, to 71.4% at D13 and to 67.9% at D15 (Figure 1). The Kaplan–Meier survival analysis showed that the BPS 0.1 and 10 µM survival curves were not significantly different from the control one (Figure 1).

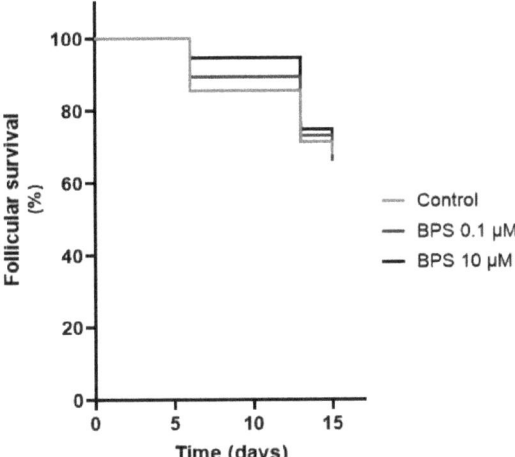

Figure 1. In vitro effects of bisphenol S (BPS) on ovine follicular survival. The survival of each follicle was assessed after 6, 13 and 15 days of treatment with or without BPS 0.1 µM or BPS 10 µM. A follicle was considered alive when there was no breakdown of the basal lamina and no extrusion of the oocyte. The oocyte had to be clear, and the follicular growth had to be measurable within 1 week. The results are representative of seven independent cultures with eight replicates per condition (n = 56 per condition). The results are expressed as percentage of alive follicles and the Kaplan–Meier survival curves obtained for the three conditions were compared using the Log-rank (Mantel–Cox) test. Differences were considered significant when $p < 0.05$.

At the beginning of the culture (D0), the diameter of the follicles (Figure 2A) was similar in the three experimental groups (216.1 +/− 2.7 µm for control, 214.6 +/− 2.6 µm for BPS 0.1 µM and 216.3 +/− 2.3 µm for BPS 10 µM, $p = 0.88$) and they presented no antral cavity (Figure 2B). After 6, 13 and 15 days of culture, the control follicles were 310 +/− 8.0 µm, 473.5 +/− 16.0 µm and 532.4 +/− 20.2 µm in diameter, respectively. There was no significant difference in the follicular diameter growth between conditions at any time point (Figure 2A).

The percentage of control alive follicles with an antral cavity increased from 4.2% at D6, to 72.5% at D13 and to 81.6% at D15 (Figure 2B). Neither BPS treatment affected the percentage of follicles presenting an antrum for each measurement day.

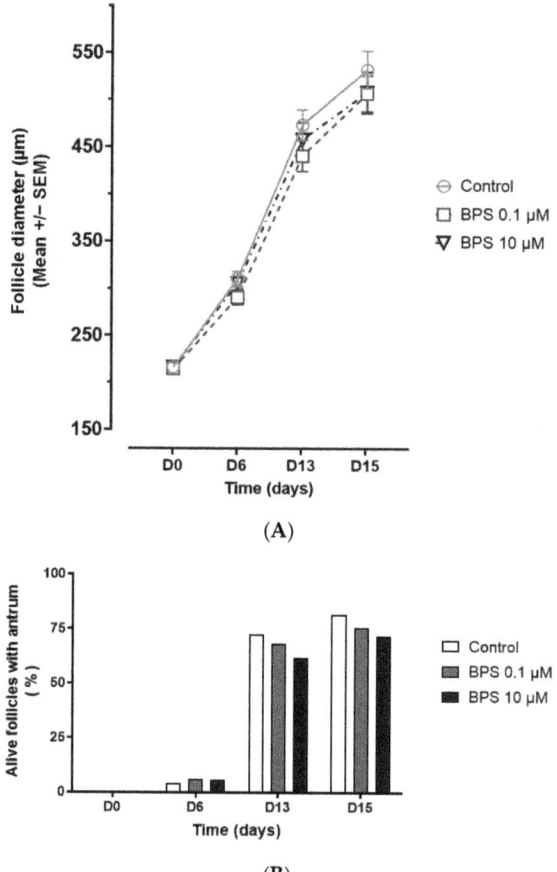

Figure 2. In vitro effects of bisphenol S (BPS) on ovine follicular growth and antrum appearance. The diameter evolution (**A**) and the antral cavity appearance (**B**) for each alive follicle were assessed after 6, 13 and 15 days of treatment with or without BPS 0.1 µM or BPS 10 µM. The results are representative of seven independent cultures with eight replicates per condition ($n = 56$ per condition at day 0, $n = 48–53$ according to the conditions at day 6, $n = 40–42$ according to the conditions at day 13 and $n = 38–39$ according to the conditions at day 15). For the diameter evolution, the results are expressed as mean +/− SEM and were analysed with a Brown–Forsythe ANOVA test at each day of measure (**A**). For the antrum appearance, the results are expressed as the percentage of alive follicles with an antrum and were analysed with a logistic regression at each day of measure (**B**). Differences were considered significant when $p < 0.05$.

3.2. BPS Effects on Ovine Follicular Hormonal Secretions: Oestradiol, Progesterone and AMH

Hormonal secretions were measured in spent culture media of alive follicles with BPS (0, 0.1 and 10 µM) for oestradiol after 13 days (Figure 3A) and for progesterone and AMH after 15 days (Figure 3B,C).

After 13 days of culture, the oestradiol concentration in the control culture medium was 108.3 +/− 11.8 pg/mL (Figure 3A). BPS 10 µM had no effect on the oestradiol concentration, but BPS 0.1 µM decreased its secretion by 48.8% compared with the control group ($p = 0.0004$, Figure 3A).

After 15 days of treatment, the progesterone and AMH concentrations in the control culture media of control group were 177.6 +/− 0.007 pg/mL (Figure 3B) and 13,943 +/− 1854 pg/mL (Figure 3C), respectively. There were no differences in these hormone levels among the three experimental groups (Figure 3B,C).

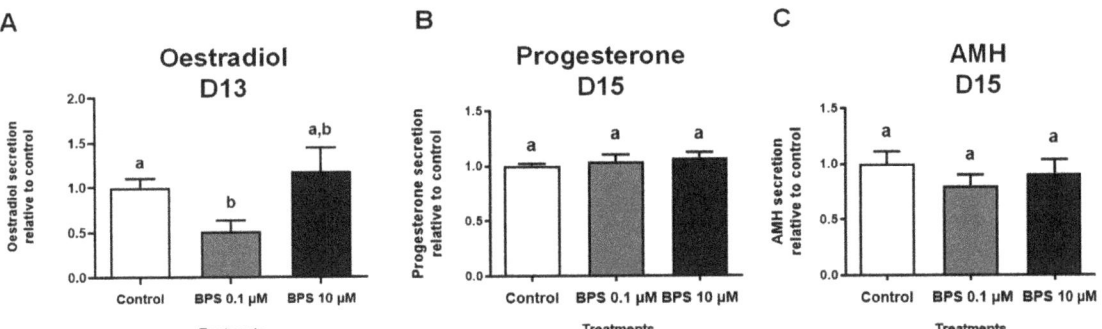

Figure 3. In vitro effects of bisphenol S (BPS) on ovine follicular hormonal secretions. Ovine follicles were cultured for 15 days with or without BPS (0.1 or 10 µM). Hormonal secretions were measured by ELISA in spent culture media of alive follicles after 13 days (D13) of treatment for oestradiol (**A**) and after 15 days (D15) for progesterone (**B**) and AMH (**C**). The results are representative of six independent cultures with eight replicates per condition at the beginning of the experiment for oestradiol (**A**), $n = 34$–37 alive follicles according to the conditions at day 13 and $n = 32$–33 according to conditions for progesterone (**B**) and AMH (**C**) at day 15. The data are expressed as mean +/− SEM relative to controls and were analysed with a Kruskal–Wallis test followed by a Dunn's multiple comparison post hoc test. Bars without at least one common letter (a,b) are significantly different ($p < 0.05$).

3.3. BPS Effects on Ovine Basal Stage Gene Expressions after 15 Days Treatment

The expression of seven genes involved in follicular development (*CYP19A1, ESR1, ESR2, FSHR, HSD3B1, BMP15* and *AHR*) and 12 genes involved in redox status (*CAT, COX4I1, COX5B, GPX3, GPX8, NDUFB4, NDUFB5, NDUFV2, NDUFAF2, SDHA, SOD1* and *SOD2*) was analysed in ovine follicles after 15 days of treatment with or without BPS (0.1 or 10 µM) (Figure 4 and Table 2). No significant differences were observed for any of the analysed genes between control and BPS conditions in this study. For the total of 64 alive follicles that were analysed for gene expression, the follicular diameter at D15 was similar for all groups: 509.4 +/− 29.0 µm, 514.1 +/− 26.9 µm and 479.6 +/− 29.4 µm for the control, BPS 0.1 µM and 10 µM groups, respectively ($p = 0.63$). In addition, the percentage of follicles with an antrum at D15 was similar among the groups: 77.8% for control, 72.7% for BPS 0.1 µM ($p = 0.71$) and 66.7% for BPS 10 µM group ($p = 0.43$).

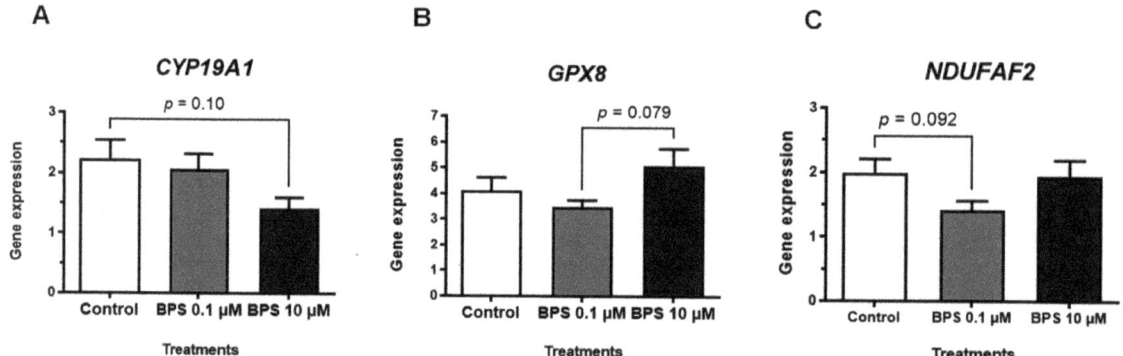

Figure 4. In vitro effects of bisphenol S (BPS) on ovine basal stage follicular gene expression. Ovine follicles were cultured for 15 days with or without BPS (0.1 or 10 µM). At day 15, the culture was stopped, and 64 alive follicles were used to assess the expression of 19 gene; they were preserved in a lysis buffer for RNA extraction and stored at −80 °C until use. The results are representative of four independent cultures, with n = 18 for control, n = 22 for BPS 0.1 µM and n = 24 for BPS 10 µM. The geometric mean of two housekeeping genes (beta-actin (*ACTB*) and ribosomal protein L19 (*RPL19*)) was used to normalise gene expression. The data are expressed as mean +/− SEM and were analysed with the Brown–Forsythe ANOVA test followed by Dunnett's T3 multiple comparison post-hoc test. In this figure, the results are presented for the 3 genes for which a p value $\leq$ 0.10 was obtained with the Brown–Forsythe ANOVA: one gene involved in follicular development, Cytochrome P450 Family 19 Subfamily A Member 1 (*CYP19A1*, p = 0.064, (**A**) and two genes involved in redox status, Glutathione Peroxidase 8 (*GPX8*, p = 0.068, (**B**) and NADH Ubiquinone Oxidoreductase Complex Assembly Factor (*NDUFAF2*, p = 0.097, (**C**). The p values $\leq$ 0.10 obtained with the Dunnett's T3 multiple comparison post-hoc test are drawn between conditions on each graph.

Table 2. In vitro effects of bisphenol S (BPS) on ovine basal stage follicular gene expressions.

Gene Name Abbreviation	Gene Expression (Mean +/− SEM)			p
	Control	BPS 0.1 µM	BPS 10 µM	
Specific genes of follicle functionality				
AHR	0.986 +/− 0.282	0.808 +/− 0.194	1.260 +/− 0.232	0.367
BMP15	3.806 +/− 0.629	3.938 +/− 0.721	5.757 +/− 1.067	0.180
ESR1	0.533 +/− 0.074	0.547 +/− 0.056	0.621 +/− 0.080	0.631
ESR2	4.487 +/− 0.666	3.784 +/− 0.468	4.745 +/− 0.691	0.505
FSHR	2.461 +/− 0.400	2.552 +/− 0.473	2.245 +/− 0.466	0.876
HSD3B1	0.039 +/− 0.011	0.034 +/− 0.009	0.047 +/− 0.012	0.691
Specific genes of redox status				
CAT	0.672 +/− 0.064	0.775 +/− 0.066	0.609 +/− 0.056	0.152
COX4I1	0.619 +/− 0.042	0.614 +/− 0.056	0.602 +/− 0.049	0.970
COX5B	1.291 +/− 0.151	1.288 +/− 0.124	1.284 +/− 0.160	0.999
GPX3	0.212 +/− 0.035	0.166 +/− 0.028	0.152 +/− 0.028	0.363
NDUFB4	7.039 +/− 0.754	6.002 +/− 0.472	7.056 +/− 0.635	0.393
NDUFB5	5.380 +/− 1.034	4.464 +/− 0.710	6.608 +/− 1.392	0.353
NDUFV2	2.205 +/− 0.264	2.085 +/− 0.248	2.118 +/− 0.233	0.944
SDHA	1.038 +/− 0.066	0.991 +/− 0.088	1.139 +/− 0.116	0.502

Table 2. Cont.

Gene Name Abbreviation	Gene Expression (Mean +/− SEM)			p
	Control	BPS 0.1 µM	BPS 10 µM	
SOD1	3.517 +/− 0.362	3.387 +/− 0.234	3.853 +/− 0.316	0.518
SOD2	0.753 +/− 0.098	0.701 +/− 0.059	0.708 +/− 0.073	0.885

Ovine follicles were cultured for 15 days with different concentrations of BPS (0, 0.1 or 10 µM). At day 15, the culture was stopped and 64 alive follicles were used to assess the expression of 19 genes; they were preserved in lysis buffer for RNA extraction and stored at −80 °C until use. The results are presented for six genes involved in follicular development (Aryl Hydrocarbon Receptor (*AHR*)), Bone morphogenetic protein 15 (*BMP15*), Estrogen receptor 1 (*ESR1*), Estrogen receptor 2 (*ESR2*), Follicle-stimulating hormone receptor (*FSHR*) and Hydroxy-Delta-5-Steroid Dehydrogenase (*HSD3B1*)) and 10 genes involved in redox status, (Catalase (*CAT*), Cytochrome C Oxidase Subunit 4I1 (*COX4I1*), Cytochrome C Oxidase Subunit 5B (*COX5B*), Glutathione Peroxidase 3 (*GPX3*), NADH Dehydrogenase Ubiquinone 1 Beta Subcomplex Subunit 4 (*NDUFB4*), NADH Dehydrogenase Ubiquinone 1 Beta Subcomplex Subunit 5 (*NDUFB5*), NADH Ubiquinone Oxidoreductase Core Subunit V2 (*NDUFV2*), Succinate Dehydrogenase Complex Flavoprotein Subunit A (*SDHA*), Superoxide Dismutase 1 (*SOD1*) and Superoxide Dismutase 2 (*SOD2*)). The results are representative of four independent cultures, with n = 18 for control, n = 22 for BPS 0.1 µM and n = 24 for BPS 10 µM. The geometric mean of two housekeeping genes (beta-actin (*ACTB*) and ribosomal protein L19 (*RPL19*)) was used to normalise gene expression. The data are expressed as mean +/− SEM and were analysed with the Brown–Forsythe ANOVA test followed by Dunnett's T3 multiple comparison post hoc test. A difference was considered significant for $p < 0.05$.

We evaluated correlations between gene expressions, D15 follicular diameter, antrum presence at D15, oestradiol secretion at D13 and progesterone and AMH secretions at D15 were studied for these 64 alive follicles (Supplementary Excel File 1, tab 'Spearman r' for the Spearman correlation coefficients and Supplementary Excel File 1, tab 'p values' for the associated p values). The results revealed several positive correlations ($p < 0.0001$) between D15 AMH secretion and D15 follicular diameter ($r = 0.84$), between FSHR expression and D15 follicular diameter ($r = 0.70$), between FSHR expression and D15 AMH secretion ($r = 0.72$), between AHR expression and SOD2 expression ($r = 0.74$) and between the expressions of several genes involved in redox status (NDUFB4–NDUFB5, $r = 0.91$; GPX8–NDUFB4, $r = 0.82$; GPX8–NDUFB5, $r = 0.78$; NDUFB5–SOD1, $r = 0.78$; NDUFB4–SOD1, $r = 0.74$; GPX8–SOD1, $r = 0.70$). There was only one negative correlation, namely between AHR expression and D15 follicular diameter ($r = −0.70$). There were no significant correlations between the presence of an antrum at D15 and the expression of the 19 genes.

4. Discussion

We aimed to evaluate the effects of BPS, currently the main substitute of BPA, on ovine follicular development and hormonal secretions during in vitro basal folliculogenesis. We have reported for the first time in a mono-ovulatory species model that a long-term exposure to a possible human exposure dose of BPS decreases oestradiol secretion by basal follicles without affecting their viability, growth and antral formation.

4.1. BPS Disrupted Oestradiol Secretion without Impairing Progesterone Secretion

We found that 0.1 µM BPS strongly decreased ovine oestradiol secretion (almost two-fold) after 13 days of treatment compared with the control. In sheep and humans, in vitro studies on the BPS effects on steroid secretions by ovarian somatic follicular cells has been conducted, but only on primary-cultured granulosa cells from antral follicles (2–6 mm) and preovulatory follicles, respectively [27,37]. At the concentration of 0.1 µM, the authors observed no effect of BPS on oestradiol secretion after 48-h exposure, but they found alteration of estradiol secretion from 10 µM BPS in ewes (an increase [37]) and for 50 µM BPS in humans (a decrease, [27]). In another mono-ovulatory species, the cow, oestradiol secretion from granulosa cells from antral follicles (3–7 mm) was also not affected after 6-day treatment with 0.1 µM BPS, whereas it was increased with 100 µM BPS [31]. These results, along with our data suggest that follicular cells could be more sensitive in vitro to a longer duration of BPS treatment regardless of the folliculogenesis phase, or they could be more sensitive to a possible human exposure BPS concentration (0.1 µM) for oestradiol secretion during basal folliculogenesis rather than during terminal folliculogenesis. They also show different responses of granulosa cells for oestradiol secretion according to species or the folliculogenesis phase. Furthermore, our results are consistent with a previous in vivo study from our team, which revealed a decreased oestradiol plasma level in ewes with food-restricted intakes and exposed to BPS (50 µg/kg body weight (bw)/day through diet, for at least 3 months; [63]). This decline in the oestradiol concentration was not observed in well-fed ewes [63]. In the present work, the metabolic status of the peri-pubertal ewes was not known, because they came from a slaughterhouse. Moreover, our data are also in agreement with a previous in vivo study conducted in female rodents with a long BPS exposure [43]. Indeed, Ijaz et al. [43] observed a decreased plasma oestradiol concentration in pre-pubertal rats treated with BPS (5 or 50 mg/kg bw; intraperitoneal administrations) for 28 days. However, these results are not in concordance with a previous study, which revealed an increased serum oestradiol level in mice after post-natal subcutaneous BPS treatment (50 µg/kg bw and 10 mg/kg bw) for 60 days [40]. These data indicate that the BPS administration route, dose, exposure period and treatment duration can influence the results on oestradiol level in females. Finally, our oestradiol secretion results are also consistent with those of Hu et al. [64], who examined human samples. They found a negative association between the urine BPS concentration and the serum oestradiol level in children (6–11 years) and adolescents (12–19 years) of both sexes (n = 1179) in the US NHANES study from 2013 to 2016. Their results were more pronounced in pubertal children. In contrast, Gao et al. [65] did not report a correlation between serum BPS and oestradiol concentrations in a population of 328 adult men and women (21–76 years) in a dense industrial area in China in 2017. These discrepancies between the studies could be linked to the age of the subjects (children versus adults) or to the level of BPS exposure, which was lower in the Chinese study (0.072 ng/mL) than in the US NHANES study (2.02 ng/mL), even if the type of biological fluid should be taken into account. An interesting point in connection with the study by Hu et al. [64] is that biological material for our experimental model of follicular development comes from peri-pubertal sheep ovaries. It could raise the question of whether there is greater BPS sensitivity of ovarian somatic follicular cells during the peri-pubertal period.

Unlike the 0.1 µM dose, 10 µM BPS (a high concentration) had no effect on oestradiol secretion after 13 days of exposure, whereas it increased 48-h oestradiol secretion from ewe granulosa cells [37] and had no effect in human granulosa cells [27], both from large antral follicles. Although these discrepancies could be partially explained by several factors (species, cellular models and exposure durations), our results highlight a non-monotonic response of BPS, as it has been described for BPA [66]. Therefore, additional experiments are required to investigate the effects of more BPS doses, including lower exposure doses on oestradiol secretion during basal folliculogenesis and whether the same observations could be made with ovaries from adult ewes.

Regarding progesterone secretion, we have shown here no effect of the two BPS concentrations during basal folliculogenesis after 15 days of exposure. In contrast, the plasma progesterone level was decreased in female rats treated with BPS during the neonatal period (50 mg/kg bw; [42]) or the adult stage (0.5, 5 or 50 mg/kg bw; [43]). In studies on cultured granulosa cells punctured from large antral follicles, there was no effect of 0.1 µM BPS in several mono-ovulatory species, namely ovine [37], bovine [31] and human [27], findings consistent with our results. However, 10 µM BPS decreased progesterone secretion in ewe [37] and human female [27] granulosa cells, whereas it had no effect on cow granulosa cells [31], as in our study. These data highlight differences related to species, study models or to exposure durations, while also suggesting that somatic follicular cells during basal folliculogenesis could be less sensitive to BPS for progesterone secretion than during terminal folliculogenesis or pregnancy. This could be explained at least in part by the fact that progesterone production is even lower during basal folliculogenesis compared with terminal folliculogenesis or pregnancy.

Our steroid hormone secretion data support that BPS at a possible human exposure dose may disrupt oestradiol secretion during basal folliculogenesis. Oestradiol is well known to be involved in feedback regulation of gonadotrophin secretions (LH and FSH). However, it also participates directly or indirectly in enhancing folliculogenesis through autocrine-paracrine modes on granulosa cells: it increases proliferation, differentiation, the expression of growth factors and receptors (Insulin-like Growth Factor-1 (IGF-1)) gonadotrophin receptors) and the number of gap-junctions, and it attenuates apoptosis [67,68]. Therefore, our results suggest that BPS could ultimately affect antral follicular development through oestradiol regulation, but a longer follow-up of our model of follicular development is required to investigate this eventuality.

4.2. BPS Did Not Impair Anti-Müllerian Hormone (AMH) Secretion

In the present study, at D15 control follicles reached the early antral follicle stage (diameter of 532.4 +/− 20.2 μm). Moreover, we found a strong positive correlation (r = 0.84) between AMH secretion and follicular diameter at D15, as expected for small antral follicles and in this in vitro model of basal follicular growth [58]. In humans as in sheep, AMH is expressed in granulosa cells from growing follicles after activation of the primordial follicle and transition to the primary follicle stage [69,70]. AMH expression being maximal in pre-antral and early antral follicles, it is considered as a marker of the small antral follicle population and plays a key role in controlling ovarian reserve [1,71].

We observed no significant changes in AMH secretion after 15 days of BPS exposure in our model of in vitro basal folliculogenesis. Such absence of effect of BPS on plasma AMH level after a 3-month exposure of BPS in diet (4 and 50 μg/kg bw/day) has already been reported in ewes [36]. Moreover, a 24-h BPS treatment during oocyte maturation (0.05 mg/mL [around 200 μM]) in bovine cumulus cells and cumulus oocyte complexes (COC) had no effect on AMH mRNA and protein expressions [72]. On the contrary, BPA decreased AMH mRNA level in COC and AMH protein expression in these bovine cumulus cells [72]. BPA exposure (5 and 500 μg/kg bw/day) also decreased the serum AMH concentration in sexually mature mice [73] and BPA concentration in urine or follicular fluid was negatively correlated with the serum AMH level in women [70,71]. However, an absence of correlation was also reported in infertile women [74]. These initial data on BPS suggest that BPS and BPA could act differently on AMH production and BPS would thus affect early follicle development, independently from AMH. Additional investigation is required to confirm this possibility.

4.3. BPS Did Not Impair Follicular Survival, Follicular Growth and Antral Formation

In our in vitro model of basal follicular development, neither follicular survival, nor follicular growth (diameter size) nor antrum appearance were significantly affected by both doses of BPS after 6, 13 and 15 days of exposure. In our in vitro model of basal follicular development up to small antral follicles (<600 μm), follicular growth is essentially due to proliferation of granulosa cells as it is the case in vivo [1].

In agreement with our results, several in vitro studies in mono-ovulatory species have shown no effect of BPS (including 0.1 or 10 μM) on the viability and/or proliferation of granulosa cells (from large antral follicles) after 48-h exposure in ewes [37] and women [27] and after 6-day treatment in cows [31]. However, regarding viability, some in vivo studies in rodents have revealed that BPS decreased the number of antral follicles (early/small and late/large) and increased the number of atretic follicles after a 28-day treatment (5 and/or 50 mg/kg body weight/day [43]) or a 10-day neonatal exposure (5 and 50 mg/kg body weight/day; [42]). We only investigated the transition between the pre-antral and early antral stages, and we did not have information about the antral-follicle stage (>550 μm). As our model enables a 21D culture of follicles that could reach up to 1 mm [58], it could be interesting to further study follicle survival in bigger antral follicles.

Finally, some studies in rodents have reported an increased number of primordial follicles after BPS exposure [35,75]. In parallel, fewer primary [41] or secondary follicles [35] have been observed. These data emphasise that it would be necessary to investigate BPS effects on earlier basal folliculogenesis (before the pre-antral stage) in mono-ovulatory species.

4.4. BPS Did Not Impair mRNA Expression of Key Markers of Follicular Development

As we observed a decreased oestradiol secretion after 0.1 µM BPS treatment, we analysed the mRNA expression of the steroidogenic enzymes, *HSD3B1* and *CYP19A1*. HSD3B1 protein is involved in synthesis of progesterone and androgens in converting pregnenolone into progesterone and androstenediol into testosterone, respectively. CYP19A1 protein is essential for estrogen production; it allows the conversion of testosterone into oestradiol and androstenedione into estrone. In our study, BPS at 0.1 and 10 µM did not significantly affect the mRNA expression of *HSD3B1* and *CYP19A1*. These results for *HSD3B1* expression are consistent with the absence of BPS effect on progesterone secretion in our model. One study found a decreased expression of *CYP19A1* in swine cumulus cells after a 48-h exposure with BPS at 30 µM [30], whereas other studies have shown no correlation between the oestradiol concentration in biological fluids or in cell culture medium and mRNA and/or protein expression of steroidogenic enzymes [37,40]. Thus, it could be interesting to measure the activities of steroidogenic enzymes, as a change in their activities could lead to hormonal imbalance. Moreover, because progesterone secretion was not affected by BPS treatment in our model, it might still be important to control the expression and activities of CYP17A1 and HSD17B, which are involved in androgen production independently of progesterone synthesis.

Here, we showed no modulation of mRNA expression of *BMP15* (a specific gene of oocyte activity [1,2]), *FSHR* (a marker of follicle maturation [1,2]) and *AHR* (a possible modulator of follicular growth and steroidogenesis [76]) in the presence of BPS. Consistently, BPS (10 nM, 1 µM) had no effect on *FSHR* expression in ewe cumulus cells from COC after 6-h in vitro maturation [77]. To our knowledge, no other studies are available on the effects of BPS on the *BMP15* and *AHR* expression. In view of the few studies available on all the expression of these genes, further investigation is required to conclude definitively on the effects of BPS on the expression of development markers of oocyte and somatic follicular cells in mono-ovulatory species.

Finally, the two tested BPS concentrations had no effect on *ESR1* and *ESR2* expression in our model of basal folliculogenesis. In agreement with our results, two studies using BPS concentrations close to those tested here found no modulation of *ESR1* and *ESR2* expression in ewe cumulus cells after 6 h of in vitro maturation [77] and in human granulosa cells from pre-ovulatory follicles after 48 h of exposure [27]. In contrast, *ESR1* and *ESR2* expression was increased in ovine granulosa cells from antral follicles after 48-h treatment but only for very high doses (50 and/or 100 µM; [37]). Oestrogen receptors play an important role in ovarian follicles in supporting granulosa cell differentiation, follicular growth and oocyte maturation [78,79]. Thus, our data suggest that BPS could not affect the possibility of follicular cells to respond to oestrogens during basal folliculogenesis. Nevertheless, we have to keep in mind that BPS can activate nuclear oestrogen receptors [80,81], leading to potential modulations of estrogen signalling pathways in addition to its alteration of estradiol secretion observed in this study.

4.5. BPS Did Not Impair mRNA Expression of Key Players of Redox Status

Several studies have focussed on oxidative stress as a potential mechanism of action of bisphenols in different cell types [54,82,83]. Thus, we measured mRNA expression of some actors in redox-status regulation, as enzymes involved in defence against free radicals (*SOD1*, *SOD2*, *CAT*, *GPX3* and *GPX8* [84]), and several enzymes of the mitochondrial respiratory chain complexes (the NADH ubiquinone oxidoreductase for complex I, namely *NDUFB4*, *NDUFB5*, *NDUFV2* and *NDUFAF2* [85]), succinate dehydrogenase for complex II (*SDHA* [86]) and cytochrome c oxidase for complex IV (*COX4I1*, *COX5B* [87]). BPS exposure at the two tested concentrations did not significantly modulate the expression of these genes in our model of basal follicular development. Few studies are available in the literature regarding the role of BPS in oxidative stress in ovarian cells. In agreement with our results, BPS (from 10^{-9} to 10^{-4} M) had no effect on 4-h reactive oxygen species (ROS) production and 24–48-h SOD1 and SOD2 mRNA expression in a human granulosa cell line (COV434; [88]). However, the other studies have shown that BPS increased ROS production and/or decreased activities of SOD and/or CAT in ovarian cells in vivo [43] or in vitro [38,55] but mainly for high doses. Thus, it could be interesting to test other BPS doses and to measure the ROS level and the activities of these enzymes of redox-status regulation in our model, to determine whether oxidative stress is really a key mechanism of action of BPS at possible human exposure doses during follicular development.

On the other hand, we did not investigate the potential effects of BPS on DNA methylation in our in vitro model of basal follicular development. However, it could be very interesting to further investigate this mechanism of action, as it was well described for BPA [49–51].

4.6. Limitations and Strengths of the Study

Some limitations occurred in this study, related to the use of this ovine model of basal follicular growth. As mentioned above, sheep ovaries came from a local abattoir and the metabolic and health status of animals was not known. However, this status may influence BPS effects on steroid secretion [63].

Nevertheless, we chose the ewe as a translational experimental model to study ovarian human basal folliculogenesis for several reasons. Unlike rodents, the appearance of primordial follicles starts at a similar time during the gestation period in both humans and ovines [56]. Furthermore, the duration of folliculogenesis, from primordial follicle to preovulatory follicular development, is similar between the two species: nearly 170 days in ewes and 200 days in women [57] versus approximatively 20 days in rodents [3,89]. More precisely, the period of antral development is about 50 days in women and 45 days in ewes [1,57,89].

On the other hand, our study model of ovarian basal folliculogenesis is somewhat far from the physiological situation in the ovary, because follicles are cultured individually without the influence of the other follicles usually present in the ovary. However, it provides a good model to study the antrum appearance [58], which is not possible to study in vivo with the same monitoring parameters as in the present study. These cultured follicles present the main features of in vivo follicles of the same size. They are able to produce steroid hormones and AMH and to express mRNA of relevant genes (*BMP15, GDF9*, Zona pellucida sperm-binding protein 3 [*ZP3*], *FSHR, ESR1* and *ESR2*) [58]. Furthermore, we observed positive correlations between D15 follicular diameter and *FSHR* expression and AMH secretion that demonstrates a consistent model of early antral follicular development for human species.

Finally, we tested in our work a long-term exposure to 0.1 µM and 10 µM concentrations of native BPS, concentrations that we have termed as a possible human exposure dose and high dose of BPS, respectively. Indeed, in human biological fluids (urine, plasma and follicular fluid), the mean BPS concentration is 10 nM, which is 10-fold lower than our lower dose. However, this dose of 0.1 µM seems to be relevant, because several studies reported BPS concentrations close to or above 100 nM for some people [19,25,59]. However, we have to keep in mind that for these people, we do not know whether their BPS exposure time is equivalent to that in our study. Furthermore, BPS is metabolised in glucuronide form in humans, which cannot be achieved in our in vitro model. Thus, human tissues could be exposed to native BPS for a shorter time than in our in vitro model. Finally, the second dose tested in our study has allowed us to compare our results with previous data—for example, studies that used the same dose for acute exposure.

5. Conclusions

In the present study, we showed for the first time in a mono-ovulatory species (ovine) that a long-term BPS exposure at a possible human exposure concentration drastically decreased oestradiol secretion during basal folliculogenesis in vitro. Antral formation, follicular survival and growth and AMH and progesterone secretions were not affected by BPS. The results suggest that BPS could impair oestradiol secretion early in ovarian follicular development in vivo. It may therefore affect the quality of the follicle in the long term. This work may contribute to raising the question of categorising BPS as an endocrine disruptor and of substituting BPA with BPS. It also underlines the necessity to assess the risk of BPS exposure for reproduction of mono-ovulatory mammals. Further investigation is required to confirm potential BPS effects during in vivo basal folliculogenesis and study the BPS effects on primordial follicle activation and on antral stage preceding terminal folliculogenesis and to elucidate its mechanisms of action in mono-ovulatory species.

Supplementary Materials: The following are available online at https://www.mdpi.com/article/10.3390/toxics10080437/s1, Table S1: Correlations between gene expression, follicular diameter, antrum presence and hormonal secretions in cultured ewe basal follicles. Ovine follicles were cultured in Petri dishes for 15 days with different concentrations of BPS (0, 0.1 or 10 µM). At day 15, the culture was stopped and 64 alive follicles were used to assess the expression of 19 genes: seven genes involved in follicular development (aryl hydrocarbon receptor [AHR], bone morphogenetic protein 15 [BMP15], cytochrome P450 family 19 subfamily a member 1 [CYP19A1], oestrogen receptor 1 [ESR1], (oestrogen receptor 2 [ESR2], follicle-stimulating hormone receptor [FSHR] and hydroxy-delta-5-steroid dehydrogenase [HSD3B1]) and 12 genes involved in redox status, (catalase [CAT], cytochrome c oxidase subunit 4I1 [COX4I1], cytochrome c oxidase subunit 5B [COX5B], glutathione peroxidase 3 [GPX3], glutathione peroxidase 8 [GPX8], NADH dehydrogenase ubiquinone 1 beta subcomplex subunit 4 [NDUFB4], NADH dehydrogenase ubiquinone 1 beta subcomplex subunit 5 [NDUFB5], NADH ubiquinone oxidoreductase core subunit V2 [NDUFV2], NADH ubiquinone oxidoreductase complex assembly factor 2 [NDUFAF2], succinate dehydrogenase complex flavoprotein subunit A [SDHA], superoxide dismutase 1 [SOD1] and superoxide dismutase 2 [SOD2]). This file includes nonparametric Spearman correlation coefficients (tab 'Spearman r') and the associated p values (tab 'p values') that were assessed between gene expression, follicular diameter at day 15 (D15), antrum presence at D15, oestradiol secretion at D13 and progesterone and anti-Müllerian hormone (AMH) secretion at D15. Correlations were considered significant when $|r| \geq 0.70$ and $p < 0.0001$.

Author Contributions: C.V. performed experiments, analysed the data and wrote the manuscript. V.C. performed experiments and helped analyse data and write the manuscript. P.J.-G. and P.P. performed experiments. O.T., A.D., S.U., A.B. and F.G. helped write the manuscript. S.E. helped analyse data and write the manuscript. V.M. conceived the study, helped to perform some experiments, analysed data and wrote the manuscript. All authors have read and agreed to the published version of the manuscript.

Funding: This study was financially supported by INRAe and the French National Research Agency (project ANR-18-CE34-0011-01 MAMBO) and by Region Centre-Val de Loire (APR IA 2019-00134937 PERFIDE).

Institutional Review Board Statement: Not applicable.

Informed Consent Statement: Not applicable.

Data Availability Statement: The data presented in this study are available only in the present article and its supplementary Table S1.

Acknowledgments: We would like to thank Albert Arnould and Thierry Delpuech for ovine ovary collection, the Endocrinology and Phenotyping Laboratory (Reproductive Physiology and Behaviors Unit, INRAe Nouzilly), Mailys Gaudet and Dominique Gennetay for the progesterone assay and Anaïs Carvalho for advice on the standardisation of gene expression analysis.

Conflicts of Interest: The authors declare that there are no conflict of interest that could be perceived as influencing the representation or interpretation of the reported research study.

References

1. Monniaux, D.; Cadoret, V.; Clément, F.; Dalbies-Tran, R.; Elis, S.; Fabre, S.; Maillard, V.; Monget, P.; Uzbekova, S. Folliculogenesis. In *Ilpo Huhtaniemi and Luciano Martini, Encyclopedia of Endocrine Diseases*, 2nd ed.; Academic Press (Elsevier): Oxford, UK, 2019; Volume 2, pp. 377–398, ISBN 978-0-12-812200-6.
2. Dalbies-Tran, R.; Cadoret, V.; Desmarchais, A.; Elis, S.; Maillard, V.; Monget, P.; Monniaux, D.; Reynaud, K.; Saint-Dizier, M.; Uzbekova, S. A Comparative Analysis of Oocyte Development in Mammals. *Cells* **2020**, *9*, E1002. [CrossRef] [PubMed]

3. McGee, E.A.; Hsueh, A.J. Initial and Cyclic Recruitment of Ovarian Follicles. *Endocr. Rev.* **2000**, *21*, 200–214. [CrossRef] [PubMed]
4. Uzumcu, M.; Zachow, R. Developmental Exposure to Environmental Endocrine Disruptors: Consequences within the Ovary and on Female Reproductive Function. *Reprod. Toxicol.* **2007**, *23*, 337–352. [CrossRef]
5. Hahladakis, J.N.; Iacovidou, E.; Gerassimidou, S. An Overview of the Occurrence, Fate, and Human Risks of the Bisphenol-A Present in Plastic Materials, Components, and Products. *Integr. Environ. Assess. Manag.* **2022**, 1–18. [CrossRef] [PubMed]
6. Geens, T.; Goeyens, L.; Covaci, A. Are Potential Sources for Human Exposure to Bisphenol-A Overlooked? *Int. J. Hyg. Environ. Health* **2011**, *214*, 339–347. [CrossRef]
7. Kim, Y.; Park, M.; Nam, D.J.; Yang, E.H.; Ryoo, J.-H. Relationship between Seafood Consumption and Bisphenol A Exposure: The Second Korean National Environmental Health Survey (KoNEHS 2012–2014). *Ann. Occup. Environ. Med.* **2020**, *32*, e10. [CrossRef]
8. Velázquez-Gómez, M.; Lacorte, S. Nasal Lavages as a Tool for Monitoring Exposure to Organic Pollutants. *Environ. Res.* **2019**, *178*, 108726. [CrossRef] [PubMed]
9. Vasiljevic, T.; Harner, T. Bisphenol A and Its Analogues in Outdoor and Indoor Air: Properties, Sources and Global Levels. *Sci. Total Environ.* **2021**, *789*, 148013. [CrossRef]
10. Liu, J.; Martin, J.W. Prolonged Exposure to Bisphenol A from Single Dermal Contact Events. *Environ. Sci. Technol.* **2017**, *51*, 9940–9949. [CrossRef] [PubMed]
11. Champmartin, C.; Marquet, F.; Chedik, L.; Décret, M.-J.; Aubertin, M.; Ferrari, E.; Grandclaude, M.-C.; Cosnier, F. Human in Vitro Percutaneous Absorption of Bisphenol S and Bisphenol A: A Comparative Study. *Chemosphere* **2020**, *252*, 126525. [CrossRef] [PubMed]
12. Hwang, S.; Lim, J.-E.; Choi, Y.; Jee, S.H. Bisphenol A Exposure and Type 2 Diabetes Mellitus Risk: A Meta-Analysis. *BMC Endocr. Disord.* **2018**, *18*, 81. [CrossRef] [PubMed]
13. Abraham, A.; Chakraborty, P. A Review on Sources and Health Impacts of Bisphenol A. *Rev. Environ. Health* **2020**, *35*, 201–210. [CrossRef]
14. Meli, R.; Monnolo, A.; Annunziata, C.; Pirozzi, C.; Ferrante, M.C. Oxidative Stress and BPA Toxicity: An Antioxidant Approach for Male and Female Reproductive Dysfunction. *Antioxidants* **2020**, *9*, E405. [CrossRef] [PubMed]
15. Zhang, Y.-F.; Shan, C.; Wang, Y.; Qian, L.-L.; Jia, D.-D.; Zhang, Y.-F.; Hao, X.-D.; Xu, H.-M. Cardiovascular Toxicity and Mechanism of Bisphenol A and Emerging Risk of Bisphenol S. *Sci. Total Environ.* **2020**, *723*, 137952. [CrossRef] [PubMed]
16. Oliviero, F.; Marmugi, A.; Viguié, C.; Gayrard, V.; Picard-Hagen, N.; Mselli-Lakhal, L. Are BPA Substitutes as Obesogenic as BPA? *Int. J. Mol. Sci.* **2022**, *23*, 4238. [CrossRef] [PubMed]
17. Flint, S.; Markle, T.; Thompson, S.; Wallace, E. Bisphenol A Exposure, Effects, and Policy: A Wildlife Perspective. *J. Environ. Manag.* **2012**, *104*, 19–34. [CrossRef]
18. European Chemicals Agency. *General Report 2017*; European Chemicals Agency: Helsinki, Finland, 2018; ECHA-18-R-08-EN; ISBN 978-92-9020-506-7. [CrossRef]
19. Wu, L.-H.; Zhang, X.-M.; Wang, F.; Gao, C.-J.; Chen, D.; Palumbo, J.R.; Guo, Y.; Zeng, E.Y. Occurrence of Bisphenol S in the Environment and Implications for Human Exposure: A Short Review. *Sci. Total Environ.* **2018**, *615*, 87–98. [CrossRef] [PubMed]
20. Liao, C.; Liu, F.; Guo, Y.; Moon, H.-B.; Nakata, H.; Wu, Q.; Kannan, K. Occurrence of Eight Bisphenol Analogues in Indoor Dust from the United States and Several Asian Countries: Implications for Human Exposure. *Environ. Sci. Technol.* **2012**, *46*, 9138–9145. [CrossRef]
21. Liu, Y.; Yan, Z.; Zhang, Q.; Song, N.; Cheng, J.; Torres, O.L.; Chen, J.; Zhang, S.; Guo, R. Urinary Levels, Composition Profile and Cumulative Risk of Bisphenols in Preschool-Aged Children from Nanjing Suburb, China. *Ecotoxicol. Environ. Saf.* **2019**, *172*, 444–450. [CrossRef]
22. Mendy, A.; Salo, P.M.; Wilkerson, J.; Feinstein, L.; Ferguson, K.K.; Fessler, M.B.; Thorne, P.S.; Zeldin, D.C. Association of Urinary Levels of Bisphenols F and S Used as Bisphenol A Substitutes with Asthma and Hay Fever Outcomes. *Environ. Res.* **2020**, *183*, 108944. [CrossRef] [PubMed]
23. Sol, C.M.; van Zwol-Janssens, C.; Philips, E.M.; Asimakopoulos, A.G.; Martinez-Moral, M.-P.; Kannan, K.; Jaddoe, V.W.V.; Trasande, L.; Santos, S. Maternal Bisphenol Urine Concentrations, Fetal Growth and Adverse Birth Outcomes: A Population-Based Prospective Cohort. *Environ. Health Glob. Access Sci. Source* **2021**, *20*, 60. [CrossRef] [PubMed]
24. Khmiri, I.; Côté, J.; Mantha, M.; Khemiri, R.; Lacroix, M.; Gely, C.; Toutain, P.-L.; Picard-Hagen, N.; Gayrard, V.; Bouchard, M. Toxicokinetics of Bisphenol-S and Its Glucuronide in Plasma and Urine Following Oral and Dermal Exposure in Volunteers for the Interpretation of Biomonitoring Data. *Environ. Int.* **2020**, *138*, 105644. [CrossRef]
25. Li, A.; Zhuang, T.; Shi, W.; Liang, Y.; Liao, C.; Song, M.; Jiang, G. Serum Concentration of Bisphenol Analogues in Pregnant Women in China. *Sci. Total Environ.* **2020**, *707*, 136100. [CrossRef]
26. Claessens, J.; Pirard, C.; Charlier, C. Determination of Contamination Levels for Multiple Endocrine Disruptors in Hair from a Non-Occupationally Exposed Population Living in Liege (Belgium). *Sci. Total Environ.* **2022**, *815*, 152734. [CrossRef] [PubMed]
27. Amar, S.; Binet, A.; Téteau, O.; Desmarchais, A.; Papillier, P.; Lacroix, M.Z.; Maillard, V.; Guérif, F.; Elis, S. Bisphenol S Impaired Human Granulosa Cell Steroidogenesis in Vitro. *Int. J. Mol. Sci.* **2020**, *21*, 1821. [CrossRef]
28. Rochester, J.R.; Bolden, A.L. Bisphenol S and F: A Systematic Review and Comparison of the Hormonal Activity of Bisphenol A Substitutes. *Environ. Health Perspect.* **2015**, *123*, 643–650. [CrossRef] [PubMed]
29. Thoene, M.; Dzika, E.; Gonkowski, S.; Wojtkiewicz, J. Bisphenol S in Food Causes Hormonal and Obesogenic Effects Comparable to or Worse than Bisphenol A: A Literature Review. *Nutrients* **2020**, *12*, E532. [CrossRef] [PubMed]

30. Žalmanová, T.; Hošková, K.; Nevoral, J.; Adámková, K.; Kott, T.; Šulc, M.; Kotíková, Z.; Prokešová, Š.; Jílek, F.; Králíčková, M.; et al. Bisphenol S Negatively Affects the Meotic Maturation of Pig Oocytes. *Sci. Rep.* **2017**, *7*, 485. [CrossRef] [PubMed]
31. Campen, K.A.; Lavallee, M.; Combelles, C. The Impact of Bisphenol S on Bovine Granulosa and Theca Cells. *Reprod. Domest. Anim. Zuchthyg.* **2018**, *53*, 450–457. [CrossRef] [PubMed]
32. Sabry, R.; Saleh, A.C.; Stalker, L.; LaMarre, J.; Favetta, L.A. Effects of Bisphenol A and Bisphenol S on MicroRNA Expression during Bovine (Bos Taurus) Oocyte Maturation and Early Embryo Development. *Reprod. Toxicol.* **2021**, *99*, 96–108. [CrossRef] [PubMed]
33. Nevoral, J.; Kolinko, Y.; Moravec, J.; Žalmanová, T.; Hošková, K.; Prokešová, Š.; Klein, P.; Ghaibour, K.; Hošek, P.; Štiavnická, M.; et al. Long-Term Exposure to Very Low Doses of Bisphenol S Affects Female Reproduction. *Reprod. Camb. Engl.* **2018**, *156*, 47–57. [CrossRef] [PubMed]
34. Prokešová, Š.; Ghaibour, K.; Liška, F.; Klein, P.; Fenclová, T.; Štiavnická, M.; Hošek, P.; Žalmanová, T.; Hošková, K.; Řimnáčová, H.; et al. Acute Low-Dose Bisphenol S Exposure Affects Mouse Oocyte Quality. *Reprod. Toxicol.* **2020**, *93*, 19–27. [CrossRef]
35. Zhang, M.-Y.; Tian, Y.; Yan, Z.-H.; Li, W.-D.; Zang, C.-J.; Li, L.; Sun, X.-F.; Shen, W.; Cheng, S.-F. Maternal Bisphenol S Exposure Affects the Reproductive Capacity of F1 and F2 Offspring in Mice. *Environ. Pollut.* **2020**, *267*, 115382. [CrossRef]
36. Desmarchais, A.; Téteau, O.; Kasal-Hoc, N.; Cognié, J.; Lasserre, O.; Papillier, P.; Lacroix, M.; Vignault, C.; Jarrier-Gaillard, P.; Maillard, V.; et al. Chronic Low BPS Exposure through Diet Impairs in Vitro Embryo Production Parameters According to Metabolic Status in the Ewe. *Ecotoxicol. Environ. Saf.* **2022**, *229*, 113096. [CrossRef] [PubMed]
37. Téteau, O.; Jaubert, M.; Desmarchais, A.; Papillier, P.; Binet, A.; Maillard, V.; Elis, S. Bisphenol A and S Impaired Ovine Granulosa Cell Steroidogenesis. *Reprod. Camb. Engl.* **2020**, *159*, 571–583. [CrossRef] [PubMed]
38. Berni, M.; Gigante, P.; Bussolati, S.; Grasselli, F.; Grolli, S.; Ramoni, R.; Basini, G. Bisphenol S, a Bisphenol A Alternative, Impairs Swine Ovarian and Adipose Cell Functions. *Domest. Anim. Endocrinol.* **2019**, *66*, 48–56. [CrossRef]
39. Bujnakova Mlynarcikova, A.; Scsukova, S. Bisphenol Analogs AF, S and F: Effects on Functional Characteristics of Porcine Granulosa Cells. *Reprod. Toxicol.* **2021**, *103*, 18–27. [CrossRef] [PubMed]
40. Shi, M.; Sekulovski, N.; MacLean, J.A.; Hayashi, K. Effects of Bisphenol A Analogues on Reproductive Functions in Mice. *Reprod. Toxicol.* **2017**, *73*, 280–291. [CrossRef] [PubMed]
41. Shi, M.; Sekulovski, N.; MacLean, J.A.; Whorton, A.; Hayashi, K. Prenatal Exposure to Bisphenol A Analogues on Female Reproductive Functions in Mice. *Toxicol. Sci. Off. J. Soc. Toxicol.* **2019**, *168*, 561–571. [CrossRef] [PubMed]
42. Ahsan, N.; Ullah, H.; Ullah, W.; Jahan, S. Comparative Effects of Bisphenol S and Bisphenol A on the Development of Female Reproductive System in Rats; a Neonatal Exposure Study. *Chemosphere* **2018**, *197*, 336–343. [CrossRef]
43. Ijaz, S.; Ullah, A.; Shaheen, G.; Jahan, S. Exposure of BPA and Its Alternatives like BPB, BPF, and BPS Impair Subsequent Reproductive Potentials in Adult Female Sprague Dawley Rats. *Toxicol. Mech. Methods* **2020**, *30*, 60–72. [CrossRef] [PubMed]
44. Cimmino, I.; Fiory, F.; Perruolo, G.; Miele, C.; Beguinot, F.; Formisano, P.; Oriente, F. Potential Mechanisms of Bisphenol A (BPA) Contributing to Human Disease. *Int. J. Mol. Sci.* **2020**, *21*, 5761. [CrossRef] [PubMed]
45. Donini, C.F.; El Helou, M.; Wierinckx, A.; Győrffy, B.; Aires, S.; Escande, A.; Croze, S.; Clezardin, P.; Lachuer, J.; Diab-Assaf, M.; et al. Long-Term Exposure of Early-Transformed Human Mammary Cells to Low Doses of Benzo[a]Pyrene and/or Bisphenol A Enhances Their Cancerous Phenotype via an AhR/GPR30 Interplay. *Front. Oncol.* **2020**, *10*, 712. [CrossRef] [PubMed]
46. Naderi, M.; Kwong, R. A Comprehensive Review of the Neurobehavioral Effects of Bisphenol S and the Mechanisms of Action: New Insights from in Vitro and in Vivo Models. *Environ. Int.* **2020**, *145*, 106078. [CrossRef] [PubMed]
47. Amir, S.; Shah, S.T.A.; Mamoulakis, C.; Docea, A.O.; Kalantzi, O.-I.; Zachariou, A.; Calina, D.; Carvalho, F.; Sofikitis, N.; Makrigiannakis, A.; et al. Endocrine Disruptors Acting on Estrogen and Androgen Pathways Cause Reproductive Disorders through Multiple Mechanisms: A Review. *Int. J. Environ. Res. Public Health* **2021**, *18*, 1464. [CrossRef]
48. Cooney, C.A. Epigenetics—DNA-Based Mirror of Our Environment? *Dis. Markers* **2007**, *23*, 121–137. [CrossRef] [PubMed]
49. Manikkam, M.; Tracey, R.; Guerrero-Bosagna, C.; Skinner, M.K. Plastics Derived Endocrine Disruptors (BPA, DEHP and DBP) Induce Epigenetic Transgenerational Inheritance of Obesity, Reproductive Disease and Sperm Epimutations. *PLoS ONE* **2013**, *8*, e55387. [CrossRef] [PubMed]
50. Faulk, C.; Kim, J.H.; Anderson, O.S.; Nahar, M.S.; Jones, T.R.; Sartor, M.A.; Dolinoy, D.C. Detection of Differential DNA Methylation in Repetitive DNA of Mice and Humans Perinatally Exposed to Bisphenol A. *Epigenetics* **2016**, *11*, 489–500. [CrossRef]
51. Beck, D.; Nilsson, E.E.; Ben Maamar, M.; Skinner, M.K. Environmental Induced Transgenerational Inheritance Impacts Systems Epigenetics in Disease Etiology. *Sci. Rep.* **2022**, *12*, 5452. [CrossRef]
52. Maćczak, A.; Cyrkler, M.; Bukowska, B.; Michałowicz, J.; Bisphenol, A.; Bisphenol, S.; Bisphenol, F.; Bisphenol, A.F. Induce Different Oxidative Stress and Damage in Human Red Blood Cells (in Vitro Study). *Toxicol. Vitr.* **2017**, *41*, 143–149. [CrossRef]
53. Wang, C.; He, J.; Xu, T.; Han, H.; Zhu, Z.; Meng, L.; Pang, Q.; Fan, R. Bisphenol A(BPA), BPS and BPB-Induced Oxidative Stress and Apoptosis Mediated by Mitochondria in Human Neuroblastoma Cell Lines. *Ecotoxicol. Environ. Saf.* **2021**, *207*, 111299. [CrossRef] [PubMed]
54. Mączka, W.; Grabarczyk, M.; Wińska, K. Can Antioxidants Reduce the Toxicity of Bisphenol? *Antioxidants* **2022**, *11*, 413. [CrossRef] [PubMed]
55. Huang, M.; Liu, S.; Fu, L.; Jiang, X.; Yang, M. Bisphenol A and Its Analogues Bisphenol S, Bisphenol F and Bisphenol AF Induce Oxidative Stress and Biomacromolecular Damage in Human Granulosa KGN Cells. *Chemosphere* **2020**, *253*, 126707. [CrossRef] [PubMed]

56. Padmanabhan, V.; Veiga-Lopez, A. Sheep Models of Polycystic Ovary Syndrome Phenotype. *Mol. Cell. Endocrinol.* **2013**, *373*, 8–20. [CrossRef] [PubMed]
57. Lunardi, F.O.; Bass, C.S.; Bernuci, M.P.; Chaves, R.N.; Lima, L.F.; da Silva, R.F.; de Figueiredo, J.R.; Rodrigues, A.P.R. Ewe Ovarian Tissue Vitrification: A Model for the Study of Fertility Preservation in Women. *JBRA Assist. Reprod.* **2015**, *19*, 241–251. [CrossRef] [PubMed]
58. Cadoret, V.; Frapsauce, C.; Jarrier, P.; Maillard, V.; Bonnet, A.; Locatelli, Y.; Royère, D.; Monniaux, D.; Guérif, F.; Monget, P. Molecular Evidence That Follicle Development Is Accelerated in Vitro Compared to in Vivo. *Reprod. Camb. Engl.* **2017**, *153*, 493–508. [CrossRef]
59. Thayer, K.A.; Taylor, K.W.; Garantziotis, S.; Schurman, S.H.; Kissling, G.E.; Hunt, D.; Herbert, B.; Church, R.; Jankowich, R.; Churchwell, M.I.; et al. Bisphenol A, Bisphenol S, and 4-Hydro Xyphenyl 4-Isopro Oxyphenyl Sulfone (BPSIP) in Urine and Blood of Cashiers. *Environ. Health Perspect.* **2016**, *124*, 437–444. [CrossRef]
60. Estienne, A.; Pierre, A.; di Clemente, N.; Picard, J.-Y.; Jarrier, P.; Mansanet, C.; Monniaux, D.; Fabre, S. Anti-Müllerian Hormone Regulation by the Bone Morphogenetic Proteins in the Sheep Ovary: Deciphering a Direct Regulatory Pathway. *Endocrinology* **2015**, *156*, 301–313. [CrossRef] [PubMed]
61. Canepa, S.; Laine, A.-L.; Bluteau, A.; Fagu, C.; Flon, C.; Monniaux, D. Validation d'une méthode immunoenzymatique pour le dosage de la progestérone dans le plasma des ovins et des bovins. *Cah. Tech. INRA* **2008**, *64*, 19–30.
62. Elis, S.; Oseikria, M.; Vitorino Carvalho, A.; Bertevello, P.S.; Corbin, E.; Teixeira-Gomes, A.-P.; Lecardonnel, J.; Archilla, C.; Duranthon, V.; Labas, V.; et al. Docosahexaenoic Acid Mechanisms of Action on the Bovine Oocyte-Cumulus Complex. *J. Ovarian Res.* **2017**, *10*, 74. [CrossRef] [PubMed]
63. Téteau, O.; Liere, P.; Pianos, A.; Desmarchais, A.; Lasserre, O.; Papillier, P.; Vignault, C.; Lebachelier de la Riviere, M.-E.; Maillard, V.; Binet, A.; et al. Bisphenol S Alters the Steroidome in the Preovulatory Follicle, Oviduct Fluid and Plasma in Ewes with Contrasted Metabolic Status. *Front. Endocrinol.* **2022**, *13*, 892213. [CrossRef]
64. Hu, P.; Pan, C.; Su, W.; Vinturache, A.; Hu, Y.; Dong, X.; Ding, G. Associations between Exposure to a Mixture of Phenols, Parabens, and Phthalates and Sex Steroid Hormones in Children 6-19 Years from NHANES, 2013–2016. *Sci. Total Environ.* **2022**, *822*, 153548. [CrossRef] [PubMed]
65. Gao, C.; He, H.; Qiu, W.; Zheng, Y.; Chen, Y.; Hu, S.; Zhao, X. Oxidative Stress, Endocrine Disturbance, and Immune Interference in Humans Showed Relationships to Serum Bisphenol Concentrations in a Dense Industrial Area. *Environ. Sci. Technol.* **2021**, *55*, 1953–1963. [CrossRef] [PubMed]
66. Vom Saal, F.S.; Vandenberg, L.N. Update on the Health Effects of Bisphenol A: Overwhelming Evidence of Harm. *Endocrinology* **2021**, *162*, bqaa171. [CrossRef] [PubMed]
67. Chou, C.-H.; Chen, M.-J. The Effect of Steroid Hormones on Ovarian Follicle Development. *Vitam. Horm.* **2018**, *107*, 155–175. [CrossRef] [PubMed]
68. Kolibianakis, E.M.; Papanikolaou, E.G.; Fatemi, H.M.; Devroey, P. Estrogen and Folliculogenesis: Is One Necessary for the Other? *Curr. Opin. Obstet. Gynecol.* **2005**, *17*, 249–253. [CrossRef]
69. Weenen, C.; Laven, J.S.E.; Von Bergh, A.R.M.; Cranfield, M.; Groome, N.P.; Visser, J.A.; Kramer, P.; Fauser, B.C.J.M.; Themmen, A.P.N. Anti-Müllerian Hormone Expression Pattern in the Human Ovary: Potential Implications for Initial and Cyclic Follicle Recruitment. *Mol. Hum. Reprod.* **2004**, *10*, 77–83. [CrossRef] [PubMed]
70. Monniaux, D.; Drouilhet, L.; Rico, C.; Estienne, A.; Jarrier, P.; Touzé, J.-L.; Sapa, J.; Phocas, F.; Dupont, J.; Dalbiès-Tran, R.; et al. Regulation of Anti-Müllerian Hormone Production in Domestic Animals. *Reprod. Fertil. Dev.* **2012**, *25*, 1–16. [CrossRef] [PubMed]
71. Pankhurst, M.W. A Putative Role for Anti-Müllerian Hormone (AMH) in Optimising Ovarian Reserve Expenditure. *J. Endocrinol.* **2017**, *233*, R1–R13. [CrossRef] [PubMed]
72. Saleh, A.C.; Sabry, R.; Mastromonaco, G.F.; Favetta, L.A. BPA and BPS Affect the Expression of Anti-Mullerian Hormone (AMH) and Its Receptor during Bovine Oocyte Maturation and Early Embryo Development. *Reprod. Biol. Endocrinol. RBE* **2021**, *19*, 119. [CrossRef] [PubMed]
73. Cao, Y.; Qu, X.; Ming, Z.; Yao, Y.; Zhang, Y. The Correlation between Exposure to BPA and the Decrease of the Ovarian Reserve. *Int. J. Clin. Exp. Pathol.* **2018**, *11*, 3375–3382. [PubMed]
74. Silvestris, E.; Cohen, M.; Cornet, D.; Jacquesson-Fournols, L.; Clement, P.; Chouteau, J.; Schneider, M.; Besnard, T.; Ménézo, Y. Supporting the One-Carbon Cycle Restores Ovarian Reserve in Subfertile Women: Absence of Correlation with Urinary Bisphenol A Concentration. *BioRes. Open Access* **2017**, *6*, 104–109. [CrossRef] [PubMed]
75. Liu, W.-X.; Donatella, F.; Tan, S.-J.; Ge, W.; Wang, J.-J.; Sun, X.-F.; Cheng, S.-F.; Shen, W. Detrimental Effect of Bisphenol S in Mouse Germ Cell Cyst Breakdown and Primordial Follicle Assembly. *Chemosphere* **2021**, *264*, 128445. [CrossRef]
76. Hernandez-Ochoa, I.; Barnett-Ringgold, K.R.; Dehlinger, S.L.; Gupta, R.K.; Leslie, T.C.; Roby, K.F.; Flaws, J.A. The Ability of the Aryl Hydrocarbon Receptor to Regulate Ovarian Follicle Growth and Estradiol Biosynthesis in Mice Depends on Stage of Sexual Maturity. *Biol. Reprod.* **2010**, *83*, 698–706. [CrossRef] [PubMed]
77. Desmarchais, A.; Téteau, O.; Papillier, P.; Jaubert, M.; Druart, X.; Binet, A.; Maillard, V.; Elis, S. Bisphenol S Impaired In Vitro Ovine Early Developmental Oocyte Competence. *Int. J. Mol. Sci.* **2020**, *21*, 1238. [CrossRef] [PubMed]
78. Tang, Z.-R.; Zhang, R.; Lian, Z.-X.; Deng, S.-L.; Yu, K. Estrogen-Receptor Expression and Function in Female Reproductive Disease. *Cells* **2019**, *8*, E1123. [CrossRef] [PubMed]

79. Chauvin, C.; Cohen-Tannoudji, J.; Guigon, C.J. Estradiol Signaling at the Heart of Folliculogenesis: Its Potential Deregulation in Human Ovarian Pathologies. *Int. J. Mol. Sci.* **2022**, *23*, 512. [CrossRef]
80. Grignard, E.; Lapenna, S.; Bremer, S. Weak Estrogenic Transcriptional Activities of Bisphenol A and Bisphenol S. *Toxicol. Vitro Int. J. Publ. Assoc. BIBRA* **2012**, *26*, 727–731. [CrossRef] [PubMed]
81. Molina-Molina, J.-M.; Amaya, E.; Grimaldi, M.; Sáenz, J.-M.; Real, M.; Fernández, M.F.; Balaguer, P.; Olea, N. In Vitro Study on the Agonistic and Antagonistic Activities of Bisphenol-S and Other Bisphenol-A Congeners and Derivatives via Nuclear Receptors. *Toxicol. Appl. Pharmacol.* **2013**, *272*, 127–136. [CrossRef] [PubMed]
82. Ullah, A.; Pirzada, M.; Jahan, S.; Ullah, H.; Shaheen, G.; Rehman, H.; Siddiqui, M.F.; Butt, M.A. Bisphenol A and Its Analogs Bisphenol B, Bisphenol F, and Bisphenol S: Comparative in Vitro and in Vivo Studies on the Sperms and Testicular Tissues of Rats. *Chemosphere* **2018**, *209*, 508–516. [CrossRef]
83. Zhang, Z.; Lin, L.; Gai, Y.; Hong, Y.; Li, L.; Weng, L. Subchronic Bisphenol S Exposure Affects Liver Function in Mice Involving Oxidative Damage. *Regul. Toxicol. Pharmacol. RTP* **2018**, *92*, 138–144. [CrossRef]
84. Lu, J.; Wang, Z.; Cao, J.; Chen, Y.; Dong, Y. A Novel and Compact Review on the Role of Oxidative Stress in Female Reproduction. *Reprod. Biol. Endocrinol. RBE* **2018**, *16*, 80. [CrossRef] [PubMed]
85. Wirth, C.; Brandt, U.; Hunte, C.; Zickermann, V. Structure and Function of Mitochondrial Complex I. *Biochim. Biophys. Acta* **2016**, *1857*, 902–914. [CrossRef] [PubMed]
86. Hwang, M.-S.; Rohlena, J.; Dong, L.-F.; Neuzil, J.; Grimm, S. Powerhouse down: Complex II Dissociation in the Respiratory Chain. *Mitochondrion* **2014**, *19 Pt A*, 20–28. [CrossRef]
87. Čunátová, K.; Reguera, D.P.; Houštěk, J.; Mráček, T.; Pecina, P. Role of Cytochrome c Oxidase Nuclear-Encoded Subunits in Health and Disease. *Physiol. Res.* **2020**, *69*, 947–965. [CrossRef] [PubMed]
88. Bujnakova Mlynarcikova, A.; Scsukova, S. Bisphenol Analogs AF and S: Effects on Cell Status and Production of Angiogenesis-Related Factors by COV434 Human Granulosa Cell Line. *Toxicol. Appl. Pharmacol.* **2021**, *426*, 115634. [CrossRef] [PubMed]
89. Monniaux, D.; Huet, C.; Besnard, N.; Clément, F.; Bosc, M.; Pisselet, C.; Monget, P.; Mariana, J.C. Follicular Growth and Ovarian Dynamics in Mammals. *J. Reprod. Fertil. Suppl.* **1997**, *51*, 3–23. [PubMed]

MDPI
St. Alban-Anlage 66
4052 Basel
Switzerland
Tel. +41 61 683 77 34
Fax +41 61 302 89 18
www.mdpi.com

Toxics Editorial Office
E-mail: toxics@mdpi.com
www.mdpi.com/journal/toxics

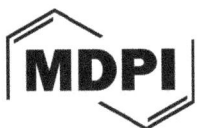